Managing the Respiratory Care Department

John W. Salyer, RRT, MBA, FAARC

Director Respiratory Care
Children's Hospital and Regional Medical Center
Seattle, Washington

JONES AND BARTLETT PUBLISHERS

Sudbury, Massachusetts

BOSTON   TORONTO   LONDON   SINGAPORE

World Headquarters

Jones and Bartlett Publishers
40 Tall Pine Drive
Sudbury, MA 01776
978-443-5000
info@jbpub.com
www.jbpub.com

Jones and Bartlett Publishers
Canada
6339 Ormindale Way
Mississauga, ON L5V IJ2
CANADA

Jones and Bartlett Publishers
International
Barb House, Barb Mews
London W6 7PA
United Kingdom

Jones and Bartlett's books and products are available through most bookstores and online booksellers. To contact Jones and Bartlett Publishers directly, call 800-832-0034, fax 978-443-8000, or visit our website www.jbpub.com.

Substantial discounts on bulk quantities of Jones and Bartlett's publications are available to corporations, professional associations, and other qualified organizations. For details and specific discount information, contact the special sales department at Jones and Bartlett via the above contact information or send an email to specialsales@jbpub.com.

The authors, editor, and publisher have made every effort to provide accurate information. However, they are not responsible for errors, omissions, or for any outcomes related to the use of the contents of this book and take no responsibility for the use of the products and procedures described. Treatments and side effects described in this book may not be applicable to all people; likewise, some people may require a dose or experience a side effect that is not described herein. Drugs and medical devices are discussed that may have limited availability controlled by the Food and Drug Administration (FDA) for use only in a research study or clinical trial. Research, clinical practice, and government regulations often change the accepted standard in this field. When consideration is being given to use of any drug in the clinical setting, the health care provider or reader is responsible for determining FDA status of the drug, reading the package insert, and reviewing prescribing information for the most up-to-date recommendations on dose, precautions, and contraindications, and determining the appropriate usage for the product. This is especially important in the case of drugs that are new or seldom used.

Production Credits

Executive Editor: David Cella
Acquisitions Editor: Kristine Johnson
Editorial Assistant: Lisa Gordon
Production Director: Amy Rose
Associate Production Editor: Wendy Swanson
Marketing Manager: Jennifer Bengtson
Manufacturing and Inventory Supervisor: Amy Bacus

Interactive Technology Manager: Dawn Mahon Priest
Cover Design: Anne Spencer
Text Design: Graphic World, Inc.
Composition: Graphic World, Inc.
Printing and Binding: Malloy, Inc.
Cover Printing: Malloy, Inc.

Library of Congress Cataloging-in-Publication Data
Salyer, John.
  Managing the respiratory care department / John Salyer.
    p. ; cm.
  Includes bibliographical reference and index
  ISBN-13: 978-0-7637-4044-3 (casebound : alk. paper)
  ISBN-10: 0-7637-4044-6 (casebound : alk. paper) 1. Hospitals—Respiratory therapy services—Administration.
I. Title.
  [DNLM: 1. Respiratory Care Units—organization & administration. WF 27.1 S186m 2008]
  RA975.5.R47S35 2008
  362.196′2—dc22
                              2007026915
6048
Printed in the United States of America
11 10 09 08 07   10 9 8 7 6 5 4 3 2 1

Table of Contents

Preface

Return My Breath

—John Salyer

So tired, but sleep cannot be found
Upon this night of gasping want
In blue green robes, arriving now
This lack of breath they come to daunt

With eyes alert and listening too
They prod, examine and prescribe
A heart so kind, and mind keen too
They touched my wheeze, it did subside

Then off it is to noisier place
Where bright lights shine throughout the night
Machines, whirring, clamorous flow
The reaper grim they came to fight

Who are these warriors, from whence they come
Carried on a comfort wind
With fluids, switching, desperate speed
Tubing and steel and gases to blend

Anonymous at times they seem
And yet, they're called to me again
Sometimes by name, but often not
They stand at the beginning, and at the end

From the forceps to the stone
In houses tall, with healing filled
From darkened rooms to stark white tile
The fluttering, fearful, they can still

Breath and flow, these are their goals
Scopes and screens their tools of trade
Hands that touch and sense and feel
The breath of life they contemplate

When asked, they often will defer
To tell you of their moral cause
For why they labor with low compense
It's what I do, they say with pause

A therapist I am they'll say
The breath of life, my expertise
I came to help you, to make relief
The symptoms of your lung disease

Well, I for one am glad they came
To render unto me this eve
Their ministrations, sound and true
I'll call them back, I do believe.

Acknowledgments

Writing a book is an adventure. To begin with, it is a toy and an amusement; then it becomes a mistress, and then it becomes a master, and then a tyrant. The last phase is that just as you are about to be reconciled to your servitude, you kill the monster, and fling him out to the public.

—Winston Churchill

It is said that to steal the work of one is plagiarism, but to steal the work of many is research. In writing this book, I have stolen the work of many. I have had the honor and pleasure to work with and learn from many wonderful, committed professionals in my short journey through this forest. I wish to thank all the people who knowingly or unknowingly contributed to this book. Some of the examples of educational material and various forms in this book were developed collaboratively with me as outliner and editor and many staff therapists, supervisors, and managers providing input. Specifically, I want to thank Dave Crotwell, Rob Diblasi, Christina Collin, Don Foubare, Ann Korn, Kevin Jacques, Kevin Cleary, Tina Whitby, Dianne Hale, David Hartman, and Cary (the bass master) Jackson. Thanks also to the respiratory leadership team at Children's Hospital, Seattle who have taught me so much and are some of the best people I have ever worked with, including Susan Nanninga, Joy Gilmore, Jenny Reid, and Dan Hernandez.

Going further back in time, there were many people from whom I learned a great deal and whose collaboration and friendship I still value even though the winds of time and fate have taken some of our respective ships in different directions. These include Rob (Master Po) Chatburn, Tom (Special K) Kallstrom, Roger Butler, Karen Kay Burton, RN, Kathy and John Davidson, Jim Keenan, J. Michael Dean, Phaedrus, Slip Kid, and Big Chief Bromden.

This book, such as it is, would not have happened without the unflinching support of my family. To my spousal unit Ellen and my children, Jeremiah, Hannah, and Joel I say mucho gracias and ain't you glad this is over (til the next one)?

I love deadlines. I particularly like the sound of them as they go whooshing by. I waved at many passing deadlines in writing this book, and I want to acknowledge the editorial staff at Jones and Bartlett, particularly Lisa

Gordon, who had the unpleasant job of trying to get me to finish this (expletive deleted) thing. Thanks to all of you for your patience. For my writing skills, for what they are worth, I have to mention my mentor and friend, Jim Gish.

I also feel compelled to thank Phil Keaggy, Pink Floyd, The Who, Johann Sebastian Bach, the Easy Star All-Stars, John Prine, Harry Chapin, Michael Hedges, The Mothers of Invention, the Chad Lawson Trio, Diana Krall, Steely Dan, Kansas, Al Di Meola, Mozart, Alice in Chains, Wes Montgomery, and G. F. Handel for providing the soundtrack for this book.

And finally, and most importantly, thanks to all the great respiratory therapists I have had the good fortune to work with. You are legion. I have been blessed to be an observer of an amazing transformation of the environment of care for those whose lives are threatened by respiratory disease. This transformation would not have been possible without the skills and commitment of that unique variant of the healthcare professional: the respiratory therapist.

Introduction

A man is known by the company he organizes.

—Ambrose Bierce[i]

Books on management principles and theories are a dime a dozen. You can find lots of them in any good book store. If you pursue a degree in business, you will be forced to buy lots of them and at least pretend to have read them. This book is intended to be more focused than all those other admirable, yet pedestrian texts; it covers the specific topic of managing a hospital department (in this case a respiratory therapy service). The principles and practices included here are sort of a quasi-concordance of my learning, both didactic and experiential, after over 30 years in respiratory therapy, 23 of which have been in various management positions.

Because this book is about managing people and processes, it will, regrettably, force us to at least touch on the topic of management theory. Let's go ahead and get this over with, and then we won't have to touch on this disagreeable topic again. Like most good theories, management theory is an amorphous, moving, ever-changing thing. It wriggles and squirms and stumbles its way from one era to another, changing with the passage of time, the accumulation of new learning, according to the culture in which it operates. Many theories of how best to manage organizations of people have been put forth. Premodern theories on management are probably to be mostly avoided because they resulted in such notable institutions as indentured servitude and slavery.

The overall history of modern management theory can be broadly divided into three phases: scientific management theory (1890–1940), bureaucratic management theory (1930–1950), and the human relations movement (1930 to today).[ii] These schools of thought have been somewhat evolutionary in that

---

[i]Ambrose Bierce (1842–1914) was an American satirist, critic, poet, short story (horror) writer, editor, and journalist who was known for his dark, sardonic views and vehemence as a critic.
[ii]It is instructive to remember that the Roman Legions had some fairly effective management theories 2100 years ago, including a very classical hierarchical structure and well-defined job responsibilities with excellent managerial controls. Of course, when their employees failed to follow policies, they were flogged with a cat-o'-nine-tails or killed outright, so we may want to be careful when applying some of their ideas to the modern workplace.

each school has built on the work of the previous school. Scientific management theory developed as human organizations grew in size and complexity, and the tasks that people did became routine and repetitive, which was a necessary evil to manufacture the wide variety of products now associated with modern life. Industrialized countries came to highly value scientific and technical matters, including careful measurement and specification of activities and results. Frederick Taylor developed the scientific management theory which promoted a careful specification and measurement of all organizational tasks. Activities were to be standardized as much as possible. Workers were to be rewarded and punished. Modern hospitals seem to have forgotten much of this.

Max Weber further developed scientific management theory with his bureaucratic theory. He focused on establishing strong lines of authority and control, dividing organizations into hierarchies. Comprehensive and detailed standard operating procedures were to be created for all routine tasks. Maybe we have forgotten some of this too?

Unfortunately, overzealous managers and supervisors used these theories in ways that had dehumanizing effects. During the human relations period, the belief has developed that the organization will prosper if its workers prosper as well. Imagine that. Human resource departments were added to organizations. The behavioral sciences helped us to learn how the needs of workers and the organization could be better aligned. Various new theories were spawned, many based on the behavioral sciences, most of which espoused a more participative management style. Current trendy management theories incorporate aspects from all of these movements. However, if someone came into today's workplace and tried to lead a group of people using management principles and practices from the 1950s, they would probably foment rebellion among the staff, develop an ulcer, and decide that maybe they should have gone to accounting school like cousin Hector. Fifty years ago, many FORTUNE 500 companies gave all prospective employees a Rorschach ink blot test. Today this is very rare.

Don't be frightened. This book will not be a turgid, painful, dry dissertation on management theory. I like my readers too much to put them through that, and I like myself too much to compose such a thing. Here is a simple summary of my management theory that might help you. Good management practices incorporate a balanced approach—not too autocratic, but not too mealy-mouthed either. A very nice acronym for developing a management theory or philosophy is ART (accountability-respect-teamwork).

We hold one another accountable for good work, we treat one another with respect, and we value the principles and practices of teamwork.

Instead of arid theoretical dissertations, this book is mostly about what I have learned, and I learned most of it the hard way. It is about trying to lead people in accomplishing difficult tasks, and as much as possible, standardizing and improving the work we do. My general observation is that it is pretty amazing that more than two of us together ever accomplish anything. Humans, and especially that particular regional variant, the Americans, are notoriously individualistic, even iconoclastic. They have their own ideas, don't want to work too hard if they don't have to, are sometimes pretty stubborn, have a practically inbred (and often well deserved) distrust of authority, and can be as easy to organize as a herd of cats. They also typically take a great deal of pride in their work, come to work wanting very much to do a good job, and desperately want to be led by people whom they trust and respect. This is why management can be so much fun. If it were too easy, it would be boring.

Some book introductions are a thinly disguised rehash of the table of contents. I am operating under the assumption that you can read the table of contents, so I won't go over it again.

Here is a warning about this book. Throughout it you will encounter my *immutable truths* (see Table I-1). These are axioms (sometimes pompous) that I have smashed into, tripped over, or have had fall on my head in my journeys through the corridors of hospital management. Let's get right to it.

Immutable Truth #1: Management and leadership are not the same thing. You can manage without leading. It is vastly more difficult to lead without managing. The Latin root for management (*manu agere*) means to lead by the hand. To lead, you first must answer the seminal question: Why in the world would anyone want to follow me? Or, more appropriately for the context of this book, why would anyone want to listen to what I have to say, do what I ask, or believe what I say? Do I have any credibility to pontificate on a given subject? Do I have any idea what I am doing? I personally have a lot of trouble putting much stock in the advice of alleged experts (the notorious "consultants") unless they clearly have a proven track record related to what they are preaching (and they are willing to hang around and help me troubleshoot the systems they have dreamed up). In my case, you will have to be the judge of my credibility. Along the way, I have taken charge of two different respiratory therapy departments that were in the deep weeds (and managed in two others). Both departments had gone

Table I-1. Immutable Truths

Immutable truth #1	Management and leadership are not the same thing.
Immutable truth #2	One way you learn to make good decisions is by making bad ones.
Immutable truth #3	Don't get too close to the people you are leading.
Immutable truth #4	The plural of anecdote is not data.
Immutable truth #5	It is a good idea to like your job.
Immutable truth #6	Good listening doesn't just happen, you have to work at it.
Immutable truth #7	No margin, no mission.
Immutable truth #8	It's all about processes.
Immutable truth #9	You cannot manage what you do not measure.
Immutable truth #10	Do not sacrifice the good for the perfect.
Immutable truth #11	The main thing is to keep the main thing, the main thing.
Immutable truth #12	*Someone* is going to be in charge.
Immutable truth #13	If you are coasting, it probably means you are going downhill.
Immutable truth #14	The law of unintended consequences is as ubiquitous as gravity.
Immutable truth #15	If a hospital can shut down your department, it should.
Immutable truth #16	Unwarranted variation is usually not good in health delivery systems.
Immutable truth #17	Not everything that counts can be counted, and not everything that can be counted counts.*
Immutable truth #18	The cycle of fear rules.
Immutable truth #19	Directors–managers are often the last ones to know what is going on in their departments.
Immutable truth #20	Sleep deprivation, derangement, and disruption makes unhappy campers.

Table I-1.   Immutable Truths *(Continued)*

Immutable truth #21	Generally speaking, most folks don't read much, if any, of the stuff you send to them.
Immutable truth #22	There is wisdom in the counsel of many.
Immutable truth #23	The burden of proof is on the advocate.
Immutable truth #24	All measurements are erroneous.
Immutable truth #25	All evidence is not created equal.
Immutable truth #26	All assumptions are suspect until proven otherwise.
Immutable truth #27	The Six P Principle: Proper Planning Prevents Piss Poor Performance.
Immutable truth #28	It is very hard to have too much training.

*OK, I admit it. I did not think this one up, although I wish I had. This has been attributed to Einstein. It is unclear to me whether he was the author or not. It is reported to have been a sign posted on his office wall. One of my favorite Einstein quotes: "Reality is merely an illusion, albeit a very persistent one."
This table contains the sometimes disturbing musings of a self-described sage. They are allegedly immutable truths. The reader will enter at their own risk and judge for themselves.

leaderless for some time before my arrival. Both departments had a lot of native talent but almost no well-designed systems for ensuring high quality patient care and business operations, and both departments experienced a substantial turnaround. Like all organizations made up of humans, they were, and remain, far from perfect, but in reshaping those operations I learned and learned and learned.

Immutable Truth #2: One way you learn to make good decisions is by making bad ones. I know this because I have made plenty of bad decisions. And through the good offices of my own suffering, I may be able to offer you some advice about how to avoid some of the same mistakes I have made. Don't worry though. If this book doesn't dissuade you from considering or continuing a career in healthcare management, then you will have the opportunity to make plenty of mistakes that you too can proudly call your very own.

Also, I have traveled around a bit and these wanderings have given me a fairly broad perspective on leadership styles and management techniques. My entry into the world of respiratory therapy began in 1975 while I was a Navy

Hospital Corpsman[iii] at the Great Lakes Naval Regional Medical Center in Waukegan, Illinois. I had noticed that some of the corpsmen had a pretty cool job running mechanical ventilators[iv] in a blood gas laboratory. I decided I wanted to try that and landed a job in the Inhalation Therapy Department. After stints as a medic with the Marine Corps and a couple of years of full-time college, I went back to respiratory therapy and never left again. I have held management positions at Kaiser Hospital in Fontana, California; Rainbow Babies and Children's Hospital in Cleveland; Primary Children's Medical Center in Salt Lake City; and Children's Hospital and Regional Medical Center in Seattle. I have also worked as a staff therapist at quite a few other hospitals, which, for the sake of decorum, will remain unnamed. Along the way, I did several years of full-time health services research, got a bachelor's degree in healthcare management and a master's degree in business administration, and amassed an extensive Pink Floyd collection. I have had the fortune to work with a lot of great clinicians and managers as well as a few who should have given thoughtful consideration to another field of endeavor. From these folks I have learned a lot about what to do, and, more importantly, what not to do to be an effective clinician, leader, and manager. As you progress through this text you will read many case studies and anecdotes. The names have all been changed to protect the innocent and the guilty. You may be tempted to speculate about which hospital these episodes occurred in. Don't bother. Not every anecdote or story you will read is from my own experience. Some were recounted to me by other managers and directors. And the episodes I did participate in have all been changed in ways that make it very hard indeed to figure out which hospital I am talking about, but not enough to change the message of the story.

The people I have had the opportunity to lead might give you a mixed message about me if you were to question them all. Some have had a high regard for me. Others do not. Some of this was undoubtedly due to my many and various shortcomings, but some was a result of my occasionally pushing the boundaries and raising the bar of what it meant to be a respiratory therapist.

[iii]The Navy Hospital Corps, the only enlisted corps in the U.S. military, is the single most decorated rating of all branches of the military. Twenty-three Hospital Corpsmen have received the Medal of Honor, the most of any single group in the U.S. Navy. Fourteen ships have been named after Hospital Corpsmen. Hospital Corpsmen performed 14 unassisted appendectomies while in a submarine in World War II. The career and skill set of Hospital Corpsmen were recognized in an article published in the *Journal of the American Medical Association* in 1961, and they were considered to be ideal students for the pilot class of physician assistants in 1965 at Duke University Medical Center.
[iv]Emerson Post-ops and a single brand new MA-I.

The fact that you are reading this now indicates that you appear to be crazy enough to be considering a job in management (or have already foolishly decided to take such a position). Those of you who are already managers will understand what I am about to ask: "*Are you nuts?*" Indeed, being a manager can be one of the most rewarding jobs imaginable. It provides you with an opportunity to make a real difference in how hospitals operate and, either directly or indirectly, improve the quality of patient care. If you do the job right, you can substantially improve the working conditions of your staff, and you can implement lasting changes of which you can be very proud. You can help people develop their potential, solve intractable problems, and, in the end, contribute to the greater good. Healthcare management is like that. It is a larger calling in a sense. At the heart of all the processes and systems and plans and procedures are sick people whom you can help to heal or at least help by easing their passage.

But here's the catch. It can also be very tough, emotionally draining, isolating, scary, infuriating, tense, boring, tiring, complicated, and sometimes very unrewarding. I think this is why they call it work. There are times when you walk down the hall knowing that you would, at that very moment, like to be anywhere else on earth doing anything but what you are about to have to do. Other times you will lie awake in the blackness of night trying to figure out what in the world to do about the latest crisis. New and incumbent managers need to expect this as part of the drill and learn to accept it. Of course, it is easy to spout such platitudes, and sometimes it is not so easy to survive in management positions.

I only bring this up to help you embrace management with your eyes wide open. If promoted to a management position, you are no longer "one of the crew." The staff will regard you differently, as well they should. This doesn't mean that you cannot have wonderful relationships with your staff; indeed, you had better have good relationships with your staff if you want to survive. But it does mean that the way you interact with other people in your department will subtly change. For new managers, this can be a very difficult adjustment, and I have known some very capable people who moved from staff into management positions only to eventually choose to go back to staff, in part because of the difficulty of this adjustment.

Here comes another rule: *Immutable Truth #3: Don't get too close to the people you are leading.* This can make doing your job much harder than it needs to be sometimes. The demands of management make it necessary at times for you to correct the behavior of others, which becomes very emotionally complicated if you are too close to them. This is a mistake I have made in the past, and it can lead to you being unable to do the tough things that your job might require. It is a continuing challenge for me, and I have to remind myself to keep some emotional distance between myself and those who report to me.

Respiratory therapy is a great field. The U.S. Department of Labor reports that there were 115,540 respiratory clinicians (therapists and technicians) employed in the United States in 2004.[1] The American Association for Respiratory Care puts the number much higher at 151,000.[2] About 78% of these therapists are employed in hospitals. There are approximately 5759 hospitals in the United States. Table I-2 lists the number of hospitals by type in the United States.

If you have the experience, education, and references needed, it is not too difficult to land a job in respiratory therapy management with one significant caveat: You must sometimes be willing to relocate. Certainly hospitals like to develop home-grown talent, but my experience is that many manager–director jobs go to people hired from the outside and often from outside the region, especially for director positions in larger hospitals.

Salary data for managers of respiratory therapy departments varies widely from region to region and is very dependent on the size of the hospital and thus the size of the staff you are managing. The interquartile range of salaries nationwide for managers is $65,838 to $83,290 with a median of $74,324 (in 2005 dollars). Just in case your statistics class was not the most inspiring and memorable episode of your college experience, I will remind you that the interquartile range describes the 25th to the 75th percentiles of a range of numbers. Half of all salaries fall within this range. Said another way, 25% of all salaries are both above and below this range. While these salary data may not make you feel particularly well paid, your pain might be eased by remembering that the median income in the United States for 2001–2004 was $44,473.[3] Not too shabby because you can get into front line clinical supervision with a 2-year degree in respiratory therapy, and you can usually get a managers job with a 4-year degree, assuming, of course, you have all the other requisite skills and experience.

There are some things that are not in this book to which other RT managers might take exception. There is not a chapter on managing blood gas labs. Approximately three-fourths of all blood gas operations are managed by respiratory therapy departments. But for the last 16 years my path has led me to work in hospitals where the blood gas labs were not part of the RT operation,

Table I-2. Numbers and Types of U.S. Hospitals

Total number of all U.S. registered hospitals	5759
Number of U.S. community hospitals	4919
Number of nongovernment not-for-profit community hospitals	2967
Number of investor-owned (for-profit) community hospitals	835
Number of state and local government community hospitals	1117
Number of federal government hospitals	239
Number of nonfederal psychiatric hospitals	466
Number of nonfederal long-term care hospitals	112
Number of rural community hospitals	2003
Total staffed beds in all U.S. registered hospitals	955,768
Staffed beds in community hospitals	808,127
Total admissions in all U.S. registered hospitals	36,941,951
Admissions in community hospitals	35,086,061
Total expenses for all U.S. registered hospitals	$533,853,359,000
Expenses for community hospitals	$481,246,587,000

Source: Data from www.aha.org as of January 2006.

and thus I have no meaningful recent experience and wisdom to offer you on this topic. I recommend to anyone who does use blood gases or manages a blood gas laboratory to read the delightful history of this technology written by Astrup and Severinghaus.[4]

This book does not contain a chapter on the Joint Commission on Accreditation of Healthcare Organizations (JCAHO). A great deal has been published by and about the JCAHO, and the interested student should have absolutely no trouble whatsoever finding some excellent material to help you be compliant with JCAHO guidelines.

REFERENCES

1. Bureau of Labor Statistics. May 2004 national occupational employment and wage estimates: healthcare practitioner and technical occupations. U.S. Department of Labor Bureau of Labor Statistics Web site. http://www.bls.gov/oes/home.htm.
2. American Association for Respiratory Care. Respiratory therapist: human resources study. *American Association for Respiratory Care.* 2005.
3. DeNavas-Walt C, Proctor BD, Lee CH. Income, poverty, and health insurance coverage in the United States: 2004. *U.S. Census Bureau.* August 2005.
4. Astrup P, Severinghaus JW. *The history of blood gases, acids and bases.* Copenhagen: Munksgaard, Radiometer; 1986.

CHAPTER 1

Preparations for Becoming an RT Manager

There is nothing more difficult to take in hand,
More perilous to conduct, or more uncertain in its success,
Than to take the lead in the introduction of a new
order of things

—Niccolò Machiavelli[i]

One of the most common reasons that people fail or have only limited success as managers of respiratory therapy departments is that they are not properly prepared. Frequently, really good clinicians get promoted to supervisory positions on the strength of their clinical skills and by virtue of their de facto clinical leadership. Unfortunately, this does not really prepare one for some of the things that will assault you in a management position. People love to tell anecdotal stories about great leaders and managers who had no formal preparation (e.g., college). These stories are usually told by folks who either couldn't or wouldn't get their college degrees themselves. *Immutable Truth #4: The plural of anecdote is not data.* An anecdote is just that, anecdote. It is a story told by an individual. It is a single observation. Another definition of anecdote: It is a research study where n = 1. While there are exceptions to virtually every rule or axiom, remember that an axiom is the axiom because it represents a larger truth. The larger truth that I am proposing here is that an undergraduate degree is a very good thing to have if you want to be a department manager in a hospital. For every story of someone in a leadership position in a knowledge industry, like health care, who doesn't have a college degree, there are 99 stories of people who have innate leadership skills but will never get the chance to develop them because they were denied management positions owing to the absence of a college degree.

---

[i]Niccolò Machiavelli (1469–1527) was a Florentine political philosopher, musician, poet, and romantic comedic playwright. He is (unjustly) remembered almost singularly for his political philosophy, which some summarize as "the ends justify the means." It was a little more complicated than that.

ACADEMIC PREPARATION

It is tough nowadays to find hospital department management-level positions that do not require a bachelor's degree. And the really great jobs are nowadays going to those who have gone on to get a masters degree. The paper chase[ii] has gotten a lot of bad press over the years and to some extent justifiably so. But if you are willing to work at it, you can get a lot out of an undergraduate or graduate degree. Or you can simply focus on getting the diploma. It is quite possible to go through the motions while in school, do the requisite work, and scrape by to get your degree. But some day you will encounter episodes where you find yourself saying, "Oh yeah, we studied that in school, but I don't remember much about it." Yes, we all know college is very tough, especially if you go back to school as a working adult. And nowadays, college can be very stifling intellectually because many campuses have become boot camps of intellectual conformity where political correctness is the new orthodoxy. But you cannot let these obstacles deter you from your goal. Believe me—not having a degree will be a much larger obstacle for you. A diploma alone won't get you a management job, but you won't get a management job without one.

There are various opinions about the best field of study to prepare you to manage a respiratory therapy department. To begin with let's assume that you have graduated from an accredited two-year program in respiratory therapy and that you hold an advanced practice credential in respiratory therapy, for example an RRT, or RRT-NPS, or RPFT issued by the National Board for Respiratory Care. The days are long gone when a respiratory therapist could get a management job while only holding a Certified Respiratory Technician's credential or being only registry eligible, not yet having sat for the examination. There are some managers who only have a CRT credential, but I haven't crossed paths with one for many years.

There are over 300 accredited two-year programs offering respiratory therapy education in the United States, a great many of them are community colleges that make it very affordable.[iii]

For the RT who is pondering a bachelor's degree, the United States has approximately 40 colleges and universities that offer a baccalaureate degree

---

[ii]An excellent novel and movie from the early 1970s.
[iii]Go to http://www.coarc.com to obtain a complete listing of the accredited schools in the nation listed by state. CoARC is the Committee on Accreditation for Respiratory Care and is responsible for granting credentials to schools of respiratory therapy nationwide.

in respiratory therapy (according to the National Board for Respiratory Care). With the advent of distance learning and online courses, access to these programs has gotten a lot easier. History will have to decide whether or not an online degree is any less credible or useful than actually attending a university in person. However, most managers of RT departments I know have an undergraduate degree in other fields, such as healthcare management or business or education. I recommend a degree in business or management. This will help you with the business processes that you will be required to manage as a hospital clinical department manager. Accounting and budgeting are important duties for the typical hospital department manager and especially so for the respiratory therapy manager. Respiratory therapy is among the few hospital departments that actually generate revenue by being able to bill and be reimbursed for their services. Respiratory therapy departments typically generate about $200 thousand to $300 thousand in gross charges (revenues) per full-time employee per year. So if you have a department of 45 full-time employees, you may be responsible for managing as much as $13 to $15 million per year in revenue.[iv] Trust me—you will be glad you have some business training. Before you get all flummoxed about the outrageous amount of cash generated by the hospital per year by respiratory therapists, remember that this is gross revenue. Direct and indirect expenses, contractual discounts of various types, bad debts, and charity care must be deducted from this revenue. Typically hospitals are actually reimbursed only about 50–75% of every dollar they bill depending on the type of hospital and the insurance environment in which they operate. In some very competitive markets, reimbursement rates are even lower. This will be discussed in more detail later.

Getting a graduate degree is also becoming more and more common among hospital department managers. I am a big fan of the masters in business administration (MBA). Of course, in some circles, the term "MBA" has become an expletive deleted. But a good MBA program will teach the student advanced financial management, analytical tools for evaluating and improving systems, and leadership principles. An MBA makes you very marketable. And let's face it—while you may love your job in many ways, you ain't exactly in it for your health. As you read the literature of healthcare

---

[iv]Welcome to your first encounter with the mind numbing confusion generated whenever you have to deal with charges, revenue, gross revenue, costs, reimbursement, discounts, expenses, etc., etc. These terms are explained in more detail in other parts of this book. Gross revenue in no way reflects the actual remuneration the hospital receives, which is affected by a dizzying array of factors.

management and health services research you see more and more authors and investigators with MBAs. One of the reasons for this is the excellent analytical training you get from an MBA program. In the operation of a clinical hospital department, you are managing lots of complex, interacting processes. To understand these, measure these, and God willing improve them, you will need some highly developed analytical skills.

CLINICAL PREPARATION

Along with a college degree or two you will have to obtain significant clinical experience to be an effective manager of a clinical department. This involves the time honored principle of rising through the ranks. If you want to be identified and eventually rewarded (promoted) into front line supervisory positions that could lead to a higher level management position, there are some things you need to attend to. *Immutable Truth #5: It is a good idea to like your job.* When I am looking for a candidate to promote to a leadership position, surprisingly, I am looking for someone who actually likes their job. The prima facie evidence of this is whether or not they are positive about their work, their organization, their colleagues, life, the universe, and everything. No one wants to follow someone who is overly negative or bitter. This is very bad form. If it is not in your personality to be generally pretty positive about the vicissitudes of daily work and life, you may want to give serious consideration to another field of endeavor, say radio talk show host or grief counselor. Of course, this does not mean that you habitually gloss over or fail to acknowledge problems. If you do that, you will eventually step on one of the mines you have laid. But in a management position, you can become so overly focused on problem solving that you can forget that lots of great things happen around you every day. Keep your vision of the good alive. Feed on it every day.

You will probably have to start as a clinical supervisor on night shift. Working through the middle of the night when sane people are sound asleep is a particularly potent form of self-abuse. Night shift work creates chronic sleep deprivation, sleep disruption, and generally makes people a bit crabby from time to time. There is now a growing body of evidence on the effect of sleep disruption and deprivation on human cognitive and physical performance.[1] It is not happy evidence. Higher reasoning skills and judgment begin to decline as do very fine motor skills, all of which are essential for clinicians operating life support equipment. Keeping mentally sharp and emotionally grounded on nights is essential for all staff, but it is particularly important for those in leadership positions. An effective leader is one who keeps his or her head together when all those around them have lost theirs (my apologies to Kipling for this paraphrase). One of the questions I ask all supervisor candidates is to describe an emotionally charged episode during which they were able to diffuse the situation and tell me about how they did it. I call this skill the "imperturbability coefficient." You want to have as high a coefficient as possible. Unfortunately, many people who have natural leadership skills don't naturally have this characteristic well developed. I certainly did not. But with awareness, coaching, and time, this skill can be developed. I am still working on it. How well you manage your life outside of work will have a significant impact on your imperturbability coefficient. If you are not getting enough sleep or play, you will have difficulty managing stress at work.

OFF TO SEE THE WIZARD

One useful way to think about the skill set you will eventually have to develop as a leader–manager is to call upon one of the greatest resources in the American pop culture lexicon—*The Wizard of Oz.* In keeping with the theme of the good wizard, you will need to develop the brains of the Scarecrow, the courage of the Lion, the heart of the Tin Man, and it never hurts to have a good pet like Toto too. Seriously, hospital management can often be a very stressful gig and there is nothing like a Toto jumping into your lap when you get home to help you unwind. I call this decompression. Cats work well too, although they are often psychotic and demanding. Remember, dogs have masters, cats have staff.

The brains of the Scarecrow are essential. The Scarecrow had all the intelligence he needed all along, but he simply had to recognize it and develop it. Admittedly, intelligence is somewhat difficult to precisely define, but most of us know it when we encounter it. The Latin root word for intelligence is "intelligo," which means "understanding." So one simple definition of intelligence is to "get it." Further analysis of "Intelligo" reveals that it is actually two words: "inter" and "ligo," that is, "I tie between." This would suggest that intelligence is the ability to see relationships among things and ideas—the ability "to put it all together."

For the purposes of our discussion, one of the more important intellectual skills you will need is the ability to process lots and lots of data. In respiratory therapy and other technical fields in health care, there is a lot of data to process, and to do a good job you need good analytical skills. Most hospitals now suffer from data glut. They essentially have too much data. They have mountains of paper and acres of servers where data is dutifully stored, cata-logued, indexed, sorted, and mostly ignored. In fact some managers are at risk of drowning in data. They are on overload, maxed out and overwhelmed by the amount of data they have to process. What is needed is good analysis, which is the process by which data are turned into information. My recom-mendation is to take every class you can on data management, statistical analysis, decision making, and research design. These courses and seminars will help you to develop skills you need to turn an ocean of data into finely crafted decisions. I cannot overemphasize computer skills as a prerequisite to successful management of an RT department. You must master the tools that computers offer to attack data. The spreadsheet and the database are your friends. Get well acquainted with them. This is discussed in a little more detail later.

Emotional intelligence is a relatively new concept that describes an ability or skill to perceive, assess, and manage the emotions of yourself and oth-ers.[2-4] One convention is to think of emotional intelligence as having four major components that include the capacity to: (1) accurately perceive emo-tions, (2) use emotions to facilitate thinking, (3) understand emotional mean-ings, and (4) manage emotions. Opinions vary about whether emotional intelligence is innate or whether it can be learned and increased.[5] For me, my ability to handle emotional conflict at work and at home has improved over the years. Whether this is because of my own efforts or in spite of them is un-clear to me. I have known folks who had a razor sharp intellect in terms of cognitive and analytical skills but were not particularly good at coping with the emotional challenges of leading people in the daunting task of applying complex technology to people who are deathly ill. Some of my most serious mistakes have been made when I was in the middle of powerful and complex emotional forces. Once again, you need a high imperturbability coefficient to be an effective leader. Without fail, the *effective* executive leaders I have worked for had a very high imperturbability coefficient, which I believe was a result of their emotional intelligence. Never let them see you sweat.

You will also be called upon to exhibit the courage of the Lion from time to time. This is particularly true if you want to be an agent of change. It will be necessary from time to time for you to act practically fearlessly, to take risks, to be bold, all of which require some degree of courage. But don't be mistaken. Courage is not the absence of fear. No indeed, history has taught us that you can be very brave and pretty much scared speechless simultaneously. Courage is acting in spite of your fear. Within the context of a hospital manager, courage can be taking responsibility when things go wrong, looking someone in the eye and telling him or her something they do not want to hear, being willing to risk your reputation by trying something new, and saying the truth at committee meetings when the emperor has no clothes. And believe me, things will go wrong.[v] Hospitals are operated by humans and as such are somewhat prone to error. You will find yourself dealing with your own errors and the errors of others. A bad habit that I have seen some managers slip into is a reluctance to admit they were wrong. There is an irrational fear that admitting error is a sign of weakness or bad leadership. I think we should embrace our errors. By holding them close and carefully examining them we can learn so much. Hiding from our mistakes is only a temporary respite.

The courage of the Lion can come in very handy when you have to make difficult decisions. Your decisions can affect a lot of people and patients. As such, a lot of courage is necessary to make and carry out such decisions. Sometimes our fear leads us to avoid risks at any cost. We over analyze issues, and in so doing we put off making a decision. We call this analysis paralysis. Theodore Roosevelt said, "In any moment of decision the best thing you can do is the right thing, the next best thing is the wrong thing, and the worst thing you can do is nothing." True leaders lead. Sometimes they are the only ones who see the vision, and they have to be willing to stand alone in their vision until others can be persuaded to follow. Of course, this has to be carefully balanced with listening to your staff, your team, and your colleagues and whenever possible, building consensus. The good news is that if you build good data and measurement systems for your operation, the number of decisions you will have to make will significantly diminish. This is because a decision is the action an executive must take when he or she has information so incomplete that the answer does not suggest itself.[vi]

You will know you have the heart of the Tin Man when you have your first experience with having it broken at work. This is inevitable working in health care. You will encounter the sick, the dying, the suffering, and all the pain and fear that go with these. If you are not moved to tears by the daily ebb and flow of the tragedy and suffering that occurs in hospitals, then you may have made a stone of your heart. You especially need a deep compassion for those who work for you. Being a clinician, especially a respiratory therapist, can be a very emotionally draining experience. We often

[v]Mistakes will happen. The key is not to make the same mistake twice. And only make one mistake at a time. Loosely translated from *The House of God* by Samuel Shem.
[vi]Arthur W. Radford, "Man Behind the Power," *Time*, February 25, 1957.

deal with patients who have life threatening illness or chronic debilitation. We attend at many deaths. We often live a high-pressured professional life. Thus we often need solace and understanding, patience and support. A highly developed sense of compassion for patients and families is also required. The suffering of patients and the burden this places on their families ought to be gasoline on the fire that drives you to work hard to make things better. If you do not feel this drive, this fire, this compassion for those we treat and those who do the treating, I recommend career counseling.

INTERPERSONAL AND COMMUNICATION SKILLS

Great interpersonal skills are absolutely essential in a manager. My thinking about this has undergone a change over the years. I initially thought interpersonal skills were overrated. I believed that first and foremost, the one thing that mattered more than anything else was being "right." I thought the power of correctness could transport you past the pedestrian obstacles in your path and lead you to the promised land where you would "get your way." Don't get me wrong, being "right" is generally a good thing. At least it is way better than being "wrong." But I have come to realize that rightness can be small comfort when you are isolated and avoided because of the way you communicate your ideas and plans. I learned the hard way that being confident is a good thing but that it can quickly transmogrify into an obnoxious smugness that sets others' teeth on edge. Learning to communicate your ideas in a thoughtful and collegial manner will help you considerably.

The single toughest thing for me to develop and one that I still struggle with, unless I really concentrate, is the practice of *active listening*. Uh oh, here comes another one: *Immutable Truth #6: Good listening doesn't just happen, you have to work at it*. Often, when I am having a conversation with someone, my mind is trying to race ahead. After only a few words, I think I know what the person I am talking to is going to say. In fact, I rush ahead and start planning what I am going to say back to them before they have finished what they are saying. This is risky business because often they will have something subtle but important they are trying to communicate to you, but you miss it, being busy as you are composing your response. Or just the simple act of concentration on the words and mannerisms of the person you are talking to can help you enormously in getting deeper meaning out of what someone is saying to you.

I like to teach the concept of "saving face." You will often find yourself in a position where logic and reason force you, regrettably, to have to disagree with someone. You should always find a way to do this while allowing others to save face. Acknowledge the soundness of other people's arguments and positions (if there is some). Appreciate their desire to do the right thing. Honor their positions and stature. This is done with words and tone and mannerisms. If possible, do not correct or reproof someone in public and never do so in the heat of the moment. If possible, walk away and let the dust settle and then speak to them privately. You will get a much better hearing. Someone once told me one of the things they liked about me was my ability to disagree without being disagreeable. This is not natural for me. It is something I have to work on all the time. I have made many mistakes in this area, having in the past dressed people down in front of others or let my temper get the best of me. I have always suffered because of this (as have those that I abused). These moments limit your effectiveness as a leader and do not help you accomplish your larger purposes.

One serious communication skill is the ability to present your ideas in a clear and concise manner. This is true during one-on-one communication and in the group setting. In the corporate life of hospitals, department managers have to routinely present their analyses, ideas, and plans to groups of people. If you do not have well-honed presentation skills, you will have trouble getting and keeping people's attention. Executives have notoriously short attention spans. You have to learn to be thorough and concise, and do it in a hurry.

Standard operating procedure in corporate life now includes the use of computerized presentation technology, such as Microsoft PowerPoint. I love PowerPoint. It has greatly simplified things since I started in the business of presenting ideas, research, and plans. Some of my earliest presentations were chiseled onto large clay tablets. However, this comes with a great big caveat. PowerPoint is a sword with two edges. I have suffered through countless presentations that were visually abysmal. Bad visual presentation aids can really screw up an otherwise good presentation. And conversely, the best slides in the world won't save you from having a weak presentation if your content and speaking style are not up to the task. The mistakes made are as predictable as they are tiresome. Table 1-1 lists some guidelines when making presentations using a program like PowerPoint.

Finally, content and visual aids are not all you need to worry about when making presentations. Your speaking skills are very important. I remember listening to an audio tape of myself giving a lecture before about 300 people at a national scientific conference many years ago. It was my first "big"

Table 1-1. Guidelines to Good Computerized Presentations (PowerPoint)

Use Lots of Data

- Charts and graphs will help present your ideas much more clearly (if done properly) than words alone.

- However don't abuse the privilege of having an audience by overwhelming them with figures and charts either.

- A good rule of thumb is 2 minutes per slide. For complex technical data, a slide needs to be up for at least two minutes for it to be analyzed properly by your audience. Thus a 45-minute presentation should not have more than 25 slides.

Use the Largest Fonts Possible

- What you see is what you get (WYSIWYG) is the idea that your computer screen shows you what your final product will look like. This is generally true in printing, but not so true in presentations.

- What looks good on your screen may project very poorly in a large room. I have sat through countless presentations where the labeling of figures, tables, and graphs could not be read in the back of the room, or when the colors and contrast chosen make the slides largely unreadable.

- With this in mind use large fonts, typically ≥ 24. In very large rooms, even larger fonts are required if you want the whole room to be able to read your slides, especially your charts and graphs. If they look too big on your computer screen, they are probably just about right.

- Never use a graphic or figure that cannot be read. I have seen many presenters put a slide in that they know cannot really be read, saying, "I know you cannot read this, but . . ." This is somehow supposed to absolve you from sin. It doesn't. Scanned images of medical documents are often unreadable in a presentation.

Minimize the Shtick*

- Limit fancy animation functions such as whirling, crawling, sliding, spinning, flashing, fading, dancing, twirling, creeping, jumping, or flying slide transitions, to name only a few. Cuteness generally is not a desired feature of slide presentations when you are trying to convince people that your ideas have merit and thus they should give you money to implement your new program.

---

*Shtick is a Yiddish term referring to a contrived and often used bit of business that a performer uses to steal attention, as in "play it straight with no shtick." Captain Beef Heart called it "Stark Media Jive."

Table 1-1. Guidelines to Good Computerized Presentations (PowerPoint) *(Continued)*

Please oh please do not give in to this temptation. Taste is a very personal thing and what you find cute, others may find tiresome. This is not to be confused with the value of humor. See below.

- Audio and video can be useful but keep it simple and short. Also, audio and video files embedded in PowerPoint are more prone to technical glitches. I have had presentations with video clips work well in one room with a projection system and take the same file to another room and with a different computer (same operating system) and had the video clips not work. Also some projectors seem to have trouble with video clips. You always want to get there early enough to test your presentation on the local technology.

Proper Use of Colors

- Keep the number of colors used to a minimum. Four is good. Three is better.

- Use colors with high contrast with one another. Forget about the gentle, subtle interplay and nuanced beauty of two different shades of magenta. First of all, most people don't care, and secondly, high contrast is necessary to make your slides readable in large rooms or rooms with high ambient lighting.

- I like dark backgrounds like dark blue with white or bright yellow text and objects.

Occasionally Wake People Up

- Rooms are often dimmed or darkened for computerized presentations. While I personally like this because it often allows me to catch a much needed nap, it is generally not helpful to you as a presenter to have your audience obtunded. The monotonous, smooth sounds of your voice can help lull the audience into near stupefaction if you don't jazz the program up a bit. Modulate the volume of your voice. Change the cadence too.

- It is very helpful to break up your presentation with humor or pictures. I will often insert a funny picture or joke periodically throughout a presentation to break up the presentation (this is not a de facto admission that my presentations are ever monotonous).

- Humor is a vital element to a good presentation. Don't underestimate its value.

- If the technology allows it, get out from behind the podium. Move around, look people in the eye. Speak right at them, as this can be very persuasive.

(Continues)

Table 1-1. Guidelines to Good Computerized Presentations (PowerPoint) *(Continued)*

Jargon Jive

- Geeky technical specialties like respiratory care or other allied health fields can be afflicted with too many abbreviations and way too much jargon. Avoid overdoing this in your presentations. It turns out there is a lot of local variation in abbreviations and jargon in the healthcare field, so not all your audience may understand your slide if it is overloaded with these.

No Reading Please

- A slide presentation should be an outline of your talk. With rare exception you should never read verbatim from a slide. This sets most people's teeth on edge and will cause you to totally lose your audience in a New York minute.

Keep Slides Simple

- Do not, I repeat, do not put too much text on a slide. Bullet points are very helpful organizing tools. But you can wound your audience with too many bullets per slide. Five bullets a slide is good, four are better.

- Do not put too much text in your overall presentation. Minimize text only slides. If all you have to share with your audience is words, skip the hassle of preparing a PowerPoint presentation. Just give a cracking good speech instead.

Keep Your Presentations to a Reasonable Length

- Remember, the mind can absorb only what the butt can endure. About 45 minutes or so is as long as you can hope to keep someone's attention, even with the best presentation possible.

Laser Pointer Boogie

- Laser pointers are nice. Especially when presenting graphs and figures. Be careful not to use it too much. Some speakers point the pointer at the screen a lot, even continuously, and wiggle it around a lot. It makes me nauseous. I drink so much coffee that I can't hold the darn things still under the best of circumstances.

lecture. I was shocked to hear myself. I talked too fast, ran my sentences together, and said "um" a lot. Good speaking skills come with practice. Find someone who is really good at making presentations and practice your presentation with them. Have them look at your slides and critique your skills. Receive their criticisms with style and wit.

MEMBERSHIPS

Another important preparation you can make to enhance your performance in a management position is membership in professional organizations. Through networking and meetings you can learn a great deal from others who are suffering your same fate. You can get so caught up and bogged down in the tyranny of the urgent that you don't attend to your participation in these forums. This can have bad long-term consequences because you may fall behind the progress made by your colleagues from other hospitals and regions and deny yourself the benefit of learning from them, many of whom have already made the dreadful mistakes that are about to overtake you.

Important associations for the respiratory therapy manager start with the American Association for Respiratory Care (AARC). This professional organization has been a constant advocate for good respiratory therapy and has one of the best scientific meetings for respiratory clinical care, management, and education that I have ever attended. I heartily encourage all my staff members to join. I have even purchased memberships for all staff members. This was done as a one time gift from the management team to encourage membership and give them first hand experience with the benefits of membership. It was and is worth every penny.

Membership in state level respiratory care societies can also be very helpful. It will connect you with the other managers in the region with whom you will be competing to recruit and retain qualified staff. Increasing membership in state societies will also increase the profession's political power, which is important in matters of licensing and regulation of respiratory therapists.

Other organizations in whose membership you might benefit as a manager of a respiratory therapy department includes medical and nursing societies. Some of these organizations (like the Society for Critical Care Medicine, College of Chest Physicians, and American Academy of Pediatrics) have long recognized the important role played by respiratory therapists and have each in their own way advocated for respiratory therapy.

A more intangible but no less important benefit of membership in professional organizations like the AARC is a sense of professional self-identity. I remember well my first AARC conference (in Anaheim in the early 1980s). I had been working off and on as an RT for about 5 years. I was stunned by how many people were there and by the high quality of the lectures and the poster presentations. I was hooked. I realized I was part of something larger than just myself. I further realized that there were a lot of people who took being a respiratory therapist very seriously and worked hard at it, including doing and presenting research.

Last but not least, one of the most important things you can do to be an effective manager of a clinical practice service like respiratory therapy is simple; read. You simply have to be conversant with the best literature on the clinical science of respiratory care practice. Managers of respiratory care services ought to be the experts on the best evidence supporting various clinical interventions used by their staff. This is not accomplished by briefly glancing at a journal now and then. I personally review the contents of 15–25 journals per month. This is a high level review, going over the tables of contents and getting reports that relate to the work being done by the respiratory care staff. Based on this review, I then go on to read 10–15 research articles per month. Even at this, it is tough to keep up. One of the easiest ways to do this is to use Internet-based medical literature search engines. My favorite is www.PubMed.com.[vii] This free program allows you to rapidly search millions of published resources related to medical science. It is easy to use and allows you to review abstracts of all these articles free. If you want the full articles, many are now available online. Most journals require a paid electronic subscription to get these full-text articles, but some are free. Also many hospitals now have institutional subscriptions that individual staff members are authorized to use. Details can be obtained from your hospital library.

ORGANIZATIONAL SKILLS

I am not the most organized person around. I am not even the second or third most organized person around. In fact, my natural state is one of chaotic entropy. The single biggest obstacle for me in accomplishing my professional goals has been staying organized and on task. I go through tremendous oscillations in my efficiency at work. I notice that when it is working the best is when I take the time to get more organized and stay organized. I like to make lists. I make lists and then rewrite them in order of priority. At first, this is a terribly debilitating experience because the lists of things I need or want to get done at work is usually longer than a Bill Clinton speech. But then I realize that there is no way I am going to get it all done anyway, so then I start concentrating on the one or two things that I can have a real hope of getting

---

[vii]PubMed is a service of the U.S. National Library of Medicine that includes over 16 million citations from MEDLINE and other life science journals for biomedical articles back to the 1950s. PubMed includes links to full text articles and other related resources.

finished any time soon. This is somewhat liberating and usually helps me get fired up. There are entire training seminars you can take to help develop your organizational skills. I recommend taking them. You will eventually have to find a system that works for you. There is a lot of extant technology to help you, like Day-Timers and organizers,[viii] Palm Pilots, personal digital assistants, BlackBerrys, and laptops. Nothing really worked well for me until I learned to take the time to be organized. This has to be programmed time. You must block time off your schedule that is unassigned. Use this time to plan, to regroup, to make lists, whatever. If you don't consciously do this, your schedule as a hospital manager can rapidly fill up with meetings, meetings, and more meetings. You will end up meeting to decide when you are going to meet, followed by meetings to decide the name of your meeting. Finally, there are many advanced computer tools designed to enhance your degree of organization. As an example, there are a number of very advanced organizational tools inside Microsoft Outlook to name only one. Learn to use them.

I personally use a laboratory notebook in which I take notes at meetings, write down ideas at Starbucks or on planes, and record all manner of things, for example poetry, reminders to myself regarding the NBA schedule, and some very artful and intricate doodles. I keep these notebooks and occasionally go back and review them. Sometimes I will have had some pretty good developmental ideas that I never got to or forgot about and I rediscover them in my notebook.

REFERENCES

1. Drake CL, Roehrs T, Richardson G, Walsh JK, Roth T. Shift work sleep disorder: prevalence and consequences beyond that of symptomatic day workers. *Sleep.* 2004;27:1453–1462.
2. Reeves A. Emotional intelligence: recognizing and regulating emotions. *AAOHN J.* 2005;53(4):172–176.
3. Herbert R, Edgar L. Emotional intelligence: a primal dimension of nursing leadership? *Can J Nurs Leadersh.* November 2004;17(4):56–63.
4. Grandey AA. Emotion regulation in the workplace: a new way to conceptualize emotional labor. *J Occup Health Psychol.* 2000;5:95–110.
5. Mayer JD, Salovey P. The intelligence of emotional intelligence. *Intelligence.* 1993;17:433–442.

[viii]Don't start on me about how old school Day-Timers are. The best technology in the world is useless if it doesn't help you do your job. Many people were highly effective with Day-Timers. Of course I wasn't one of them, but I knew people who seemed to work pretty well with one. I could never seem to keep track of mine. Also, they were way too trendy for my taste.

CHAPTER 2

How Hospitals Are Organized

The trouble with organizing a thing is that pretty soon folks get to paying more attention to the organization than to what they're organized for.

—Laura Ingalls Wilder

I won't belong to any organization that would have me as a member.

—Groucho Marx

Hospitals are places of great contrast. Much good is done in hospitals, and the overwhelming majority of people have positive experiences. But we are also learning that hospitals, being operated by humans who are infected with the regrettable disease of fallibility, are places where lots of errors are made. I am certain that hospital operations are substantially better now than they were when I first started working in them. We have improved the training and preparations of our staff, vastly increased the quality (and complexity) of our technology, and learned a great deal about the right and wrong things to do for and to patients.

We have also improved our ability to measure how well (or sometimes not so well) hospitals work. This has given us a chance to greatly improve things because we have learned that there is a great deal of room for improvement, notably in the areas of patient safety and error management. The old school of hospital culture suggested that good clinicians didn't make errors. Thus, when patients were injured or had near misses from staff errors, there was a tendency to fire staff and blame these mishaps on individual human error. We are now learning that the design of our hospital systems can contribute greatly to the likelihood that someone, anyone, might make an error. There is an emerging view that suggests that many, if not all, staff members make errors and that the "good" staff members report their errors and help the organization learn from these mishaps.

I am bringing all this up because the data about quality and safety in hospitals has revealed that the scope of the problem is troubling indeed. The Institute of Medicine issued a watershed report in 1999 that shook the foundations of the healthcare system in its suggestions that between 48 thousand and 98 thousand patients die every year in United States hospitals from preventable medical errors.[1] Others have estimated that the combined impact of errors and adverse effects of treatment total 225 thousand preventable patient deaths per year.[2] I would caution the reader that these are estimates (extrapolations) based on sampling relatively small numbers of admissions and studying the error rates that can be found in the medical record. These rates are then projected to the entire population of hospitalized patients (approximately 37 million per year). It is not hard to imagine that problems with research methodology cast some doubt on the quality of these data. However, the degree of precision of these figures is not nearly as important as the acknowledgment that our system has large, pressing problems with patient safety. Why discuss this here in a chapter on the organization of hospitals, you ask? Because the design of our systems plays a very large contributory role in creating a safer system for our patients. As you read this chapter on hospital organization, keep in mind that it is not simply an arcane management topic.

The systems and structures of organizations can be enabling or disabling. Enabling structures help the individual accomplish the tasks before them in the best way possible. The argument goes like this. Some suggest that bureaucratic structure is sometimes an impediment to actually getting anything done in many organizations. I can testify that this has certainly been true in a lot of my experiences.

But in some organizations and systems, bureaucratic structures can be very enabling. The design of the system can make the accomplishment of given duties easier. Case Study 1 is an example of disabling versus enabling structures in a respiratory therapy department.

Case Study 1: Disabling Versus Enabling Structure

The Respiratory Therapy Department at St. Elsewhere Hospital had a policy and procedure manual, but if the manual had been put on trial for being useful, it would have been hard to find any evidence to convict it. It was printed and mounted in a couple of binders and loosely organized alphabetically by title, and much of it was outdated. It contained about 20 policies that had mostly been generated in response to problems in the past. Somebody would screw something up, so a policy or procedure was written in hopes that the mistake didn't happen again. The usual modus operandi was that many members of the staff never consulted the policy manual, mostly because they could never find one when they needed one. If they were lucky enough to find one, they would dust it off, try to find something helpful, and often give up. They would occasionally need to look at a device operating manual, but almost without fail, when one was needed it couldn't be found either. Then a new manager came on board and started to examine this system. She quickly realized that the manual was almost, but not entirely, useless. She put together a team of staff and management to expand, update, and rewrite the manual. She planned to make the manual entirely electronic, reasoning that this would use the ubiquitous computers in the hospital for the purpose to which they had been intended. She insisted that, as much as possible, the policies and procedures should be evidence-based, referenced, and highly visual, including pictures, diagrams, and figures whenever possible. In addition, she either obtained or created PDF files of all device-operating manuals and created computerized linkage (hyperlinks) to these manuals inside every policy and procedure in which these devices were mentioned. The whole enchilada was then packaged up and loaded onto the hospital's intranet Web page, making it accessible from any hospital workstation. Suddenly, the structure of the system for creation and distribution of policies, procedures, and manuals changed from disabling to enabling. You could get access to any existing policy, procedure, or device-operating manual as easily as logging on to any hospital computer, which St. Elsewhere had in abundance. Staff actually starting using the policy and procedure manual. Imagine that.

HOSPITAL STRUCTURE

In searching for a term to describe hospital organizational structure, the word Byzantine comes to mind. This term was first applied to the eastern Roman Empire (whose capital was Byzantium) and is used to describe any work, law, or organization that is excessively complex or difficult to understand. Don't misunderstand me. I am not suggesting that hospital organizational charts are *unnecessarily* complex. The scientific, financial, regulatory, legal, and cultural intricacies that govern hospital operations require a very elaborate organizational structure. Figure 2-1 shows a typical organizational chart of a hospital.

The single largest functional area of any hospital is the nursing service. They are typically organized into units by medical service lines, or by the level of care necessary, or both. The rationale behind this kind of organization

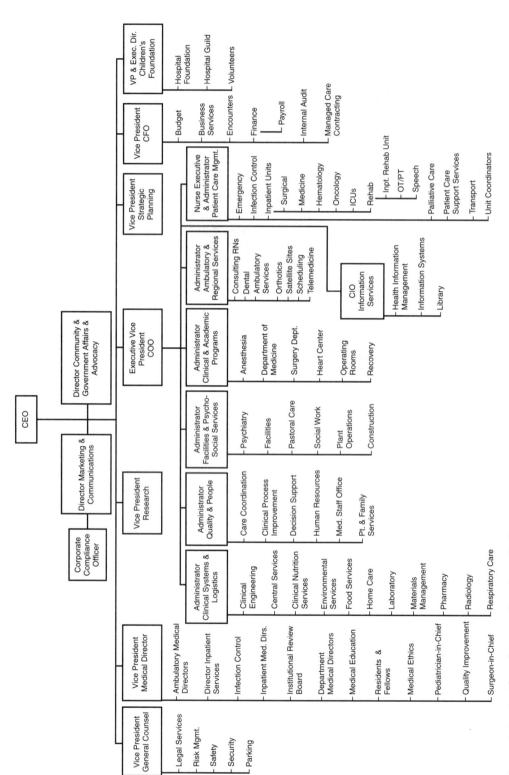

Figure 2-1. St. Elsewhere Regional Medical Center Organizational Chart

A typical hospital organizational chart. These charts, while useful, can be somewhat misrepresentative, since they do not visually describe the relative scope and size of various operations. For example, the inpatient general medical unit of this particular hospital has more than 200 nurses, while the pastoral care department has 8 staff members. This disproportion in size of staffs cannot be represented by such a chart.

is that nurses gain experience and therefore develop more specialized skills by caring for only similar types of patients. As our technology and interventions have grown increasingly complex, this has become more and more true and important. There is a definite relationship between skill at doing complex procedures and the frequency at which they are performed.[3] Hospitals that have a higher frequency of these complex procedures have better outcomes. Thus many hospitals have developed units where patients of similar disease processes or severity of illness are concentrated. Examples of this include service line intensive care units, such as cardiovascular or cardiothoracic intensive care, surgical intensive care, chronic ventilation units, and neonatal intensive care.

Another typical organizational grouping includes the ancillary service departments, which are usually comprised of the allied health professions of radiology technologists, laboratory technologists, pharmacists, and physical, occupational, and speech therapists. Respiratory therapy is often included in this type of an organizational grouping with the department manager reporting to an assistant administrator that does not include any nursing departments in his or her reporting chain. However, the alternate is also true. Some hospitals are organized with the respiratory therapy service reporting inside the nursing structure. There is grumbling by some directors who don't like reporting to nursing administrators. I have worked in all kinds of reporting relationships both within and outside of nursing services. I have reported to some great nursing administrators and some not so great ones. The quality of these reporting relationships is much more dependent on the leadership abilities of the person you are reporting to than on their work history or clinical affiliations. It is also quite true that poor reporting relationships can be caused by the person doing the reporting as well as the person being reported to. If you don't like your relationship with your boss, assume some responsibility for this and work on your end of it. Be patient and honest. Practice self-examination, difficult as that is sometimes.

In the 1990s, some hospitals embraced "business process reengineering," one definition of which is critical analysis and radical redesign of existing business processes to achieve breakthrough improvements in performance measures. Reengineering (which will be discussed later in more detail) resulted in the dismantling of some departments, the elimination of the RT management team, and had the respiratory therapist being "decentralized," for example being paid by and reporting to the nurse managers who were in charge of the units where the therapists worked. This allegedly provided for reduced costs and gains in other efficiencies by reducing or eliminating the need for the management and administrative costs of a "centralized" respiratory department. It was also supposed to smooth out care processes because staff members were cross trained across disciplinary lines (silos). In other words, therapists were going to be trained in some nursing duties, and nurses were going to be trained in some respiratory therapy duties. It looks as if this trend toward decentralizing departments has largely been abandoned, although we are still feeling its effects in some places (regrettably). I know of hospitals that tried it, and after a few years of turmoil and low staff retention, they abandoned the idea and recentralized their departments. One of the more common complaints was that the respiratory therapists became "nurse extenders," for example they got trained in various routine nursing duties and were expected to perform them whenever directed to by bedside nurses. Conversely, while the nurses got trained in some routine respiratory therapy duties, they rarely if ever performed them. Mostly, nurses were accustomed to being in charge of the care of their patients and were unaccustomed to being told what to do by respiratory therapists. It was mostly a one-way street. This became a major source of job dissatisfaction for RTs. I know of a hospital where 50% of the respiratory staff quit in the first year of the implementation of such a program on one large nursing unit.

In my experience, respiratory therapists do much better when they have a sense of group identity, as in belonging to a separate department. They have more professional pride, better training, and higher recruitment and retention when they are working out of a centralized respiratory department structure (as long as it is run well).

IT'S THE ECONOMY, STUPID

For the most part, hospitals are businesses. Allow me to rephrase. For the most part, hospitals make an attempt to operate like businesses—sort of. They have products and services that they offer their clients for which they receive remuneration. But unlike most businesses, hospitals also have secondary, nonpaying clients called physicians. This is a fairly complicated relationship. Physicians typically do not work for hospitals (although this is beginning to change). They bill patients separately for their services. They are only loosely governed by the employment and labor relations practices of hospitals. They get all the best parking spaces and in some places they even have their own private dining rooms. The reason hospitals treat physicians like customers is that hospitals need doctors to refer their patients for admission. This is a fundamental part of the business equation of hospital operations. Thus doctors are generally treated pretty well by hospitals. Sometimes hospital managers gnash their teeth while problem solving and realize that they need to change physician behavior. Because the doctors don't work for the hospital, there is the (often false) assumption that you cannot change their behavior because you have no authority over them. This has not been my experience. For the most part, physicians are invested in the success of the hospital. They also tend to be pretty analytical because of the decades of education they are forced to endure. Thus they usually respond very well to thoughtful, well articulated, data-driven arguments.

Another difference between hospitals and most other normal businesses is that clients don't actually pay their own bills. If they did, large demographic segments of the population would have long ago gone bankrupt. No, instead the bills are generally paid for by insurance companies or state and federal governments. Medicare is the federal entitlement program that pays for the health care of elderly Americans. Medicaid is a state-level program that includes federal funds and pays for the hospital and nursing home care of the uninsured poor. People often get these confused.

Whenever anyone tells you that there are 40 million Americans without medical insurance, you might want to remind them that most of these people are covered by Medicaid, on which the state and federal governments spend about $300 billion *per year*. This is actually more than is spent on Medicare. Approximately 17% of all hospital-related healthcare costs are paid by Medicaid. In some hospitals, the proportion of all funds received by Medicaid is nearly 40%. The magnitude of the future funding problem for Social Security is dwarfed by the size and immediacy of the Medicaid and Medicare funding problems.

The cost of running hospitals has typically grown much faster than the overall inflation rate. You could line a thousand million bird cages with what has been written about why this is happening. The cost of drugs and new complex, expensive technology certainly contributes to this. I have become increasingly convinced that the main reason is a lack of real market forces. If patients actually had to pay their medical expenses directly instead of having the pain of it attenuated by having costs filtered through insurance companies or the government, I think they would start protesting in earnest. They would also start shopping—something that doesn't happen much in the system now. Also the government puts an enormous regulatory burden on hospitals, which costs hospitals, and thus patients, plenty.

Hospitals can be divided into two groups: for-profit and not-for-profit operations. In some circles, "profit" is a dirty word. In other circles, "not-for-profit" is a wonderful excuse to keep wages and benefits low. Both of these business models have something in common. They must take in more money than they spend to keep the doors open. From my perspective, the main difference between for-profit and not-for-profit operations is one of terminology. For-profit hospitals call the difference between revenue and expenses "profit." Not-for-profit operations call the difference between revenue and expenses "margin." Whatever you call it, this difference helps make the world go round. *Immutable Truth #7: No margin, no mission.* Whether you are sending profits off to stockholders or pouring your margin back into capital development, you still need sound business practices. Lots of hospitals have traditionally struggled with this, for example clean, tight, efficient production and supply operations. It has gotten better lately, but much remains to be done.

Some people have theorized that the market forces associated with for-profit hospitals should drive down costs through efficient business practices. It turns out that this is not true. Per capita Medicaid costs have been shown to be higher in areas served by for-profit hospitals than in areas served by not-for-profit hospitals.[4] This is almost certainly because these for-profit hospitals have found ways to maximize reimbursement from their various sources of funding. Here is a brief primer on sound business practice. There are two principal components that contribute to profit (margin): revenue and expense. You need to either raise revenue or decrease expense, or both, to improve profit (margin). This is important to hospital department managers because they sometimes focus on the wrong thing. At the department management level, the best thing you can do to contribute to margin is to control expenses. You have very little control over revenue. The relationship between what you bill for and what you receive payment for is very tenuous and will be discussed in more detail later. Just remember that hospitals generally do not have a revenue problem, they have expense problems. Their operations are very costly, and the effective manager should be very focused on managing expense and less focused on revenue. I know of some respiratory managers who liked to think that the large amount of revenue their departments generated was so important to the hospital that they were off the hook when it came to managing expenses. Some of them have gone on to other forms of employment.

COST ACCOUNTING STRUCTURE

The real geographical and functional distinctions of hospital structure are not always clearly defined on the organizational chart. A much clearer road map would be the number and assignment of cost centers. Every department has at least one cost center. This is the accounting identifier that tells the accountants where to post expenses in the general ledger. Cost centers are where management responsibility really lands. There are usually cost centers for every functional service area and department listed in Figure 2-1. Inside each cost center are expense accounts. Department directors are charged with managing the expenses associated with operating their departments. These expenses include labor, supplies, equipment repair and maintenance, administrative supplies, computer costs, training, utilities, and lots and lots of other costs. In addition, departments that include billable services also manage their revenue stream, for example they create and manage a billing system that allows their staff to bill for the services they deliver. The departments listed in Table 2-1 are those usually associated with billed services.

There are also lots of departments that do not directly bill the patients for their services, such as security, engineering, library, housekeeping, food services, payroll, information technology, and others. Some hospitals account for the cost of these operations by billing the revenue generating departments internally using cost transfers. These transfers are expenses that are generally unmanageable by department directors who have these transfers land in their cost centers. But these cost transfers help to remind you that the cost of the respiratory therapy department is not just the expenses of the

Table 2-1. Departments in Hospitals That Usually Have Billed Services

Anatomical Pathology	Chest Clinic
Anesthesiology	Dialysis
Apnea Study Program	ECMO
Audiology	Emergency Room
Blood Bank	Gastroenterology Laboratory
Cardiology	Hematology/Oncology Unit
Cast Room	Intensive Care Unit
Cath Lab	Interventional Radiology
Central Services	IV Team

(Continues)

Table 2-1. Departments in Hospitals That Usually Have Billed Services *(Continued)*

Laboratory	Radiation Therapy
Medical Surgical Unit	Radiology CT Scanner
Medical Transport Team	Radiology Diagnostic
Microbiology	Radiology MRI
Neonatal Intensive Care Unit	Radiology Nuclear Medicine
Nephrology Clinic	Radiology Ultrasound
Neurology	Recovery Room
Nutrition Services	Rehab Unit
Occupational Therapy	Respiratory Therapy
Orthotics	Speech Pathology
Pediatric Intensive Care Unit	Surgery
Pharmacy	Surgical Unit
Physical Therapy	Various Outpatient Clinics
Psychiatric Unit	Virology
Pulmonary Function Lab	

department but also includes the services you receive from other hospital departments like payroll. Payroll is good. On a side note, become friends with the payroll director. Someday it may really payoff.

SILOS

Look again at the organizational chart shown in Figure 2-1. Note that the divisions of the service areas and functions are all aligned vertically. They are essentially stacked into what many management theorists like to call silos, for example missile or grain silos.[5–6] Nursing is in one silo. Ancillary services are in another silo, as are information technology and business practices. This convention is about as old as humanity. It is basically hierarchical, as were the Roman legions, which when you think about it were fairly effective organizations. However, it can lead to structural problems. "Hand-offs" are what happens when patients move through our silos horizontally. From the patient's perspective, they do not come into and go through our systems in a single silo. They move across the horizontal axis of our systems and cross from silo to silo. Figure 2-2 demonstrates this idea visually.

As patients move from silo to silo (figuratively and literally), there are hand-offs, for example responsibility for the patient is handed from one service to another or one clinician to another. And like a hand-off in a football game, there is always a chance for a fumble during a hand-off.[7] Fumbles during hand-offs can also occur vertically within a silo. This is particularly true for shift to shift report in clinical services like nursing and respiratory therapy. A lot is being written about hand-off failures and

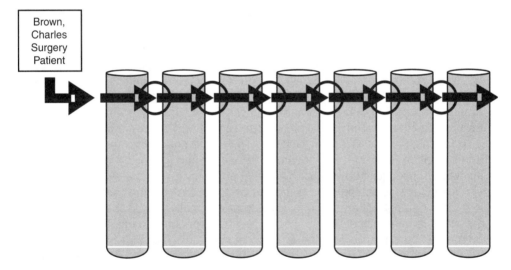

Figure 2–2. Functional Silos at St. Elsewhere Hospital

Mr. Brown is a typical surgical patient. As he moves through the system at St. Elsewhere Hospital he is frequently "handed off." Medicine (his admitting physician) hands him off to nursing and respiratory therapy. Nursing takes him to radiology for a study and hands him off to radiology. When he goes to surgery he is handed off to the operating room, who then hands him off to the nursing service again after his surgery. It goes on and on. The arrows represent his movement through the silos (systems) or processes. The circles represent potential places to fumble the hand-off.

possible solutions,[8–9] and the JCAHO has issued National Patient Safety Goals[i] that include the development of standardized methods of handing off patients.

Examples of fumbles abound. Patients have their personal effects lost when they are transferred around the hospital. Wrong tests and studies are done because the hand-off between medicine and radiology was fumbled. After surgery, patients' treatments and therapies can be wrong or delayed because of the hand-off between the operating room and the medical surgical ward. For the sake of brevity I will ask you to trust me, we could fill this entire chapter with examples like this.

Case Study 2: Fumbling the Hand-Off

Charles Brown is a 2-year-old who was being treated at the Heavenly Gates Children's Hospital for his asthma. He was receiving aerosolized bronchodilator therapy. This duty was shared between nursing and respiratory therapy. Sometimes the RN did the treatments and sometimes the RT did them. Administered medications were supposed to be recorded in a computerized medication administration record as well as on nursing and respiratory flow sheets, respectively. Gladys Wratchet, RN gave Charlie his regularly scheduled treatment at 0800. Just as the treatment ended, she got called away to go to Mr. McMurphy's room. Meanwhile Eigotta Kough, RRT came to the room at about 0820 and thoroughly and methodically evaluated the patient, gave the regularly scheduled 0800 treatment, and went to the computer and logged the treatment in the medication administration record and on his flow sheet. A few minutes later Nurse Wratchet went to log her treatment into the medication administration record and discovered the patient had received two treatments instead of one. Luckily, albuterol is a fairly benign drug, and the patient suffered no ill effects from getting two treatments at approximately the same time. This is a classic fumble of a hand-off. It is also an example of a disabling structure, for example here was a system whose design contributed to creating this error by having shared (and therefore unclear) accountability for these treatments. It also demonstrates how much poor (or in this case nonexistent) communication can contribute to errors and fumbles. Had the RT stopped to talk with the RN, this mishap could have been avoided.

---

[i]Joint Commission on Accreditation of Healthcare Organizations, 2007 National Patient Safety Goals Hospital Version, Goal 2E, which states, "Implement a standardized approach to 'hand off' communications, including an opportunity to ask and respond to questions."

Respiratory therapy departments have (to varying degrees) been using standardized forms for passing along information about patients from shift to shift. Figure 2-3 is an example of a shift report form used for tracking patients and giving reports in an RT department. It was developed in a spreadsheet.

Note the local jargon and abbreviations in the column headings. This widespread practice of making up terms and abbreviations makes my teeth ache. There is a dizzying array of arcane abbreviations in clinical documents in hospitals. And they are different from hospital to hospital. In fact, they are different from department to department. Okay, they are actually different from RT to RT, RN to RN, MD to MD, nutritionist to nutritionist, pharmacist to pharmacist. We have learned that this is not a harmless quirk in the constellation of human expression. These inconsistent abbreviations can be dangerous and are known to have contributed to patient deaths. Use of abbreviations has become a major focus of the JCAHO efforts to improve patient safety.[ii]

Some hospitals have had modest success at changing their structures so that there is less vertical integration and more lateral integration in care processes. Uh oh, here comes another one. *Immutable Truth #8: It's all about processes.* The entire operation of the hospital is a process. It can be broken down into lots and lots of smaller processes, which themselves can be further deconstructed into subprocesses. Managing a department of 50 or 60 employees can seem overwhelming. One good way to keep it intellectually manageable is to break the operation into its various processes. When this is done you can begin to analyze which parts of the processes are working and which are not. This is done using measurement. Speaking of truths, *Immutable Truth #9: You cannot manage what you do not measure.* In my experience, the number one, top dog, most common, ubiquitous mistake made by managers is to fail to build sufficient measurement systems into their processes.

Come to think of it, the patients have their own processes. A patient being admitted, studied, treated, and released is a process. In fact, it is the single most important process a hospital has to manage. All our managerial activities ought to be in some way related to lubricating this process.

MEETINGS AND ELECTRONIC MAIL

Most large organizations like hospitals are addicted to meetings. They have bad cases of meetingitis. They meet to decide when they are going to meet. It is said that there are two major kinds of work in modern organizations:

[ii]JCAHO 2007 National Patient Safety Goal 2B, http://www.jointcommission.org.

Date	Shift	RT:				Mode/LPM	F_1O_2	RR / HZ	V_T / AV	PIP AMP IPAP	PEEP MAP EPAP	PS	Blood Gas	Retape & Trach Size & Change	Equip. Change/ Sx'n Size
Room #	Patient	Diagnosis	Intervention	Comments											
ICU-1															
ICU-2															
ICU-3															
ICU-4															
ICU-5															
ICU-6															
ICU-7															
ICU-8															

Figure 2-3. Shift Report Form

A sample of a document used for tracking and "handing off" patients. These systems are only as good as the discipline of those using them. Note the use of local, arcane abbreviations.

(1) taking phone messages for people who are in meetings, and (2) going to meetings. Everyone likes to gripe about meetings. And God knows there are way too many. But when you start analyzing the phenomenon of meetings carefully, you will soon understand why this is so. People are desperately trying to communicate. They want to promote their ideas and plans. They want to solicit input. They want to persuade and influence others. These are all good things. Dilbert might come up with a different list of reasons why people have meetings—to get free donuts, to have a mechanism for blame-sharing if things go wrong, to avoid doing any real work, etc.

I have come to the conclusion that the single largest barrier to selling ideas or changing paradigms or implementing changes for the greater good is getting the players in the same room at the same time. The politically correct term for players is "stakeholders," that is, anyone who has an interest in the process that you are working on. This is principally the reason administrative assistants exist. Administrative assistants (formerly called secretaries) used to be around to answer the phone, take messages, create documents (letters), and do filing. Most of this activity has been automated or at least seriously reduced. Now administrative assistants basically manage meeting schedules. It takes a great deal of time to find a date and time when most people, if not everyone, can attend and then find a place to have a meeting. Believe it or not, one real impediment to this process in most hospitals is an insufficient number of conference rooms. There has been competition for conference rooms in every hospital I have worked at. This is an example of why thoughtful advance planning is good. Get your meetings set up early. You will have a greater chance of getting people together and finding a conference room. Early, in the context of hospital meeting scheduling, is two to three months in advance. Anything less than that and you will have trouble getting busy administrators, doctors, and nurse managers together.

Some meetings are way cool. Especially those where a group is working on a specific task, like a project team. If run properly, these can be great sessions that actually accomplish real work. The worst meetings are standing committee meetings where you go around the table and talk about what is going on in your departments. These have a very low signal-to-noise ratio.

All this notwithstanding, meetings are a vital part of corporate life. It is often where you start building relationships with other members of the hospital's leadership team, like nurse managers and physicians who have administrative duties. You will be very much tempted to skip meetings. I do it. Everyone does it. But you can't do it too much. You will miss important information, and you may not have a chance to contribute to the discussion of ideas and plans. If you are organizing a meeting yourself (which you should avoid unless absolutely necessary), you may want to use the basic guidelines in Table 2-2.

E-mail was supposed to help with the process of corporate communication (which itself is actually an oxymoron). I cannot quite figure out whether it has helped or not. For individual, person-to-person communication, e-mail is very helpful and convenient. It is a great way to share documents and other types of files. It allows me to get access to lots of work-related communication from anywhere I can get access to the Web because most hospitals now have remote access to the hospital e-mail system through a Web portal.

In my opinion, for group communication, e-mail has turned out to be less useful than hoped for. A person is less likely to really concentrate and read

Table 2-2. Guidelines for Setting Up and Running a Good Meeting

Guideline	Details
Avoid meetings	• If at all possible, don't schedule meetings.
	• Think hard about why you are calling this meeting.
	• Is it really necessary? Can you do it via e-mail or a Web-based meeting or in a conference call?
	• If you really hate meetings, then guess what, so do most other people.
Keep it short and small	• Most people's eyes glaze over after about 60–90 minutes of meeting.
	• I have violated this principle from time to time but only when I have lots of data to share or when the meeting was for a specific team that was working on a definable project or task. Keep your meeting size as small as possible.
	• Very little real work gets done if there are more than four to six people involved.
Avoid deforestation	• When we use presentation technology at meetings, we tend to hand out printed materials that

Table 2-2. Guidelines for Setting Up and Running a Good Meeting (Continued)

Guideline	Details
	are wholly or in part duplicates of what we are showing on the screen.
	• Skip this because it just contributes to deforestation.
	• Offer to send everyone at the meeting a copy of your presentation.
	• If they want to take notes, they should have brought their notebooks with them.
Have an agenda	• This sounds stupidly obvious, but not nearly enough time goes into developing well honed meeting agendas.
	• Without one, even if you have a good idea in your head of what you want to happen at these meetings, you stand a good chance of floundering around and getting off track. Some draconian meeting facilitators assign a time period for each agenda item and when the time is used up they stop the discussion and move on.
Take charge	• Meetings have to be facilitated. This is a politically correct way of saying someone is in charge and keeps things moving along.
	• This may require you to intervene when the conversation wanders. Good facilitation is a real skill and must be learned. There is formalized facilitator training. You should take it. I have.
	• If you are meeting to solicit input from others about plans and ideas, you may want to poll the jury. In other words, go around the table and specifically ask each individual what he or she thinks.
	• There is an old adage, "Silence equals agreement." Good luck with that. This is not an

(Continues)

Table 2-2. Guidelines for Setting Up and Running a Good Meeting *(Continued)*

Guideline	*Details*
	effective way to develop consensus. Also don't let certain loud mouthed individuals (like me) dominate the conversation.
Morning has broken	• My experience is that mornings are generally better times for meetings.
	• People are sharper and usually in a better mood than they are by the afternoon. The day has not yet had a chance to beat them down. By the afternoon, most folks are a little worn.
	• After years and years of day shift work, I actually prefer really early meetings. I have worked in hospitals that have executive level meetings at 0700. Of course, there are those who think this is somewhat uncivilized.
	• I think the best times are between 0900 and 1300.
Attendance	• Don't assume anything about attendees. Just because you sent out an invitation, don't assume all invited parties will show up, even if it is on their computer calendars.
	• For important stuff it does not hurt to send out a friendly and gentle reminder one or two days before the meeting.
	• If there are people whose attendance is essential, I make a phone call to be sure they are coming.
Types of meetings	• Standing meeting—A regularly scheduled gathering, such as a weekly one-on-one with a boss or a department, or a project meeting taking place at intervals until the project is over. Because these meetings recur, their format and agenda become relatively well established.
	• Topical meeting—A gathering intended to address one subject.

Table 2-2. Guidelines for Setting Up and Running a Good Meeting *(Continued)*

Guideline	Details
	• Conference—A highly structured, moderated meeting, like a presentation, where various participants contribute following a fixed agenda.
	• Emergency meeting—A meeting called to address a crisis, whether internal or external. Such meetings are often arranged with very little notice, but attendance is mandatory. If the emergency meeting conflicts with another appointment, the emergency meeting typically takes precedence.
	• Seminar—A structured meeting with an educational purpose. Seminars are usually led by people with expertise in the subject matter.
Ground rules	• It's a good idea to have ground rules for standing meetings to help participants curb their more erratic and antisocial behaviors. Here's a list of ground rules for meetings I attend.
	• Arrive on time and begin the meeting promptly (within 5 minutes of the scheduled start time)
	• End the meeting on time
	• Listen openly
	• Avoid side conversations
	• Set pagers and phones to vibrate
	• Say "We're off track" to others in the group to get the conversation back on track
	• In interactions, assume that everyone wants what's best for the patient
Minutes	• Minutes are a pain. I generally avoid them, knowing as I do that hardly anyone ever reads them. There are exceptions. Some standing committee meetings must keep minutes to meet regulatory guidelines.

(Continues)

Table 2-2. Guidelines for Setting Up and Running a Good Meeting *(Continued)*

Guideline	Details
	• Minutes are also useful when work is being passed out at meetings. Minutes can be a record of what folks agreed to do.
	• When I check the minutes of meetings it is mostly to make sure there is not something that I am supposed to do that I have not yet done. Typically, I do this 15–30 minutes before a meeting that was scheduled several weeks ago. Because it is unlikely that I will get any real work done in the brief time that remains, I usually use it to formulate excuses for why I didn't get things done.

an e-mail that is addressed to 46 other people as well (or 460). This is especially true if the e-mail did not come from someone above you in the food chain. This may sound terribly cynical, but it is a harsh reality. E-mail is a blessing and a curse. Sometimes you can be so overwhelmed by the volume of e-mails that you are reduced to a sort of quasi-hierarchical ranking of messages that you use to decide who to respond to first, if at all. There are many sources of e-mail for the typical department director–manager to deal with. Here is a list, sort of in order, maybe:

- From your boss—Far be it from me to tell you what to do, but it is generally a good idea to read your e-mails from your boss ASAP. It is also advisable to actually respond to the e-mail too, dealing with whatever he or she wanted you to deal with.
- From your staff—I have made the mistake of failing to follow up on e-mails from my staff. This usually happened when I opened the e-mail, read it, and fully intended to respond or reply and take care of whatever it was that the person wanted from me. But my mistake was not doing it right away. I got busy, went for coffee, checked the Drudge Report, got 65 other messages that day, and lost track of the e-mail. Two weeks later I had a very unhappy staffer who thought I didn't care about his or her issues. Keep track of the e-mails you need to respond to. A good rule of thumb (but very difficult to follow) is the "handle it once" rule. For

paper documents and e-mails alike, try to handle them once. Deal with them right then if possible. Dispose of the documents or e-mails the first time you read them. This is very challenging and cannot always be done, but it is a good goal to aim for.

- From other directors–managers—These might be e-mails from nursing managers or directors or physicians or pharmacists or whatever. You can easily fall into a pattern of not dealing with these right away. If you want to have good relations with nursing management, which you should, then respond to their e-mails right away.
- Global e-mails—Global e-mails come from all over the hospital. Human resources departments have a marvelous habit of sending you lengthy, turgid e-mails on the latest thing they have thoughtfully conjured up for you to do. Ditto the regulatory affairs folks. Add to this growing list marketing, compliance, budgeting, accounting, training and development, and many others, and you start to see how many e-mails you can get. I try to read these, I swear. But usually, after a couple of paragraphs, I nod off. I got into a bad habit for a while. I would read only the first couple of paragraphs of a message and then assume I had gotten the essentials of the message. Turns out this was not always true. I also have been accused of ignoring these until the second round shows up, for example when they send you a reminder that you did not do what they asked in the first global e-mail they sent out to so very many. I categorically deny this accusation, and on the advice of my attorney (A.L. Dewitt), I decline to discuss this further.
- From Listservs—Many clinical managers belong to Listservs related to their clinical specialty.[iii] These are e-mail groups of like-minded clinicians from across the country and sometimes around the globe that share stories and ask questions of their colleagues. These can generate lots of messages every day, and sometimes they are even interesting. However, there is a serious caveat here. Some people post so often to these forums that I wonder how and if they actually do any work. I went through this period myself and would save you from

---

[iii]RC_World—A list for respiratory therapy issues (http://ourworld.compuserve.com/homepages/hannigan/).
NICU-list—A list for neonatal intensive care issues (https://mailman.usm.edu/mailman/listinfo/nicu).
PICU-list—A list for pediatric intensive care issues (http://www.vpicu.org/forum.php).
CCM-L—A list for adult critical care issues (http://www.ccm-l.org/index2.html). And many more.

this self-destructive behavior. Luckily, none of my previous bosses ever read the Listservs I was subscribing to. If you are passionate about what you do, you will find yourself occasionally disagreeing with postings, and some of us feel a need to correct pretty much everybody we ever meet that is suffering from being incorrect. This will exact a heavy burden. Don't bother because hardly anyone ever has their mind changed by the incisive logic of your arguments. I tend to use these lists to find out what others are doing or distribute interesting information or articles about the latest clinical issues. Remember, Listservs in no way can be thought of as a cross-sectional representation of the RT community. The reasons for this are beyond the scope of this chapter, but trust me, asking RC_World posters what their opinion is about a topic is just like talk radio. You may get some very good advice, but then again you may not. Like I said, it is a low signal-to-noise ratio. A simple rule that works for me: Delete 90% of Listserv postings without reading them. Read only those that have a subject line that is incredibly interesting.

- Family and friends—In reality, these are pretty much at the top of your hierarchy, but I put them down here in case my boss reads this book, which I seriously doubt.
- Your bank—FYI, banks never send e-mails about your account except to inform you that your online statement is ready to view. If you get one from (supposedly) your bank asking you to respond with sensitive account information, it ain't your bank.

I can get 50–75 e-mails some days. I (and most other managers I know) have repeatedly deleted important messages without reading them. Typically, we were zipping along and accidentally deleted something we should have read. If you want to avoid having others do this with your e-mails, put something in the subject line that will grab their attention, like "Free Money" or "From your old high school sweetheart." On second thought, don't. The hospital's spam-blocking software might dump such messages, thinking they were spam. Our information technology department runs a spam blocking program that helps us by limiting the spam that gets through to users inside our intranet. They told me that 75–80% of all e-mails coming into the hospital's e-mail servers from outside are spam, and thus they are blocked. Table 2-3 lists some basic guidelines that should help you when using e-mail.

Table 2-3. Guidelines for Effective Use of E-Mail*

Good	Not good
• Keep messages short. • Use bullet points and short statements as opposed to long narrative or declarative rhetoric. • Put something about the contents in the subject line, especially if it is someone who gets a lot of messages. Otherwise, you will not get their attention and they might accidentally delete the message, as you sometimes do. • Respond as quickly as possible to e-mails from your staff. This can be very tough to accomplish for a busy manager, but nothing is as disempowering as having a staff member e-mail you and not get a response from you. I have had some staff people get very very mad at me because they thought I did not care about them or their issues. • As much as possible, handle e-mails once. Open them, read them, respond to them, and delete them all in one setting. There is a tremendous temptation to open an e-mail, read it, and decide to deal with it later. I cannot speak for everyone, but this sometimes has caused me trouble because I don't get back to the e-mail soon enough. • Minimize the number of e-mails. Most folks are on information overload. Between the Internet, cell phones,	• Never ever send an e-mail when you are really mad. You will almost certainly live to regret it. Feel free to write a viscious, slashing screed, but for God's sake don't send it. Save it, go home, play with the kids, kiss the spousal unit, and/or hold the basset hound on your lap. Go back to work, open the e-mail you saved, and reread it. You will, without fail, significantly edit the message. • Don't use e-mail to avoid an unpleasant conversation. This is a powerful temptation on par with Jack Daniels or Kobe beef or other temptations that I shall not at this time elaborate on. Do not give in to this. Do I give in occasionally? Yes, in a moment of weakness I have been known to use e-mail instead of talking to someone. I have almost always paid a price for this. Usually it involves ineffectuality, for example not really accomplishing what I wanted by way of changing people's hearts-minds-behaviors. • Don't hurry when doing e-mail. I have sometimes sent the wrong information, sometimes very sensitive information, to the wrong people because I was in too much of a hurry when doing e-mails. Proofread your e-mails, double check your distribution lists or addresses. I have (more than once) meant to send a global e-mail to my

(Continues)

Table 2-3. Guidelines for Effective Use of E-Mail *(Continued)*

Good	*Not good*
cable TV, radio, podcasts, and all the other distractions, we end up getting way more information than we can possibly process. Your messages to your staff will begin to become "noise" if you send too many. The hope of e-mail as the panacea that would solve our communication problem has been bitterly dashed on the rocks of the reality that e-mail is just another form of communication to be ignored and/or abused.	staff and accidentally sent it to 800 respiratory therapists around the world via an erroneous address to a Listserv. Sigh.
• Be careful. The "reply" command is subtly different than the "reply to all" command. Slow down, check your distribution lists, make sure you don't include someone you shouldn't or overlook someone (both equally serious crimes).	• Use humor and sarcasm with care. As you have probably figured out by now, humor is a vital part of my whole shtick. But be careful with humor, especially sarcasm, as it is sometimes lost on some Philistines. Make sure you know the recipients well before you journey too far down this road. • Don't dis. If you trash someone in an e-mail, there is always a chance it will get around. This happens and can result in your comments ending up in the mailbox of the victim of your disrespect, which is almost always not a good thing.

Caveat. There is a great Latin phrase that we would all do well to keep fresh in our minds. *Cave quid dicis, quando, et cui,* which translates: beware what you say, when, and to whom. Each company will have its own set of e-mail guidelines. You should become familiar with them. Remember that any e-mails you send or receive on a company computer or company network are technically the property of the company and thus you have no legal expectation of privacy. I thoroughly love getting and receiving funny e-mails including pictures and video clips. Just know that if they are questionable in content, you could be in the unemployment line before you know it if (1) they violate company policy, (2) the company decides to enforce its policies, or (3) you get caught or someone rats you out. Speaking of humor, for some excellent satire on netiquette, go to http://www.faqs.org/faqs/usenet/emily-postnews/part1/.

Case Study 3: The Lure of E-mail

Ira Newby, RRT was an excellent clinician. He worked at his own professional development, had lots of energy, and was highly engaged at work. So, naturally, he was eventually promoted to a leadership position. Having recently been in a staff position, he knew where all the bodies were hidden. He wanted very much to make a difference and had high expectations for standards of performance. As a supervisor, Ira started right in trying to clean things up. He soon surmised that the best way to change the behaviors of the staff was to identify a problem area, formulate a solution, which usually involved getting the staff to change their behaviors, and then sending out an e-mail to the staff outlining this problem, what our policy was, and asking everyone to comply. There was only one problem. It wasn't working. The same problems kept popping up. So Ira sent out more e-mails with more explicit directions. He attached copies of the policies involved or included hyperlinks to the policies in the e-mail. While some things got better, it was clear that this method of process improvement was not very effective. He talked to the director who suggested that he conduct an experiment. He showed Ira how to request an e-mail notification when the staff opened his e-mails. There were approximately 50 staff members on Ira's e-mail distribution list. The next time Ira sent out a message, he set his e-mail program to send him a notice of when each staff member opened the message. Within the first 48 hours he got about 15 notifications that his e-mail had been read. After that it slowed way down and he got about one to two per day for the next 10 days. He also got a few messages indicating that his e-mail had been deleted without being read. Three weeks after sending out the original message, Ira was still getting an occasional notification. It was obvious that the cycle of work schedules, time off, vacations, apathy, and indifference combined to cause a serious delay in how long it took folks to read his e-mails. Further investigation showed Ira that some RTs had worked a number of shifts between when Ira had sent out his message and when they finally got around to reading it or deleting it unread.

After fuming about this for a while, he went back to his director and asked, "What's up with that?!"

"It is the boy who cried wolf phenomenon," the director said. "Too many e-mails have the effect of diluting the importance of any single message," he pointed out. "Plus, in an attempt to be thorough, you tend to write long, dense messages. The truth is that most folks won't take the time to read them. I suggest you trim the number and lengths of e-mails you send out," he said as he headed out the door to his fifth meeting of the day.

Ira's story illustrates a vital point. E-mail is an important tool and cannot and should not be overlooked as an essential part of communication. But depending on it as the only method of communication is risky. Most of the time it doesn't work, especially when you wish to influence others and change behaviors. E-mail must be done in conjunction with other forms, including posted flyers, notices, graphs, and of course, face time.

RELATIONSHIPS WITH OTHER DEPARTMENTS AND GROUPS

As a department manager, there is a risk that you can descend into a sort of siege mentality with regard to other departments in the hospital. Circling the wagons and digging a moat are always fun. They are manifestations of our natural instinct to enter the "cycle of fear."[iv] But like a lot of other natural instincts we have, you must resist this one too. At times I have personally allowed myself to become too isolated in the hospital. The thinking goes like this. "What the hell do other managers know about how tough it is to run an RT department? Usually they just complain at me about the poor quality and quantity of RTs, and who needs that?" So you avoid them. You skip meetings and hide out. This is not good. The truth is that other managers have all the same troubles and fears and hopes that you do. Too often, the respiratory-nursing interface becomes adversarial. And from the outside, it might look like other department directors have it made. Why, after all most of her staff are in one place and do the same tasks every day in a controlled environment. How hard can that be to manage? This can be very destructive thinking. You have to rise above this as a leader and stay focused on the things that are important. Other department directors–managers can be a great help and encouragement to you. Invite one to lunch. Call them up. Send them a funny e-mail joke from time to time (do not overdo this, as people will wonder, appropriately, if you have too much time on your hands). If your natural state is to have self-confidence bordering on arrogance (as is mine) then you might figure no other managers have anything that you can learn from them. You (and I) need to be disabused of this illusion. Try to be open for learning every day.

Good relationships with other departments will help facilitate problem solving and enhance communications. Invite other department representatives

---

[iv]The cycle of fear is discussed more in Chapter 4. This term refers to a recognizable pattern of human corporate behavior exhibited when we are frightened.

to your staff meetings. Invite nursing supervisors to your supervisor meetings. They may not come, but you should invite them anyway. Keep them in the loop about what is happening in your department. Real communication between and within departments in a hospital are surpassingly hard to achieve. You can work and work at it, do all your due diligence, and still find holes in the system.

Case Study 4: Communications Fallacies

The respiratory therapy department at Heavenly Gates Children's Hospital worked for nearly 18 months developing a new model of care for the administration of routine respiratory therapy procedures outside the intensive care unit. The labor market was as tight as a snare drum head, and it was not possible to get enough RTs on board to manage the seasonal demand for nebulizer treatments and oxygen therapy during the height of the viral season. Demand for RTs was also growing in the intensive care units. A team of nursing and respiratory managers had developed a model in which the nurses would be cross trained to administer certain high-volume, low-risk respiratory procedures, like pulse oximetry, oxygen administration, and aerosolized bronchodilator therapy. A lot of training and attempted communication took place in the respiratory department and between the respiratory and nursing management teams. Posters and flyers were developed, distributed to the RTs, and given to the nursing managers. Questions were asked of the nurse managers about whether the nursing staff knew about these fundamental changes that were coming. The teams were assured that staff nurses had been kept in the loop. On the second day of the rollout of the new plan, the respiratory director ran into two different staff nurses on day shift who said they had no idea that there was a new care model, having never heard a peep about it (no pun intended). No training, no memos, zip, nada. The RT director exercised near Herculean self-control and said nothing. He left the floor and went to the gym during lunch and worked out on the body bag.

This director told me he learned some important lessons from this episode. He learned that, shockingly, nursing managers had trouble communicating with all their staff in spite of their good intentions. This is certainly true for all directors–managers. He also learned that it is almost impossible to over-communicate about important systemic changes. From then on, along with usual e-mail missives, he developed his own paper memos to nurses and had them hand delivered to all the nursing mailboxes on the various units. Good relations between respiratory therapy and the inpatient nursing units are vital and will help prevent these kinds of communication mishaps.

Physician relations are pretty vital too. As a respiratory department manager you will be working a lot with clinical practice guidelines and protocols. These are tools designed primarily to improve the quality of respiratory care procedural intervention. One of the reasons health care is so expensive is that we tend to do a lot of things that have no discernable benefit to patients. We over treat much more often than we under treat patients. Protocols and practice guidelines help improve utilization management, which is a fancy way of saying that we only do things to patients when they need things and/or they show a benefit from receiving things, such as treatments.

What all this does is set up potential conflict with the medical staff who have been the principal (but not the only) drivers of this over utilization. When you get together with groups of respiratory directors–managers you hear a lot of grousing about physicians being obstacles to improving utilization management and the development of clinical practice guidelines. This has not been my experience. I have rarely been unable to get physicians to agree with our efforts to develop and implement protocols and practice guidelines. One reason might be that we do lots of thorough research and apply good scholarship to the development of our protocols. Physicians are scientifically trained and respond very positively to well crafted and referenced arguments. Of course, they must be approached and dealt with in a deferential and collegial fashion, which is nothing more than they deserve considering their abusive educational preparation and the scope of their responsibilities. Of course, there are exceptions. But my advice is to work around these obstacles as opposed to trying to go through them. *Immutable Truth #10: Do not sacrifice the good for the perfect.* You will never really be able to obtain the perfect, and usually, the good is quite good and probably good enough and certainly better than what you have now. With regard to getting physicians to agree to practice guidelines and protocols, if you have 80% or 90% compliance, you will achieve considerable improvements. You may want to design your documentation of protocol compliance so that you can identify physicians who habitually ignore practice guidelines and protocols. This information can then be forwarded to the department medical director. Let him or her deal with it. That is usually what they are supposed to do (and are getting paid for).

Another important part of maintaining good relations with the medical staff is collaboration. It is easy to go off on your own and develop plans and ideas for improving clinical care. But these must be run through a review with your medical staff. The sooner you defer to this truth and get them involved, the happier they will be. And everybody likes happy doctors.

REFERENCES

1. Kohn LT, Corrigan JM, Donaldson MS, eds. *To Err is Human: Building a Safer Health System.* Washington, DC: National Academy Press; 2000.
2. Starfield B. Is U.S. healthcare really the best in the world? *JAMA.* 2000; 204(4):482–485.
3. Halm EA, Lee C, Chassin MR. Is volume related to outcome in health care? A systematic review and methodologic critique of the literature. *Ann Intern Med.* 2002;137:511–520.
4. Silverman EM, Skinner JS, Fisher ES. The association between for-profit hospital ownership and increased Medicare spending. *N Engl J Med.* 1999;341:420–426.
5. Chinnis A, White KR. Challenging the dominant logic of emergency departments' guidelines from chaos theory. *J Emerg Med.* 1999;17:1049–1054.
6. Begun JW, Tornabeni J, White KR. Opportunities for improving patient care through lateral integration: the clinical nurse leader. *J Healthc Manage.* January-February 2006;51:19–25.
7. Patterson ES, et al. Handoff strategies in settings with high consequences for failure: lessons for health care operations. *Int J Qual Health Care.* April 2004;16:125–132.
8. Alvarado K, Lee R, Christoffersen E, Fram N, et al. Transfer of accountability: transforming shift handover to enhance patient safety. *Healthc Q.* October 2006;(9, theme issue):75–79.
9. Arora V, Johnson J. A model for building a standardized hand-off protocol. *Jt Comm J Qual Patient Saf.* 2006;32(11):646–655.

CHAPTER 3

Structuring a Department

Alice: Would you tell me, please, which way I ought to go from here

Cheshire Cat: That depends a good deal on where you want to get to

Alice: I don't much care where

Cheshire Cat: Then it doesn't matter which way you go

Alice: So long as I get somewhere

Cheshire Cat: Oh, you're sure to do that . . . if you only walk long enough

—Through the Looking Glass by Lewis Carroll

Most hospital department directors or managers inherit the structure of their departments. And one of the worst things you can do is jump right in and tear things up too quickly. First you must learn how the department really works, which is almost certainly distinctly different than how it looks on paper or how you might have been told it works. Organizations like hospital departments have a sort of dualism to their nature. There are formal and informal leaders as well as formal and informal pathways of communication. There are formal and informal rules, and there are spoken and unspoken cultural norms, all of which have a great deal to do with how the department really functions. And of course there are real policies and procedures and then there is urban myth. The urban myth takes the form of policies that, like the Pentateuch, were passed along orally during the early part of their history. But unlike the first five books of the Old Testament, these oral traditions in your RT department were most probably not authored by the hand and/or inspiration of God.[i]

---

[i] I realize that discussing religious beliefs is no longer acceptable in civilized society, and soon any tangential reference to spiritual or religious matters will probably simply be outlawed altogether. Please consider the Old Testament comment to be essentially humorous in nature. It is not necessarily representative of my own beliefs, but it could be.

No, instead these oral policies have no real discernable origin and often no logical reason behind their creation. Nevertheless, they are very powerful. It takes time to learn the subtleties of these operations.

But after a thoughtful period of study and meditation, and in spite of continual attempts to avoid having to do so, the director–manager will eventually face the question of whether the department is properly structured. As I have stated earlier, the structure of organizations is pretty important. It can be enabling or disabling. Eventually you will have to ponder reasons why you might want to restructure a department. You will be tempted to put forth any of the following reasons:

- To reduce inappropriate utilization of respiratory care interventions
- To streamline operations
- To reduce cost per unit of care (this will be explained in detail later)
- To improve staff morale
- To improve the accuracy of the billing system
- To get a good performance review from your boss

All of these are cracking good reasons to restructure a department. But they are not the very *best* reason for changing the structure of a department. *Immutable Truth #11: The main thing is to keep the main thing, the main thing.* Why in the world should I restate the obvious, you ask? Because so many people forget the main purpose of a clinical hospital department. When this is learned–relearned, the systems and structure can be built around that main thing. So what is the main thing in operating a clinical hospital department like respiratory therapy? It is giving the right patient the right treatment at the right time in the best possible fashion. Everything else in the department ought to be designed, planned, built, implemented, wrapped up, compressed, and sent down the line with the single goal of putting qualified clinicians at the bedside of the patients who need them. Funny as it may seem, this can and does get lost in the calculus of decision making and rigors of daily life in a management position. When you forget about this being the number one thing, it can cause you to lose drive, focus, passion, and compassion. Do not let the rest of it interfere too much with what your overarching purpose ought to be.

This does not mean that managing finances and human resources and other vital systems are not important. But they are not ends in themselves. They are tools for achieving a larger purpose, for example ridiculously high quality patient care. At a staff meeting once, I was showing the staff the results of a study that demonstrated how poor our billing accuracy was, and I was trying to persuade them that *they* were responsible for producing an accurate bill for their services. One very gifted clinician stood up and announced, "I don't really care about billing, I came into this field and took this job at this hospital to do patient care and help people. Billing ain't important to me." My initial, fleeting reaction was a nearly overpowering desire to knock him to the floor and cause him some dyspnea by applying pressure to his crycothyroid notch with my lower extremity. I abstained. This was not an uncommon sentiment in the RT field for a while, and it is still prevalent (if unspoken) in some circles. The general feeling of some was that patient care was our lofty calling and that billing was a sort of money grubbing, pedestrian activity suitable for others. After he said this, I took a deep breath and told him that billing was an important tool to generate the funds we needed to hire and train qualified RTs and to buy the best clinical equipment possible. Thus, billing was a vital part of the process of providing high quality clinical care. He eventually came around. But this only happened after we began to measure individual billing accuracy.

MANAGING PROCESSES

It can be very helpful when thinking about the structure of a department to construct a high-level process map. This will visually describe the flow of people and materials in your operation. Figure 3-1 shows an example of a high-level process map for a respiratory department.

Process maps help illustrate an important point. The most effective managers realize that they are not managing people, they are managing processes. People are part of the process, but so are materials, facilities, ventilators, computers, pagers, phones, knowledge, training, competency, paper, ink, stethoscopes, refrigerators, water coolers, staple removers, and lots of other stuff. Construct your thinking around the processes you manage and build your structure to support those processes.

Consider Figure 3-1 again. Note that the main process runs horizontally from left to right starting with a request (or demand) for respiratory therapy services, and it flows through notification to deployment and ends up at the patient-therapist interface. Feeding into this main process are subprocesses, for example the process of training, acquiring supplies, using protocols and guidelines, staffing, and so on. You should build your measurement systems around those processes as well (see Chapter 4). All processes have outcomes. Something goes in one end of a process and something comes out of the other end. Along the way, important things happen. Some of these points in the process are conditional, for example additional things further along in the process cannot happen unless the conditional thing happens first. A respiratory therapist cannot give an aerosolized bronchodilator treatment if the patient's medication is not available. An anesthesiologist cannot induce

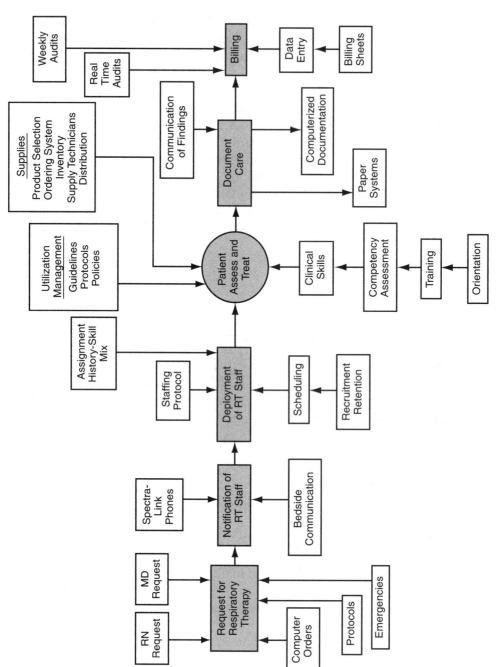

Figure 3-1. High-Level Process Map: Respiratory Therapy

High-level process map for a respiratory therapy department. At the center of the process is the assessment and treatment of the patient. Everything else flows towards or from this central thing. In fact, it is the "Main Thing."

anesthesia in a patient if the proper preoperative medications have not been given. Thus as you start analyzing the processes in your operation, you must identify key points of the process that need to run very smoothly. These are what you should focus on improving through measurement and action. Remember, *you cannot manage what you do not measure.*

A convenient convention is to categorize processes. There are clinical processes, business processes, and supply chain processes. All of these intersect at one point or another. All are vital to a department's operation.

Examples of clinical processes include ordering therapies, assessing patients, diagnostic procedures, administering ordered therapies, managing mechanical ventilators, patient monitoring, and documentation. Business processes might include scheduling, staffing, staff development, billing, recruiting, hiring, performance appraisal, and policy and procedure development. Supply chain processes could include ordering supplies, invoice management, product selection, contracting, equipment maintenance, inventory control, and supply distribution systems.

THE LEADERSHIP TEAM

Organizational charts have an interesting life. *Almost* all directors–managers can produce one for their departments. If you were to ask the staff to find the organizational chart, well, that dog might not hunt at all. These charts are very useful for presentations to people above you in the food chain to illustrate how your department is supposed to operate. Beyond that, they are mostly used for various forms of assignment, notably guilt, responsibility, and on rare occasions, congratulations. These charts lead a mostly lonely life. The actual duties of organizational charts seem to be mostly related to dust collection. This is too bad because they can be very useful when thinking about how your department is structured and how it should operate. I have looked at a lot of RT departments' organizational charts. Figures 3-2, 3-3, 3-4, 3-5, and 3-6 are examples of organizational charts that I have accumulated from other directors–managers over the years. Don't complain to me if they seem screwed up. I didn't create them. I did edit them ever so slightly for formatting purposes and to remove any unique identifiers that would allow individual hospitals to be identified. The names have been changed to protect the innocent (and the not so innocent). Note that some of these charts include the people above the director or manager, which is usually a very good political move.

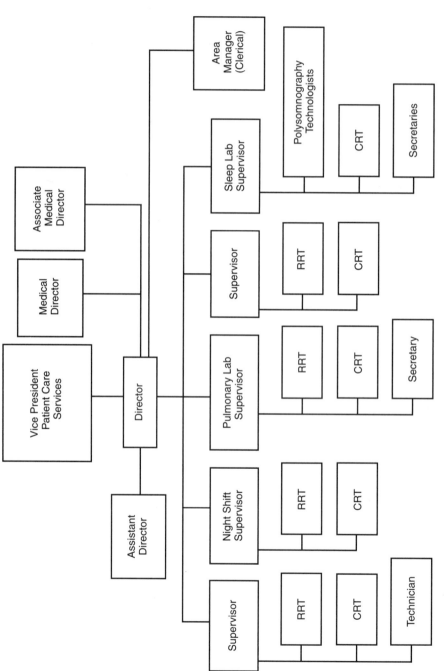

Figure 3-2. Example #1 of a Respiratory Organizational Chart

This chart represents an organizational responsibility that includes in-patient respiratory therapy, pulmonary function lab, and sleep lab (Polysomnography). Most departments have only a medical director, but this one sports an associate medical director as well. This usually represents a subspecialty, e.g., a physician who specializes in an area where respiratory therapy has a large presence, e.g., intensive care. Note the assistant director hanging out there all by his/her lonesome. When the next round of severe cost cutting approaches, people with "assistant" in their titles typically get nervous. Also, note the distinction between RRT and CRT positions. Some departments make distinctions in job duties between different levels of credentials, while others do not.

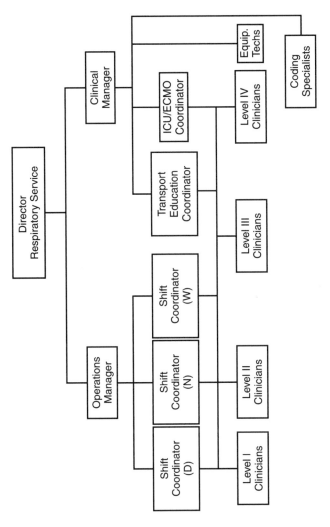

Figure 3-3. Example #2 of a Respiratory Organizational Chart
Here the department is divided administratively along lines of functional responsibility. Again, this department has what is typically called a clinical ladder. There are different levels of respiratory therapists. These typically have increasingly complex job duties and require more training and/or higher credentials.

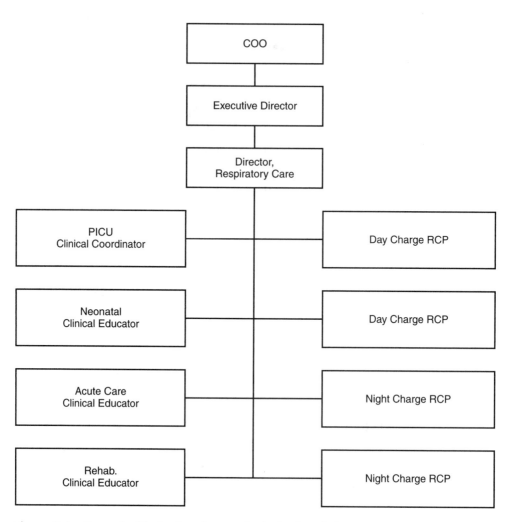

Figure 3-4. Example #3 of a Respiratory Organizational Chart
This is a "high" level organizational chart, in that it does not show any "staff" positions. While it might be useful for administrative work, I might avoid showing it to anyone in the department below the level of supervisor (or in this case "charge").

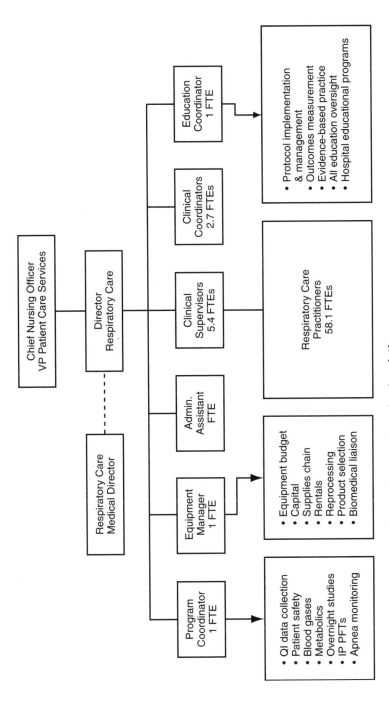

Figure 3-5. Example #4 of a Respiratory Organizational Chart

This chart begins to incorporate other important information for evaluating the structure of a department. The chart's designer included the number of FTEs in each position or area. Also included were some functional duties under the coordinator's boxes. This is typically done, because the more cynical and heartless observers (both internal and external) of the department have been known to sniff, "What the hell do coordinators do anyway?"

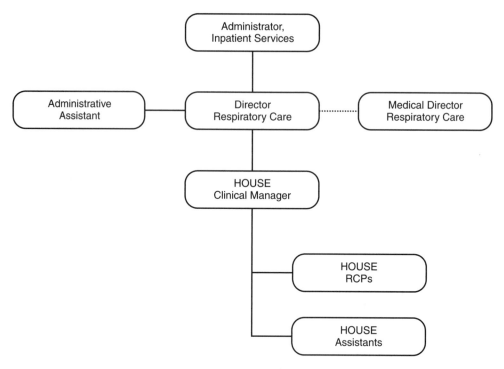

Figure 3-6. Example #5 of a Respiratory Organizational Chart
You have to admire anyone who would produce and distribute this chart. It is elegant, simple, clean, and doesn't clog up our analysis with a lot of pesky details about the department.

The people in positions of managerial authority in respiratory therapy departments have variously been called:

- Director
- Manager
- Educator
- Coordinator
- Supervisor
- Lead therapist
- Charge therapist
- Management team
- Supervisory team
- Charge group
- Lead team
- Leadership team
- Useless

I like the term "leadership team." I want my team to do more than manage and supervise. These are vital functions, but I hope they are part of the larger picture, for example leadership. As I stated earlier, leading and managing are not the same thing.[1-2] Management is focused on making sure tasks are done properly, that resources are in place, that things are run efficiently. Leadership is more focused on setting the proper goals, setting the correct vision, sharing the vision, staying focused on the mission, and helping get everyone on board about sharing the goals of the organization. It is said that managers manage tasks and leaders lead people. Table 3-1 lists statements and ideas about the difference between leadership and management that I have gathered over the years, mostly from management training seminars and in my masters program.

Table 3-1. Comparisons Between Leadership and Management

Management/Managers	Leadership/Leaders
Execute	Direct
Might be leaders	Have to be managers
Is a set of responsibilities	Is a creative act
Provide resources	Provide vision and influence
Is a function	Is a relationship
Accepts reality	Investigates reality
Maintains	Develops
Concentrates on systems and structures	Concentrates on people
Relies on control	Inspires trust
Asks how and when	Asks what and why
Focuses on the bottom line	Focuses on the horizon
Accepts the status quo	Challenges the status quo
Administers	Innovates
Has subordinates	Has followers
Push	Pull

This is not to suggest that one of these functions is any better than the other. They are both vital ideas without which an organization cannot be as effective as it should. Leadership would be empty and impractical without management. Management would be shallow and tedious without leadership.

Consider the administration of an aerosolized bronchodilator treatment. *Management* accountabilities include making sure that the RT who gives the treatment is properly trained, the treatment is done on time, the methods of giving the treatment are the most efficacious possible, a complete patient assessment is performed that includes descriptions of the effectiveness of the treatment, the cost of the treatment is kept as low as possible, and the treatment is properly documented and billed. *Leadership* accountabilities include an investigation of whether this treatment should have been given to begin with or if after given was of any discernable benefit to the patient. The sad truth is that a great deal of what respiratory therapists have done in the past have been shown to be of little value to patients. In some circles, this is heresy of the highest order, and saying that this emperor has no clothes has cost me more than one job I was seeking and well qualified for. I estimate that 25–50% of all respiratory therapy interventions are of little value to patients. By this I mean that they could not possibly have helped patients and never should have been done, or after they were done, there was no discernable patient response. The effective leader of a respiratory therapy department must attend to the management accountabilities and must also challenge the status quo and investigate whether the respiratory interventions are of value to patients. If not, systems and programs must be developed to begin to reduce the unnecessary and ineffective respiratory therapy. These have traditionally been called therapist-driven protocols and are part of a larger trend in health care toward "evidence-based practice" wherein therapeutic interventions are limited to those that have been proven to benefit patients. Historically, in autocratic, physician driven healthcare systems, doctors could order anything they thought would have the slightest possible chance of helping patients without any controlled scientific data proving that their interventions were of benefit to patients. This will be discussed in much more detail later. Just consider that it matters little, when you are doing something that is of no value to patients, whether or not you do it particularly well.

Case Study 5: But it Was the *Best Butter*

The [Mad] Hatter was the first to break the silence. "What day of the month is it?" he said, turning to Alice: he had taken his watch out of his pocket, and was looking at it uneasily, shaking it every now and then, and holding it to his ear.

Alice considered a little, and then said "The fourth."

"Two days wrong!" sighed the Hatter. "I told you butter wouldn't suit the works!" he added looking angrily at the March Hare.

"It was the best butter," the March Hare meekly replied.

—*Through the Looking Glass* by Lewis Carroll

There is a de facto convention to the structuring of respiratory therapy departments. A careful examination of various department organizational charts reveals that they almost all have the same fundamental structure, at least with regard to the types of positions in the department. Some of this is dictated by regulatory requirements and some is dictated by functional reality. The size of a hospital and thus the size of the department also have a large influence on the structure of a department. What I describe below are generalizations and may not apply to all departments.

Director–Manager

I was once offered a position as a codirector of a department. It so happened that the department of interest had an interim director and this administrator was trying to deftly plot a course that would bring me aboard and yet not alienate the person who was currently attempting to run the department. I pondered it for a while, about 15 minutes or so. I then responded to this offer with a polite and respectful rejection. I reminded the administrator who made the offer that every ship has a captain and it was somewhat risky to have more than one hand on the helm at a time. I appreciated their attempt to plot a course that would navigate those waters, but if they wanted me to come, it would only be under the conditions of a clear understanding of who was in charge. All the really effective departments or units or organizations that I have ever experienced had the indelible imprint of their leader stamped on them. People want to be led. They don't necessarily want a dictatorial, authoritarian jerk, but they do want someone they trust to represent them to the hospital and to challenge them to be the best that they can be. Appendix E lists some common mistakes made by directors–managers.

The role of the director–manager ought to be just such a person. Some hospitals are structured so that they have classified the leader of the respiratory department as a manager instead of a director. Most of these distinctions are driven by internal hospital culture, policy, and politics. Often the distinction between a manager and a director is one of scope. Some hospitals limit the title of "director" to someone who has authority over a certain number of employees. In reality the best title would probably be "department head." In one group of 19 Children's hospitals respiratory therapy departments that belong to a benchmarking group for pediatrics, I found the following distribution of titles for the leader of the respiratory therapy department: three department heads, nine directors, six managers, one chief.[ii]

For the sake of clarity I will combine all these various titles and use the generic term director–manager. Whatever the title, the leader of a department has overall responsibility for all functions of the department. In the end, the buck has to stop on someone's desk. If you don't take responsibility personally, you probably should find something else to do. If you don't own the functions in your department, who will? Most directors–managers assume direct responsibility for budgeting, both capital and operational, policy development, department performance measurement and management, recruiting and hiring staff members, technology selection, clinical practice guideline development, disciplinary action, and planning and error management. Various aspects of these duties are shared and/or delegated with others depending on the size of the department and leadership team.

One of the dangers incumbent with being a director is disconnection with your staff. I have always struggled with it. It is a constant battle not to get officeitis and spend more time than you should staring at the computer screen. The tyranny of the urgent can draw you into being increasingly isolated doing what you think are vital and mandatory duties. While all that is true, good relationships with your staff are nevertheless equally important. It is said that the best directors have an MBWA degree (management by walking around). While this phrase suffers from terminal cuteness, it also is a great reminder of an important aspect of being a leader. You cannot have a relationship with your staff if they rarely see you. E-mails are important. Memos and notices are nice too. But these alone will not save you. Don't get the impression that I have this all

---

[ii]Medical Management Planning, Inc. is a consulting and benchmarking firm that provides benchmarking data and consulting services to member hospitals. Go to www.mmpcorp.com.

figured out. I struggle with it and have to consciously renew this operating principle on a regular basis in my daily management life.

We will now enter into a wandering narrative on my thoughts about the various positions and titles in the typical respiratory therapy department. More dispassionate and detailed information can be found in Appendix B, which contains many examples of job descriptions for different kinds of positions in a respiratory care department. Job descriptions also have many names as you will see in Appendix B. Don't be fooled by the mumbo jumbo. A "Work Content Description" is a job description, as is a position description, as are the other various titles.

Medical Director

Medical directors are often an overlooked resource for the department director. All departments are required by JCAHO regulations to have a medical director, and thus all departments have one, at least on paper. Regrettably, for many departments, it is in fact just on paper. There is a medical director, but sometimes he or she has little involvement in the regular operations of the department. And most department directors put up with this because they are happy that their medical director is not "bothering" them. A capable department leader will find a way to work out a good relationship with a medical director and use his or her expertise to improve the quality of clinical care by drawing him or her into regular department operations. Admittedly these are lofty goals but I always believe in aiming high.

Various medical specialties hold these positions including internists, pulmonologists, intensivists, surgeons, neonatologists, and others. Some departments have a medical director and an associate medical director. One example of this would be a department with an internist as a medical director. Typically about 50–75% of respiratory therapy resources are consumed in the intensive care units. If the department medical director does not have a large clinical presence in the intensive care units, the hospital might feel that it needs an associate medical director who has a large clinical practice in the intensive care unit. He or she would be better prepared to understand and deal with clinical issues that are unique to intensive care. Such an associate might be an intensivist or a surgeon with lots of intensive care experience.

The medical director usually shares the regulatory responsibility with the respiratory department director for the overall quality of the respiratory care administered. He or she is usually a cosigner of the policy and procedure manual. One important duty of the medical director is to assist the respiratory therapists in the development of clinical practice guidelines and protocols. Another is the management of medical staff relations. From time to time, respiratory therapists (at least the good ones) will cross swords with a physician colleague. In the process of learning that they have divergent views about a particular clinical question, there may be the potential for a slight amount of conflict. This is particularly true as hospitals and respiratory care departments continue in their efforts to reduce unwarranted variations in processes of care. This is the politically correct version of saying that they are moving toward "protocolized" care, or evidence-based practice. The respiratory therapy community has helped lead the way in the protocol movement. This can put RTs in conflict with a small segment of medical staff members who are not always happy campers about the protocol movement. The medical director should play a large role in helping the RT director–manager maintain good relations with the medical staff. There will be more about how to implement protocols in a later chapter.

Selecting a medical director is not often something that RT department directors get to do. Often this post is filled by folks above you in the food chain. In some of the more enlightened environments I have worked in, I have interviewed candidates and have been asked to opine, but the ultimate decision is usually made by the hospital medical director. I like someone with a research background because high-performing RT departments do a lot of protocol development and utilization management, and they need someone to help champion their ideas and also to help them evaluate and develop evidence-based practice guidelines. Good communication skills and a willingness to take risks are nice too. I think some medical directors are very involved, and some RT department directors like it that way. My experience is that if the medical director is not as involved as he or she should be, it is probably the RT director's fault for not setting clear expectations for the medical director. Regular meetings should be set up. Medical directors should come to RT staff meetings and sometimes to supervisors' meetings.

Supervisors

When you move into a department director-level position, you soon come to realize that without good clinical supervision, it is difficult indeed to manage or lead or change or improve a clinical department like respiratory therapy. I have taken over two RT departments as a director. In both cases, they did not have round the clock clinical supervision seven days per week. In both cases the very first thing I did was create 24/7 clinical supervisory positions. These supervisors typically create and manage the department schedule. They often run staffing protocols that help determine how many staff members are needed and where they are needed each shift. They assign where therapists are going to work for the shift. I have always held them jointly accountable (with myself and the RTs) for the quality of clinical care on their shifts. They form the nucleus of the department leadership team. A supervisor should be on duty at all times. Whatever scheduling system you devise for your supervisory team, I suggest a working supervisory system, for example supervisors should take a clinical load. Either they take a partial load during each shift or they have scheduled shifts where they are not supervising but are taking a full clinical load. In a complex care environment, they cannot otherwise maintain their clinical skills.

You can cook up all the grand ideas in the world, but if you don't have your leadership team behind you, none of these ideas will come to fruition. I repeat, none. Father forgive me for I have sinned in the past by not being careful enough in the selection of clinical supervisors. I, and the staff, have paid for this mistake. I hope I don't make the same mistake again.

Changing all the labels is a trendy management idea. Supervisors aren't called supervisors anymore. Instead they are called lead therapists, or team leads, or clinical specialists, or charge therapists, etc. This is a vain attempt to beguile the staff into thinking they are really mostly self-directed. For reasons that escape me, the culture has slowly changed over the years in some large organizations so that it is not good form to suggest that someone is actually in charge and must be obeyed. I like the word supervisor because this is exactly what I expect them to do. This is what needs to be done—supervision. Of course, they have other duties, for example coaching, teaching, mentoring, counseling, and recognizing the contributions of the staff. But my experience has taught me a simple thing. *Immutable Truth #12: Someone is going to be in charge.* If you don't develop a formal structure where someone *you want* is always in charge, an informal system will develop where you have informal leaders *whom you did not choose.* These are usually the strong. In this type of system, the weak often get eaten by the strong. It is the director's job to create as equitable a system as possible. This is much easier to achieve if you develop a clear supervisory structure and make it clear to the staff that supervisors are in charge and indeed speak for you in your absence.

Case Study 6: The Strong Eat the Weak—Organizational Food Chains

Jubal Harshaw CRTT worked nights at the Shangri-la University Hospital as a staff RT. There were typically four to six RTs on duty on nights, and there was no supervisor. The choice assignment for RTs was the intensive care unit, and the least desirable assignment was the chronic ventilator unit. Anyone who wanted to could be the lead therapist for the night. The lead was assumed by whoever got there early enough to lay claim. This temporary title didn't give you much except for one important thing: you got to make out the assignments. Knowing this, Jubal often got to work early and assumed the lead position. This allowed him to avoid working the chronic ventilator unit, which turned out to be one of his primary objectives. He was strong willed and interpersonally intimidating and, thus, most often got what he wanted. Most of the other staff members didn't bother to take him on because it wasn't worth the hassle to them.

Enter Gillian Boardman CRTT. She was new to respiratory therapy and new to the University Hospital. She had completed her orientation to the intensive care unit but had not yet begun her training for the chronic ventilator unit. On the night in question, Jubal showed up early, made out the assignments, and true to form, put himself in the intensive care unit. He assigned her to the chronic ventilator unit. She arrived in the crowded staff room, looked at the assignment board, and shook her head. She walked up to Jubal and said, "You can't assign me to the chronic ventilator unit. I have not even started my orientation to that unit. You should put me in intensive care and take the chronic ventilator unit yourself."

Jubal got up in her face and said, "I can't assign you to the intensive care unit. Everyone knows you're incompetent to work there."

The room got very quiet. He stomped out of the room and announced on the way out the door, "You're going to the chronic ventilator unit."

Gillian stood there a moment, tears welled in her eyes, and she walked out. She paced the hallway for a few minutes and then called him on the phone and said she was so upset she could not work and so she was going home, and before he could comment, she hung up and left the building.

Jubal called the (recently recruited) director at home immediately and ranted and raved about this therapist's unprofessional conduct in not taking her assignment and unceremoniously leaving the hospital. The director listened carefully and then said one of the most important things a director can learn to say, "I'll look into it." He did not comment one way or another on who he thought was right or wrong.

The next day, Gillian called the director and gave him her side of the story. The director interviewed people who witnessed the exchange and came to the conclusion that Gillian had been pretty badly treated and that Jubal had abused his position, informal though it was.

The director met with Gillian, told her that she had not been treated properly and that Jubal had been wrong to assign her to an area that she was not trained to work in. "But," he said, "it is totally unacceptable to simply refuse to work and leave the hospital because you do not like your assignment. This cannot happen again. Call me or another one of the managers first before you do such a rash thing, or it could cost you your job."

The director met with Jubal. He pointed out that it was unprofessional to call Gillian "incompetent" in front of other staff members and that it was risky to assign someone, especially a recent graduate, to an area that she had not yet been trained in. Jubal was a deeply troubled man and was often referred to as the guy who put the "fun" in "dysfunctional." He did not receive this reproof very well and within a year he no longer worked for the director.

This episode illustrates how poor leadership selection, training, and structure can cause serious problems. It is also a great example of how the strong can prey on the weak. Not long after this, a formal supervisor's job description was developed, positions were posted, and new supervisors were selected. Within 3 years, 13 individuals had resigned under duress, left or were fired, and new staff members had been hired and trained. Someone has to be in charge, and it better be someone that you (as a director) have selected and mentored.

There are important traits you want to look for in a clinical supervisor. Lots of people think you have to be a clinical wizard, a master clinician, a hotshot therapist to be a candidate for a clinical supervisory position. I disagree. I want solid clinical skills and experience in a supervisor, but they do not necessarily need to be Hawkeye Pierce to be a good candidate. Their clinical skills are important, but some other things are even more vital. These include communication skills, patience, maturity, emotional stability, self-direction, compassion, toughness, and an ability to admit their mistakes and grow and learn from them. Of course this sounds like a pretty tall order, since Jesus is not likely to be applying for a supervisory position in your department any time soon. Thus the likelihood of you finding candidates who have *all* these traits is somewhat remote. So what are the two or three most important traits? I would list them as, in no particular order, (1) communication skills, (2) emotional strength and maturity, and (3) self-direction. The possession of these skills can forgive a lot of other shortcomings.

In most departments, individuals who have good clinical skills and ambition get promoted to supervisory positions. They typically get a brief orientation to the basics of the position, and then the front of the landing craft flops down and they are expected to lead the platoon onto the beach. Sadly, they are seldom properly prepared. Basic skills like conflict resolution, coaching, and mentoring are often absent or severely underdeveloped. More advanced organizations have some formal in-house training for new supervisors and managers but the majority of organizations do not. There are growing Internet-based training resources for managers and supervisors. It is yet unclear to me how effectively some of these complex and subtle skills can be taught at a computer terminal. A lot of one-on-one mentoring between the director and the supervisory staff is the most effective way to develop front line supervisory skills. A particularly good technique is debriefing or case review. When news of an unhappy exchange between a staff member percolates up to the director, it is a very good thing to sit down with the supervisor involved and debrief. You should review what happened in detail. Let the new supervisor do most of the talking. Most of the time they will be much tougher on themselves than the director would be (if they are any good).

Coordinators–Educators

I highly recommend the development of a clinical coordinator–educator position. These types of positions have various names, including clinical specialist, clinical coordinator, clinical educator, quality coordinator, clinical manager, and others. The pace of technological advancement and the complexity of the environment of care have made orientation and training a very large deal in RT departments. When I was Navy corpsman with the Marines I learned an important axiom. *Immutable Truth #13: If you are coasting, it probably means you are going downhill.* This is especially true of the education of clinicians in an RT department and any other hospital clinical department too. If you are not pushing the envelope in the training environment, you will have trouble keeping your clinical staff finely honed. New technologies and procedures are coming down the pike with an increasing frequency. If you aren't devoting significant time to studying the literature, attending scientific conferences, and networking with other departments, your department will stand still while the rest of the industry moves ahead. One day you will awaken and realize that your ship came in but has, regrettably, since departed. And as a director–manager, unless you have some very special powers, your time will be consumed by enough other things to make it difficult to keep on top of the pace of technological change. This is customarily the duty of the clinical coordinator–educator. The other important duty of the clinical coordinator–educator is staff training and competency. This will be discussed more later on. And finally, clinical coordinators are also frequently in charge of quality. Don't worry, by "quality" I do not mean some Dilbertesque management terminology that is as fleeting as the flavor of the month. Instead I mean the quality of the clinical care administered by respiratory therapists (or radiology techs or lab techs for other departments). Obviously, overall clinical quality is the ultimate responsibility of the department director and medical director, but many departments are structured so that processing of incident reports, ensuring patient safety, and ensuring staff competency are large parts of the portfolio of the clinical coordinator–educator.

This would be a good time to discuss the difference between training and competency. Training is what you do to and for a new staff member who comes on board or an incumbent clinician who is being introduced to new equipment. Training is exposing the staff to information and skills. Competency assessment is evaluating whether or not a clinician is able to perform a given task or procedure with sufficient skill and quality. You can train all day long, but if you aren't assessing competency, you cannot be sure that your staff members are "getting it." Consider the train engineer or the airline pilot or the nuclear power plant operator. You want them to be trained indeed, but you also want to know that the training worked and that they are competent at their jobs. This requires them to demonstrate this competency by actually doing things while someone watches and assesses how well they do the tasks. This probably sounds simple and pedant, but historically we have not done a very good job of this in the RT community (or the healthcare community in general). The good news is that this is getting better. More departments are setting up competency assessment programs where a clinician's skills are verified through direct observation by other clinicians or through clinical simulation.

COMMITTEES AND COUNCILS

As a director, you can choose to closely oversee your department, pay attention to every detail, do all the important stuff yourself, engage in lots of problem solving, assume responsibility for practically everything, and begin a path to assured self-destruction by working yourself into an early grave. Or you can try to structure the department so that responsibility for various processes in the department is delegated and shared between management and staff through a series of department councils. I like the term "councils" better than "committees."

Case Study 7: The Stigmatization of Committees

There was trouble in river city at Our Sister of Dysfunction Community Hospital. Committee attendance was down to dangerously low levels. Vital committee members were simply *not showing up* for meetings. Administration was in an uproar. Battalions of nonclinical coordinators, trainers, nurse practitioners, staff development specialists, PhD nurses, analysts, research associates, assistant directors, and others were growing increasingly concerned that the committees that they were chairing were not being attended, which they assumed was required by law and divine proclamation. Of course, a committee was formed to study the problem. Their first order of business was to select a committee name, which, after 2 hours of deliberation, they aptly decided should be The Committee on Committees. After a month of meeting weekly for 2 hours during which they worked feverishly on a mission statement, some kind soul decided that the members of this committee were way too uptight, and he anonymously posted the following list of committee jokes on the wall of the intensive care staff bathroom right next to the commode where it was sure to be read by one and all. Shortly the list was posted next to the commode in every staff bathroom in the facility, including the executive washrooms in administration. The committee jokes went as follows:

- Committee: a group of people who individually can do nothing but as a group decide that nothing can be done.
- A camel is called a horse created by a committee.
- Committee: a body that keeps minutes and wastes hours.
- A committee is best composed of three people with one who is always sick and another who is always absent.
- A committee is a dark alley down which good ideas are enticed and then slowly strangled.

The seditious nature of these jokes was discussed at the next meeting of The Committee on Committees. They formed a subcommittee to analyze the cultural implications of these jokes, which of course is named The Working Subcommittee on Committee Dysfunction. Their tentative plan was to develop a series of mandatory staff training sessions focused on building an increased understanding, and eventually a consensus, on the value and utility of committees. Also, a search for the perpetrators who distributed this seditious list is currently underway. Film at 11.

See what I mean? Committees have gotten a bad name. It is beyond the scope of this book to discuss the many and various reasons why this is well deserved. The interested student is directed to study the works of Scott Adams. But by whatever name you call it, groups of people *can* come together and accomplish things. But it doesn't happen without careful planning and hard work. In a tribute to Dilbertesque hypocrisy, I prefer the term "councils." What is probably an even more appropriate term is "team." There is a very interesting body of literature regarding the performance of work teams. I highly recommend studying this literature starting with one of the most famous texts on the subject, *The Wisdom of Teams*.[3] One of the more common conventions of describing team performance is forming, storming, transforming, and performing. Teams form followed by the inevitable storm of coming together and aligning purposes and ideas. Then, God willing and the creek don't rise, they may be transformed into a performing team and actually accomplish something. More than likely they will not accomplish anything unless leadership is strong. These periods or phases have very recognizable patterns, and the effective leader will learn what he or she can do to promote the passage through these phases into a high performing team. They cannot, and indeed should not, be avoided.

Whether they are called teams or councils or committees, a very effective department structure can include some standing councils that help develop department plans, process department problems, and help create a more participative management structure. In nursing circles this is often called shared governance, which as the name implies is designed to share the duties of governing the operations of the department between management and staff. Some cynics might have some doubts about how much is really shared because in the end, budgeting responsibilities always remain firmly in the grasp of a nurse manager. But the good thing about this model is that lots more staff members participate and become more actively engaged in furthering the overall goals of the department and the hospital.

A model that I like includes two councils: a quality management council and a resource management council. The quality management council is generally in charge of clinical quality issues. Duties of this council include oversight of the department's training and competency program, measurement of the quality of care, and patient safety activities, for example error management.[iii] It is

---

[iii]Of course this is terribly shocking to the uninformed or naive, but on rare occasions, people do make mistakes. Until we come up with a way to have a whole bunch of those computerized, holographic doctors like in Star Trek *Voyager*, hospitals will continue to be staffed by people. The magnitude and frequency at which serious mistakes are made is a point of great controversy. Current estimates of the number of people who die as a result of preventable medical errors in hospitals in the United States per year range from 48,000 to 225,000. Kohn L, Corrigan J, Donalson M. *To Err is Human: Building a Safer Health System*. Washington, DC: National Academy Press; 1999. Starfield B. Is US health really the best in the world? *JAMA* 2000;4(284):483–485.

usually made of the department director, medical director, clinical coordinator, leadership team, and several staff members whose seats often rotate. These groups can meet as often as monthly, but I prefer quarterly. The resource management council oversees the departments' consumption of resources, for example labor costs and supplies as well as other business operations like billing, scheduling, and staffing and human resource functions.

If you are just starting these councils, they will not happen without a lot of effort. If they initially are not well attended, don't give up. Just relentlessly promote them better and try to create incentives for people to participate.

THE SAGA OF DECENTRALIZATION

Immutable Truth #14: The law of unintended consequences is as ubiquitous as gravity. In the 1980s and 1990s, healthcare costs rose at two to three times the rate of inflation. It was getting scary because prognosticators were drawing trends lines on graphs that looked to the future. They realized that, if unabated, before too long all the money everywhere would be spent on health care. Something had to be done. One response of some parts of the healthcare industry was to bring in business "experts" who introduced the concept of reengineering. These consultants got rich convincing hospitals (and other businesses) that if they were bold enough to radically redesign their business processes, they could anticipate a 15–20% reduction in operating costs.[4] "But," they warned, "you have to be radical." You have to throw out your old ideas and reengineer a new system. A lot of hospital CEOs took the bait. And some hospitals made gains in efficiency and reduced costs, but in my experience, nowhere near the amounts that were forecast. One study of reengineering in health care concluded that overall hospitals did not really reduce operating costs with reengineering, although there were exceptions.[5] Other studies suggest that reengineering negatively affected the quality of care.[6–7] Table 3-2 is a bibliography of reengineering and restructuring references. It has been estimated that 66% of reengineering projects fail. Table 3-3 lists common reasons why reengineering fails according to Robin Reid and Associates, a firm specializing in organizational development.

One of the favorite techniques of the reengineers was to dismantle hospital respiratory departments. The theory was that if you decentralized RT departments, you could get rid of the overhead of an RT department administrative structure, for example managers and supervisors, secretaries, clerks, etc. Decentralization meant that RTs would be split into groups and assigned permanently to the existing nursing units. They would be paid and supervised

Table 3-2. Reengineering and Restructuring Bibliography

1. Ghoshal S, Bartlett CA. Changing the role of top management: beyond structure to processes. *Harvard Business Review.* 1995;73(1): 86–97.
2. Arndt M, Bigelow B. Reengineering: deja vu all over again. *Health Care Management Review.* 1998;23(3): 58–66.
3. Champy J. *Reengineering Management: The Mandate for New Leadership.* New York, NY: Harper Business; 1995.
4. Dixon JR, Arnold P, Heineke J, Kim JS, Mulligan P. Business process reengineering: improving in new strategic directions. *California Management Review.* 1994;36(4): 93–108.
5. Hammer M. Reengineering work: don't automate, obliterate. *Harvard Business Review.* 1990;68(4): 104–112.
6. Lathrop JP. *Restructuring Healthcare: The Patient Focused Paradigm.* San Francisco, CA: Jossey-Bass; 1993.
7. Leatt P, Baker GR, Halverson PK, Aird C. Downsizing, reengineering, and restructuring: long-term implications for healthcare organizations. *Frontiers of Health Services Management.* 1997;13(4): 3–37.
8. Pierson D, Williams J. Remaking the rules: hospitals attempt work transformation. *Hospitals & Health Networks.* September 1994;5(68): 30.
9. Schweikhart S, Smith-Daniels V. Reengineering the work of caregivers: role redefinition, team structures, and organizational redesign. *Hospital and Health Services.* 1996.
10. Walston SL, Kimberly JR. Reengineering hospitals: experience and analysis from the field. *Hospital and Health Services Administration.* Summer 1997;42:143–163.
11. Walston SL, Bogue RJ. The effects of reengineering: fad or competitive factor? *Journal of Healthcare Management.* November/December 1999;44(6): 456–472.
12. Walston SL, Burns RL, Kimberly JR. Does reengineering really work? An examination of the context and outcomes of hospital reengineering initiatives. *Health Services Research.* February 2000;34(6):1363–1388.
13. McCloskey BA, Diers DK. Effects of New Zealand's health reengineering on nursing and patient outcomes. *Med Care.* November 2005;43(11):1140–1146.
14. Woodward C, Shannon H, Cunningham C, et al. The impact of re-engineering and other cost reduction strategies on the staff of a large teaching hospital: a longitudinal study. *Med Care.* 1999;37(6):556–569.
15. Walston SL, Chou AF. Healthcare restructuring and hierarchical alignment: why do staff and managers perceive change outcomes differently? *Med Care.* September 2006;44(9):879–889.
16. Trinh HQ, O'Connor SJ. Helpful or harmful? The impact of strategic change on the performance of U.S. urban hospitals. *Health Serv Res.* February 2002;37(1):145–171.

(Continues)

Table 3-2. Reengineering and Restructuring Bibliography *(Continued)*

17. Pepicello JA, Murphy EC. Clinical reengineering. Integrating medical and operational management. *Physician Exec.* October 1996;22(10):4–9.
18. Walston SL, Lazes P, Sullivan PG. Improving hospital restructuring: lessons learned. *Health Care Manage Rev.* October-December 2004;29(4):309–319.

Table 3-3. Common Barriers to Reengineering Success, Their Estimated Percentages, and Common Reengineering Errors

Common barriers

- Indicated resistance to change—60%
- Limitations of existing systems—40%
- Lack of executive consensus—40%
- Lack of a senior executive "champion"—40%
- Unrealistic expectations—30%
- Lack of cross-functional project teams—28%
- Lack of team skills—25%
- Late staff involvement—18%
- Project charter too narrow—15%

Common errors

- Trying to fix a process instead of changing it.
- Not focusing on the business process.
- Ignoring everything except the process design.
- Neglecting people's values and beliefs.
- Being willing to settle for minor results.
- Quitting too early.
- Placing constraints on the definition of the problem and the scope of the reengineering process.
- Trying to make reengineering happen from the bottom up.
- Assigning someone who does not understand reengineering to lead the effort.

Source: Robin Reid and Associates (www.improve.org).

by nursing managers. The logic went like this: Because virtually all inpatient respiratory care was done on nursing units anyway, it was an obvious fit to have the RTs paid for and managed by nursing units. Exact numbers are not available on the total number of United States RT departments that experienced (endured) this redesign fad. I know of several large examples.

Thus as a result of reengineering, some RT leadership teams experienced an involuntary RIF (reduction in force). Serious savings in healthcare costs almost always involve a RIF because about two thirds of the cost of running a hospital are salaries. There are two types of RIF, voluntary and involuntary. The voluntary RIF typically offers incumbents an incentive (severance) package if they will voluntarily quit, usually somewhere between 3 months and 1 year of salary and benefits. Involuntary RIF is a euphemism for layoffs. Sometimes involuntary RIFs also involved a severance package, which is a farewell check for the victim that ranges from 3 months of salary (and insurance) to one year.

Case Study 8: One Flew over the Decentralized Department

Corn-Belt Children's Hospital was experiencing tremendous financial pressure and was looking for ways to cut expenses. They hired CRC (the Cut and Run Consulting Firm) which, after about 15 minutes of studying the design of a mind-numbingly complex operation like a hospital, recommended a decentralized respiratory model. The RTs were informed that the department was being restructured and they would have to bid for jobs either in the intensive care units or the nonintensive care (general floors) units where they would be paid by and managed by the nursing managers. In addition, to get (keep) their RT jobs, they would have to also obtain an additional credential, the Certified Nursing Assistant credential (CNA). Thus in addition to two years of college and two professional credentialing exams (CRTT and RRT, and for some the NPS), they would also have to obtain a nursing assistant credential to practice as an RT. There would be a selection process run by the nurse managers, and RTs would be picked for each unit. At the end of this process, the RT leadership team would go the way of all flesh. It turns out that many more RTs wanted to work in the ICU than the general care floors. At the end of the selection process, many disgruntled RTs ended up in general care units. The nurse managers had no experience managing RTs, who have a significantly different professional identity and culture than nurses. One of the alleged efficiencies to be gained was the cross training of RTs and nurses to do high volume, low risk procedures, thus reducing overall labor hours by filling the "downtime" of both disciplines by helping each other out. RTs were to be trained in rudimentary nursing duties, and nurses were to be trained in rudimentary RT duties. The model was put into place, and the RT leadership team either left voluntarily or returned to staff positions. Shockingly, the cross training train appeared to run mostly in one direction. Nursing managers and bedside nurses tended to expect RTs to do nursing duties and frequently directed them to do so. But nurses were usually "too busy" to do routine RT duties, and thus RTs did most of those too, not having the supervisory authority to direct nurses to do RT duties. Within about 18 months of the implementation of the model, 50% of the general floor care RTs had quit, and what followed was several years of inability to recruit staff RTs and heavy reliance on temporary contract and agency staff, which were much more costly than the regular RT staff. Recruitment problems persisted and, lacking a department director advocate for the RT staff, RT salaries became stagnant and as a result effectively dropped compared to the rest of the local labor market, which kept pace with inflation. Finally, disgruntled and discouraged, the RT staff (and some other departments) began union organizing activities, and within 4 years of the introduction of the decentralized RT department model, the staff voted to certify the International Brotherhood of Broke Healthcare Workers as their bargaining unit representatives (IBROKE Local 999). The hospital eventually abandoned the decentralized model, recreated a centralized RT department, hired a director, and eventually saw their recruitment and retention improve to levels comparable with other hospitals. No one in RT ever saw a single piece of data one way or the other about whether the model had or had not saved money. But the heavy reliance on agency and contract staff that followed the decentralization of the RT department suggests that maybe, just possibly, there was a chance that the new model actually cost more money than the old one in the long run.

Another alleged cost savings of decentralization was "gained efficiencies." These savings were to have been realized by having RTs and nurses cross trained into one another's high volume, low risk procedures. The obvious, though not often stated, assumption was that both disciplines were not 100% efficient and thus had downtime or what some people called "marginal" time. Cross training and its illegitimate child, gained efficiencies, were intended to stamp out this marginal time.

One of the flies in the cross training ointment involved breathless misinterpretations of the licensure laws combined with a visceral territoriality on the part of nursing leadership. Even though RTs and RNs have very similar scopes of professional academic preparation, there were some who thought that RTs could not possibly do any nursing duties, and if they did, they would have to get a nursing credential of some sort or another. Such an incursion into the kingdom of nursing would be outside of the RT "scope of practice." Speaking of cyanosis, I turn blue almost every time I hear this argument. Having very carefully examined the licensure laws for

RTs and RNs from a number of states, I can tell that they have usually been intentionally crafted so that the law governing practice of RNs cannot be used to limit the practice of RTs, and the law governing the practice of RTs cannot be used to limit the practice of RNs. My experience is that quite often, the nursing managers who start citing "scope of practice issues" have not actually studied the laws and related regulatory literature. When scope of practice issues involving the borders between RT and RN practice are trotted out by nursing leadership, this is almost always a defensive response by those who fear an erosion of nursing power and prestige. Certainly, hospitals need to operate within the defined boundaries of the regulatory environment, but almost without fail, hospitals over interpret the regulatory literature.

Thus in some decentralized models like the one previously described, RTs had to obtain some type of nursing credential, in this case a CNA, to get cross trained into nursing duties. RTs would then be able, or more correctly, *allowed* to perform low complexity nursing procedures. Once again, the train seemed to run only in one direction. By this I mean that no additional credentialing of nurses appeared to have been required. I know of no example where any nurses had to get an RT credential, such as a CRT, to get cross trained into some RT procedures.

The story of decentralization is best told in the words of those who experienced it. There is much to be learned from some excellent narratives of those who went through reengineering that are posted at the AARC Web site (www.aarc.org).

As far as I can tell, the outcomes of decentralization have been pretty much negative. I have not yet talked to an RT who liked decentralization. Those RTs who experienced decentralization began to lose their sense of professional identity. And when they started being supervised and managed by nurses, they began to feel like no one was advocating for them. The dismantling of their departments made them feel devalued. I know of no published, controlled evidence that these decentralizations ever saved a dollar. Another fly in the ointment was another "one-way" street on which the cross training buses often ran. RT's were often expected to do all that they had previously done, *AND* to pick up additional nursing duties. Like the mines of Moria, the passage through decentralization was pretty dark for most RT departments. Those who emerged from the other side point out that in the trenches the reality was that the nurses often did very little respiratory therapy, but RT's were expected to do a fair amount of "nursing." My experience with human nature leads me to say that this should have been very predictable. Nurses were now supervising RT's and thus had the operational authority to assign them work. The RT's had no operational authority to assign work to nurses. In an ideal, well tuned, balanced, team-oriented, fantasy island-type environment, this might have worked. In the real world, populated by imperfect folks, this design left lots to be desired.

Another obvious truth here is that for decentralization to have saved money via this cross training, nurses and/or RTs should have been laid off after the implementation, otherwise you are just moving people around inside the cost structure. Or at least there should have been a reduction in peak demand for RT and RN hours and thus a reduction in overtime utilization. My experience has been that there were just as many nurses after decentralization as before, but there were fewer RTs in mostly management and supervisory positions.

Another fault was in assuming that RTs *wanted* to work *only* in these units. There were some places that almost all RTs liked to work, for example critical care. There are many, many fewer RTs who want to work only on general care floors. Many RTs would not want to come to a hospital where they had to take a position where they provided care only on the general medical surgical floors. Thus there was generally a mass exodus of staff in the months after decentralization because those who did not get positions in intensive care units would not stay and work only the (gasp) "floors." I am compelled to point out that the above statements should not be construed as an endorsement on my part of the suggestion that it is harder or easier to work in one area of the hospital or another. It is just a statement of the observable truth that there is a preponderance of RTs who would prefer to work in intensive care.

I try, whenever possible, to remind everyone that the patients in general medical surgical beds deserve equally high quality care as do intensive care unit patients. And I generally prefer models where all RTs rotate to all areas of the hospital. This helps develop a wide range of assessment skills in RTs because they see a wider variety of patients when they rotate through all areas of the hospital. It also gains you an economy of scale. You have much more flexibility in moving staff around to different assignments in the hospital to cover shortages and accommodate over staffing if all staff members are qualified to work everywhere. There are obvious exceptions to this. Some areas of responsibility for RTs are so complex and technically demanding that the quality of care cannot be maintained if too many staff members are trained and rotate through these assignments. Examples of this include ECMO and interhospital transport of critically ill patients.

Decentralization models typically diminished economies of scale. The larger a system is (like a staffing model), the easier it is to shift resources around within a system. The smaller numbers of decentralized RTs on each different nursing unit made it difficult for staffing models to accommodate episodic unplanned sick leave and vacations. Thus some decentralized models kept a small centralized department that acted like a float pool of RTs to deploy to the units that had unit-based therapists when those RTs called in sick or took vacation. Or they made RTs float out of their home units to cover another area when someone called in sick or was on vacation. Of course, this may have happened infrequently enough that the RTs who had to float between units were unfamiliar with the subtleties of working on other units. The nurses and the doctors on those units didn't really know those RTs well and didn't have a relationship with them.

Finally, the pace of technologic advancement requires a great deal of ongoing training, product assessment and testing, competency verification, new employment orientation, and the development of new RT policies and procedures. To my knowledge, these things simply did not happen very well, if at all, in decentralized models because there was often no central RT department to be responsible for these duties. I know of one hospital that decentralized their RT department so that all of the PICU and NICU RTs reported to the nursing managers of those units. But they kept a management team and a centralized department to cover nonintensive care RT demands, training, competency, new product assessment, etc. It is unclear how this saved a dime because they basically had the same number of RTs around.

We come to another moment of clarity. *Immutable Truth #15: If a hospital can shut down your department, it should.* Before you run for your hog leg Colt, consider this. It may be that many departments were decentralized because administration did not see a lot of value in the services provided by the centralized department staff, for example the RT management staff. Sure, they thought RTs were important, and thus they had to have them, but they were less sure about whether they really needed an RT management staff. But why weren't they sure? I suggest that if RT management teams had been doing a better job and providing a vital service for the hospital, administration never would have given serious thought to dismantling the centralized RT function. I suspect some decentralized RT management teams had it coming.

To summarize, I have not run into a single therapist that went through decentralization and thought things were better afterward. Everyone I know who went through it thought it made things worse—some thought way worse. And most of them are still angry about it. And there continues to be a dearth of literature describing "make good" analyses of the impact of decentralizing.[iv] I am happy to announce that in spite of the furor over decentralization in the industry, it did not appear to catch on. The AARC reports that 95.7% of RT departments continue to be structured as traditional centralized models.[8]

SUPPLY CHAIN LOGISTICS

Another major issue in RT department design is supply chain logistics. Respiratory care practice is technology driven, and thus respiratory care departments require a lot of supplies and equipment. Quite often people rise into the ranks of supervision and management and do not pass through a secret garden where they eat fruit from the tree of knowledge of supply chain management. But this aspect of the operation of an RT department is a fertile soil where you can harvest serious improvements in cost savings through using fewer and more inexpensive supplies. Poor supply chain management also can make the daily lives of RTs more difficult because your supply chain is what helps to ensure that RTs have the equipment and materials they need to do their jobs.

Historically, hospitals have not had very well designed and operated supply systems. Quite often supplies were billed directly to patients, and thus many managers thought the more supplies used, the more revenue was generated. The expense of these supplies, the wastage, the excessive inventory, the storage costs, and other unpleasant realities of supply chain management were generally overlooked. There will be a whole section on supplies and equipment selection and utilization later in the book. I bring it up here to point out that the managerial structure of a department should be carefully considered with regard to efficient delivery systems and managing these costs. Many departments have an equipment manager, some-

---

[iv]"Make good" is a term used by analysts, accountants, and other luminaries to describe the process of going back and checking to see if the original assumptions of an improvement project turned out to be true. In other words, if you redesigned your system in hopes that it would result in a reduced cost structure, did anyone ever go back and carefully examine whether or not costs were actually lower? As crazy as it sounds, this is often not actually done in systems redesign projects. Often, after a project has been completed, the redesign team moved on to other things, and no one has the time, energy, or inclination to stop and reassess the fundamental metrics that drove the project in the first place. A great example of this is a hospital that decided to implement an intravenous (IV) team comprised of specialists who did nothing but insert IVs and catheters. The assumption was that IV care was insufficient, and if a team was put into place, IV care would be better. So clinicians were hired, a manager was put in place, and the IV team was created. Three years later no one had ever gone back to actually measure to see if IV care had improved. No data had been collected on the number of IV sticks it took to get IVs started, no average duration of IVs, no extravagation rates, nothing, zip, nada. I had my doubts.

times called a technical manager. This is a very good idea. This person is typically responsible for technology evaluation, contract negotiation, supply acquisition and distribution systems, and vendor management. Sometimes it is useful from a structural perspective to create an organizational chart that is based on functional responsibility as opposed to a traditional chart that is based on managing people. Figure 3-7 shows a fictitious example of such a chart.

CARE DELIVERY MODELS

If you make a careful study of how respiratory care is administered in different hospitals and different regions, you will find tremendous variation. And most of it is what we would describe as unwarranted. *Immutable Truth #16: Unwarranted variation is usually not good in health delivery systems.* There is a very large body of literature on the subject of unwarranted variation.[9–11] One of the most useful and eye-opening publications is the *Dartmouth Atlas of Health Care.*[12] In this fascinating work, the team of health services researchers from the Dartmouth Medical School's Center for the Evaluative Clinical Sciences demonstrates the degree to which the utilization of health services varies across the country. One example: In immediately adjacent counties in the United States, there are four-fold differences in rates of utilization of coronary artery bypass graft surgery even after adjustment for population differences. There are lots of other examples in the atlas. None of the explanations for these variations are good.

If some costly and risky procedures are used a lot more in some regions than others, why is this? Are there important differences in the health of the populations in these different regions? Sadly, the answer is generally no. Thus you have to ask why we use these costly and risky procedures as much as we do. Of course, a cynical answer might be because these procedures generate revenue for hospitals and physicians. Indeed it turns out that about 50% of the variation in the utilization of some procedures is explained by the number of specialists available in those regions to do (and bill for) those costly procedures.[10] I like to think the reasons are more complex than this, but followers of the Adam Smith school of economic theory would disagree with me.[v] Because the consumers in health care are not actually operating in

---

[v]Adam Smith (1723–1790) was a Scottish political economist and moral philosopher who argued that within the system of capitalism, individuals acting in their own economic interests also tend to (inadvertently) promote the overall interest of the community.

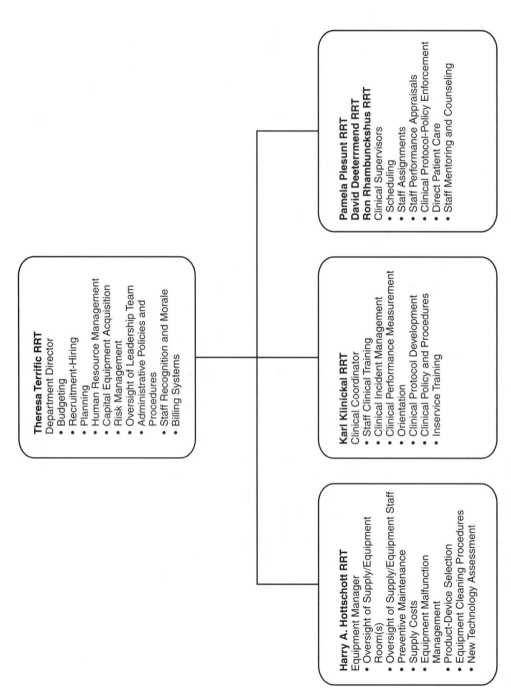

Theresa Terrific RRT
Department Director
• Budgeting
• Recruitment-Hiring
• Planning
• Human Resource Management
• Capital Equipment Acquisition
• Risk Management
• Oversight of Leadership Team
• Administrative Policies and
  Procedures
• Staff Recognition and Morale
• Billing Systems

Harry A. Hottschott RRT
Equipment Manager
• Oversight of Supply/Equipment
  Room(s)
• Oversight of Supply/Equipment Staff
• Preventive Maintenance
• Supply Costs
• Equipment Malfunction
  Management
• Product-Device Selection
• Equipment Cleaning Procedures
• New Technology Assessment

Karl Klinickal RRT
Clinical Coordinator
• Staff Clinical Training
• Clinical Incident Management
• Clinical Performance Measurement
• Orientation
• Clinical Protocol Development
• Clinical Policy and Procedures
• Inservice Training

Pamela Plesunt RRT
David Deetermend RRT
Ron Rhambunckshus RRT
Clinical Supervisors
• Scheduling
• Staff Assignments
• Staff Performance Appraisals
• Clinical Protocol-Policy Enforcement
• Direct Patient Care
• Staff Mentoring and Counseling

Figure 3-7. Functional Organizational Chart
An example of a "functional organizational chart," that is, one in which incumbents are listed with the "titles" and their "duties."

a free market, the normal forces that would bring clarity and efficiency to the utilization of healthcare procedures are not able to affect the system as they do in the general economy. Thus treatments and interventions are over utilized, especially in places where there is an excess of practitioners and infrastructure able to provide these services. The point is that there is variation in practice, and a lot of it is unwarranted.

Respiratory care suffers from the same problems. If I send three different RTs into a patient's room to do chest physiotherapy, there is a pretty good chance that I will get three different versions of the procedure. This inconsistency is evident within departments and between departments. Adding to the lack of clinical consistency is considerable variation in care delivery models. In some hospitals, all inhaled medications are delivered by RTs. In some hospitals, these duties are shared between RTs and RNs. In a very large survey that a colleague and I conducted of 3800 hospitals (with nearly 1100 responders), we discovered that nearly two thirds of hospitals had already or were about to train non-RT personnel to do respiratory therapy procedures[13] (see Table 3-4).

Thus in some hospitals, you might get your nebulized albuterol treatments from an LPN, an RN, or an RT. Of course, if you are a patient with chronic lung disease, you self-administer your inhaled medication treatments at home. This is an interesting phenomenon because patients are encouraged to self-administer their treatments at home where, admittedly, it is a bit difficult for us to monitor them. But when they come to the hospital, where keeping an eye on them is a teensy bit easier than when they are at home, we will not allow them to self-administer treatments. Go figure.

Different respiratory care delivery models include:

- Anything remotely associated with respiratory therapy being administered only by RTs, including simple oxygen therapy, incentive spirometry, coughing and deep breathing, or even attaching a pulse oximeter to a patient's finger, a mind bogglingly complex task.
- High volume, low risk, low complexity procedures are shared between nursing and RT, such as simple oxygen setups, pulse oximetry, and administration of inhaled medications. These models usually developed out of necessity in hospitals that simply could not or would not have enough RTs on board to administer all these therapies in a timely fashion. This was often related to the chronic shortage of RTs in many parts of the healthcare industry.
- High volume, low risk, low complexity procedures are all done by nursing, and RT concentrates most of its resources in the management of

Table 3-4. Results of a Survey of Hospitals and Their RT Care Delivery Models[13]

Care delivery models	% of all responders
Currently or about to start cross training RNs/LPNs to do respiratory procedures	44.9%
Currently or about to start cross training nonlicensed staff to do respiratory procedures	18.0%
Currently or about to start cross training RCPs to do nursing procedures	58.2%
Hospital has brought in outside consultants to significantly redesign hospital operations	38.0%
Respiratory department has experienced a reduction in force in past 18 months	37.4%

Source: Data from 1093 hospitals in all 50 states, Canada, Guam, and the Virgin Islands. These data are from the mid 1990s and are thus some what "aged."

artificial airways, alternative airway clearance techniques, mechanical ventilation, and other life support technologies. Again, this usually grew out of the inability or unwillingness to have RT departments that were large enough to deliver all the respiratory therapy.

The point here is that there are many different care models. I have seen all three of the models listed above in action, and I have experienced each of them working very well, and conversely, not working very well. This has been a tremendous controversy in the respiratory community for many years. This is understandable because job security and professional identity are very much influenced by the model of care chosen. Many RTs are threatened by the idea of nurses administering respiratory treatments of any kind, even something as simple as oxygen therapy. The truly insecure argue that nurses are not qualified to do many of these procedures. That dog won't hunt as far as I am concerned.

I have met some RTs that weren't terribly well qualified to do what they were doing either. I am less interested in who is delivering care than I am in having care delivered properly. This requires that hospitals have well designed and executed systems of training and competency assessment for the administration of procedures that have been traditionally thought of as "respiratory." If nurses are properly trained, have their competency adequately assessed, and do procedures with sufficient frequency to maintain their skills, then there is very little in the armamentarium of the RT that nurses could not accomplish. This is also true for RTs doing nursing procedures. Unfortunately, many nurses are a bit confused about the reciprocal nature of this truth. There remain many RTs and nurses who deeply disagree with this principle. I'm still working on them.

The model you end up choosing will depend on the complexities of the system in which you are operating. Factors that will influence your choice of care delivery model include:

- The market for RTs
- The market for nurses
- The culture of the RT department
- The culture of the nursing department
- Medical staff support
- Financial environment
- Patient population
- Resources available for training

Whatever model you wish to propose, you will have to address the influence these factors will have on your potential success and the impact your proposal will have on these factors.

REFERENCES

1. Muller PA. Leadership versus management: a matter of focus. *J Post Anesth Nurs.* October 1991;6(5):361–363.
2. Zubialde JP. Leading change versus managing care: the role of change agent in family medicine. *Fam Med.* February 2001;33(2):133–136.
3. Katzenbach JR, Smith DK. *The Wisdom of Teams: Creating the High-Performance Organization.* New York, NY: Harper Collins; 2003.
4. Hammer M, Champy J. *Reengineering the Corporation, A Manifesto for Business Revolution.* New York, NY: HarperBusiness; 1993.
5. Walston SL, Burns LR, Kimberly JR. Does reengineering really work? An examination of the context and outcomes of hospital reengineering initiatives. *Health Serv Res.* February 2000;34(6):1363–1388.

6. McCloskey BA, Diers DK. Effects of New Zealand's health reengineering on nursing and patient outcomes. *Med Care.* November 2005;43(11):1140–1146.

7. Woodward C, Shannon H, Cunningham C, et al. The impact of re-engineering and other cost reduction strategies on the staff of a large teaching hospital: a longitudinal study. *Med Care.* 1999;37(6):556–569.

8. Salyer JW, Baldesare-Burton K. A sub-set of findings from a survey of respiratory care services: clinical practice guidelines and restructuring. *Respir Care.* 1998;43:866.

9. Fisher ES, Wennberg JE, Stukel TA, Gottlieb DJ, Lucas FL, Pinder ÉL. The implications of regional variations in Medicare spending. Part 1: the content, quality, and accessibility of care. *Ann of Intern Med.* 2003;138(4):273–287.

10. Wennberg JE. Variation in use of Medicare services among regions and selected academic medical centers: is more better? The Commonwealth Fund. 2005. http://www.commonwealthfund.org/publications/publications_show.htm?doc_id =326732.

11. Wennberg JE, Peters PG Jr. Unwarranted variations in the quality of health care: can the law help medicine provide a remedy/remedies? *Spec Law Dig Health Care Law.* 2004;305:9–25.

12. Wennberg JE, McAndrew Cooper MM, eds. *The Dartmouth Atlas of Health Care in the United States.* American Hospital Publishing Inc.; 1996.

13. Salyer JW, Baldesare-Burton K. A sub-set of findings from a survey of respiratory care services: clinical practice guidelines and restructuring. *Respir Care.* 1998;43:866.

CHAPTER 4

Measuring Department Performance

If you torture data sufficiently, they will eventually confess to something . . .

—Dr. David Kleinbaum

The one with the most data wins

In my experience, the most common mistake made by hospital department managers and directors is failure to develop systems for the measurement of the performance of their departments. There are reasons why so many people fail to develop such measurement systems. Often they don't know how, or they feel as if they don't have time. And admittedly, building measurement systems is always time consuming, often frustrating, and always somewhat abstract because the benefit of building these measurement systems is, like the Bismarck, out of sight over the horizon. But if you don't take the time to build these measurement systems, then the Bismarck may very well hove into view and you may be looking down the barrel of 16-inch guns.

By default, directors–managers sometimes leave other people in the hospital to develop measures of the performance of their departments. This is a bad move. No one should know better than a department director–manager what the important things are that ought to be measured in a hospital department. Do not let someone else define what is important for your department. If you do, you may end up not liking the measures they develop. There is an old political axiom that is sooooo true. Do not be the one who reacts. Have your adversary be the one who is reacting. Don't react to administration, medical staff, and nursing.[i] Have administration, medical

---

[i]Let me not be accused of fomenting an adversarial relationship with nursing and administration. This is not healthy. I am incredibly competitive and tend to frame things within the context of conflict. And I use a lot of military metaphors. But if you regard your relationship with nursing and administration as principally adversarial, you will end up less happy than you might otherwise be. Don't hesitate to take on a tough battle, but at every opportunity, you should build relationships and trust with your administrative and nursing colleagues. Of course, this does not include the occasional hopeless cause, who is so obnoxious that you hide in a closet when you see him or her coming down the hall.

staff, and nursing reacting to you. Be proposing ideas and plans and such. Don't be the one who is always reacting to their ideas. Of course, it is somewhat helpful if, on occasion, your ideas have merit. This takes a lot of energy, and I have not always pulled it off. In my low times, I have cruised along with no agenda of my own and have been deep into reactionary mode. This will not do. Usually some rejuvenating event occurs, like a river rafting trip, or going to a scientific conference, or a righteous butt-chewing by my boss, and then I am all energized again and ready to engage the warp drive. When you are coasting it usually means you are going downhill.

To be a really good director you have to function as a process analyst. These are folks that look at systems and processes and figure out how to measure them and improve them. Like statisticians and attorneys, they have their own language. What us normal folks call measures, they call metrics. Don't ask me why. "Measures" seems like a perfectly good word to me. But the cool new term is metrics, so metrics it is. Throughout this chapter we will focus on the metrics of department performance. If you go to committee meetings or sessions with your boss and start using the word "metric," they will all be very impressed. Just don't get carried away.

The most commonly available metrics in RT departments are financial and productivity measures. All hospitals have these kinds of metrics to varying degrees, and they are used to varying degrees for the ritualistic flogging of directors–managers. Generally, I like to divide metrics into four fundamental categories: financial, productivity, clinical quality, and business operations. Typical financial metrics are usually subdivided into revenue and expense. To one uninitiated in the subtle mysteries of hospital finance, at first glance revenue would appear to be defined as what the hospital charges the patient and thus gets paid for their services. But alas, one would be wrong. Gross revenue is the sum of all billed charges. What the hospital actually *receives in payment* is affected by a wide range of factors. These include contractual discounts with payers, charges that are disallowed by payers, bad debt, and managed care payment schemes such as per diem rates and capitation. There is an arcane and dizzying lexicon associated with reimbursement. Appendix C is a glossary of terms related to insurance and reimbursement.

Most respiratory therapy departments are revenue generating departments and thus can bill for their services. Well, actually, *any* department can bill for its services. The distinction of the revenue generating department is that there is some remote hope of being reimbursed by payers for these charges. Payers are mythical creatures. They are the sources of all goodness and light. It is from them that hospitals get paid (mostly). Payers can be public or private, public being the government (county, state, or federal) and private being the insurance companies and those on the bottom of the financial food chain, the patients. Payers wield vast influence on the life of hospitals, and yet the overwhelming majority of all hospital staff never sees one of these elusive creatures.[ii]

Of course you have heard the endlessly repeated statistic that there are 44 million uninsured Americans. I have grave doubts about the validity of this number as I do of all numbers used in political debate. In reality, most states have very liberal definitions for what constitutes poverty, and if you are in *poverty*, you qualify for state paid health care in the form of Medicaid in almost all states to some degree or another. So when someone says there are so many uninsured, don't be fooled. Anyone in the United States with even the most modest capabilities can get urgently needed health care in any hospital in the United States regardless of their ability to pay. Indeed, this is required by law, specifically the Emergency Medical Treatment and Active Labor Act (EMTALA). What we *do* have in the United States is an administrative mess in the distribution and application of private and public insurance, which I also have grave doubts will ever be fixed by government fiat. It turns out that a great number of the so-called uninsured choose to be uninsured, and the real number of uninsured is unknown but probably much lower. The 44 million figure is from the current population survey (CPS), but two other sources of government survey data put the numbers at 31 and 21 million.[1] Funny how this never gets mentioned in news reports.

As a metric of performance for departments, revenue is difficult to manage and is not frequently something managers are held accountable for. The factors that bring patients of various kinds to the hospital are largely outside the control of the department director. But you might periodically be asked to explain why revenue is above (good) or below (bad) the anticipated amounts (budgeted). This is usually caused by a change in the "mix" of patients. I will say more on patient mix shortly. A common mistake made by department managers and directors is to focus excessively on revenue. The conversation typically goes something like this. "Yes boss, I know our costs are way over budget, but gee, look at our revenue." For the most part,

---

[ii]Hospitals give some large insurance companies large contractual discounts. This is done to get the insurance companies to direct their clients to the hospital. Some of the larger payers may get a discount of 30% or more from billed charges. But private pay patients in the same hospital getting the same therapy will not receive this big discount. This practice has been regarded by some as unethical, and class action lawsuits are grinding through the courts right now related to civil damages being sought against hospitals for this practice.

hospitals really don't have a problem with revenue. The problem is with costs (expenses). The fact that an RT department is revenue generating will not save you from doom if you cannot get your costs under control. Focus on expenses and productivity if you really want to become a Jedi Knight among directors–managers.

The old "filthy lucre" is the coin of the realm in the calculus of department financial performance. There are lots and lots of ways to slice up and report costs. Typically there will be amounts that you are projected or budgeted to spend for various categories. One of the most basic metrics is the difference between what you were budgeted to spend and what you actually spent. This is typically called budget "variance." It seems on the surface like such a pleasant word. But you may come to loathe and fear the utterance of "variance." But not all variance is bad. You've got your favorable and unfavorable variance—you either under spent or over spent an account. Table 4-1 lists a typical set of budget categories and definitions for those categories. Much more will be reviewed regarding budgeting and finance in another chapter.

Productivity metrics are defined as those that measure, to some degree or another, how much labor it takes your department to deliver the care being administered. Most departments have some form of productivity calculation system against which your performance will be measured. Because productivity analysis is typically part of the budgeting process, I will save a more detailed discussion of these systems for the budgeting chapter. I am not a big fan of measuring staff productivity in an acute hospital environment. It is too variable. Sometimes you are so crazy busy that if we could accurately

Table 4-1. Typical Budget Categories*

Category	Definition
Inpatient revenue	Total gross charges posted to inpatients' accounts. This is only slightly related to what reimbursement the hospital actually receives.
Outpatient revenue	Total gross charges posted to outpatients' accounts. The relationship between this and actual remuneration is even more tenuous than inpatient charges.

Table 4-1. Typical Budget Categories (Continued)

Category	Definition
Salaries staff	Total salary dollars paid to all nonmanagement staff. For respiratory therapists, usually not nearly enough. If you don't believe me, just ask them.
Salaries management/ Supervision	Total salary dollars paid to all management and supervisory staff. For managers and supervisors this is usually too much. If you don't believe me, just ask the staff.
Contract/Agency staff expense	Total salary dollars paid to agency staff (travelers). This is definitely usually too much; usually 50–75% higher than staff salaries (including benefits).
Employee benefits	The cost of Social Security, Medicare, and employee benefits, such as medical and dental insurance. Typically somewhere between 28 and 35 cents for every salary dollar spent. Take up any grievances you have here with state and federal governments.
Oxygen and other gases	Costs of all medical gases. Can include the cost of inhaled nitric oxide, which is typically about 5–10 times more costly than all other medical gases combined. No, there is no stock currently available in companies that produce and sell nitric oxide.
Minor medical equipment	Non-disposable and non-capital medical equipment. Capital equipment is usually defined as an item that costs $1000, but this varies from hospital to hospital. Examples of minor medical might include a gauge or a cable for a monitor.
Medical supplies	These are typically consumable, disposable medical supplies. In RT they are typically tubing, masks, sensors, connectors, tubes, catheters, etc. This is always a nice area to go hunting for cost savings.

(Continues)

Table 4-1. Typical Budget Categories *(Continued)*

Category	Definition
Other minor equipment	Non-disposable, non-capital, non-medical equipment that costs less than the capital budget limit. Examples include that nice stereo you are thinking about buying for your office.
Office supplies	Duh.
Computers	Duh again.
Equipment maintenance and repair	This is typically what you pay to have your equipment maintained and repaired. This can include internal and external costs since some hospitals have internal biomedical departments that actually charge other departments for this service. This is, of course, funny money since no dollars actually leave the organization. Unfortunately, these funny dollars can still land in your budget.
Administrative physician	The fee you pay for your department medical director. It is not entirely uncommon to not get your money's worth here, but that is usually the director's fault for not holding the medical director's feet to the fire.
Other purchased services	Any contractual services you purchase from outside the hospital that does not involve the servicing of equipment.
Equipment rentals	The cost of renting clinical and non-clinical equipment. Can be a lot of expense for some departments that do not have sufficient capital equipment or extremely volatile demand for services. This is a fertile ground to cultivate cost savings for the savvy manager.
Other miscellaneous	Slush fund for everything else, including food for meetings and special events and staff recognition activities.

Table 4-1. Typical Budget Categories *(Continued)*

Category	Definition
Travel/Conference	An essential budget category. Often overlooked and underfunded. Fight for this budget account. It is worth it.

*This is just one example of a budget categorization system. There are many variations to this with each hospital having different category names and sometimes subtle and not so subtle differences in the definitions for similarly named categories.

measure the work you are doing, you would appear to be Superman, moving faster than the speed of light and able to leap tall buildings at a single bound. Other times, like a firehouse, there just isn't much to do. But of course you cannot just send everyone home when it is slow for the same reason they cannot send firemen home when it is slow at the firehouse.

Finally, metrics of business operations can be thought of as measures of the business processes, such as the supply chain, billing systems, scheduling, staff retention, and recruitment, to name a few. This is often an overlooked aspect of department performance. The hospital industry in general is a bit behind the curve in adapting sound business practices to hospital operations. This is largely due to the fact that the government began routinely delivering wheelbarrows full of money to hospitals in the 1970s because of the passage of the Medicare act in 1965.[iii] Without market forces at work and little real competition, hospitals were not forced to improve their business operations to survive. This is much better now than it was; competition has improved and indeed many hospitals have not survived. However, this is often a result of their inability to maintain market share, and hence revenue stream, as opposed to their competitors having more efficient operations.

[iii]The federal government will spend $395 billion (with a "b") on Medicare and $276 billion (also with a "b") on Medicaid in 2007. This does not count what the *states* will spend on Medicaid, nor does it include private insurance spending on health care, nor out of pocket expenses. It is estimated that total healthcare spending in the United States is approximately $1.9 trillion (with a "t") yearly, or $1,900,000,000,000. This amounts to about $6200 per person in the United States (based on 2004 data). While the government has worked very hard over the last 20 years or so to curb the growth in Medicare spending, this is still a 12% increase over Medicare spending from 2006. It appears that soon all money everywhere will be spent on health care. Works for me because I work in the industry. Although I must admit that I seem to notice a hefty chunk of my income going to taxes and insurance.

BENCHMARKING AND INDEXING

The whole point of metrics is comparison. Any measure by itself isn't particularly useful. If you are a 6'2" power forward, you probably are going to have a short lived career unless you are playing junior high school basketball. Thus, if you have a metric, it may very well get lonely unless you have another metric to compare it to. Then you can make graphs and charts, develop PowerPoint presentations and, if you are really gifted, draw some conclusion or make a judgment about the quality or efficiency of your operation. The healthcare industry is rife with attempts to build comparable metrics systems. Benchmarking is a new racket, oops, I mean cottage industry in health care. Benchmarking can be defined as taking lots of (allegedly) comparable metrics from lots of hospitals and showing you where your hospital or department ranks among the other hospitals or departments. The benchmark is a term that refers to the hospital or department with the best metric in any particular category. The theory is that if you are not the benchmark, maybe you could learn something from the benchmark hospital or department to improve the efficiency of your operation.

But there is a hole in the dike. The emperor may not be naked, but he is certainly scantily dressed. It turns out that comparing cost and quality data from different hospitals and departments is very difficult. We are finding out that metrics aren't very comparable after all unless some special precautions are taken.

Case Study 9: Out of This Maze

Joe N. Fection RRT had just quaffed his fourth cup of Starbucks' Sumatra (venti) and it wasn't even 0900. He was trying to figure out what to do with the data his boss had just sent him. According to the report he held in his trembling hand, the intensive care unit had 12 lower respiratory tract infections (LRIs) in ventilated patients in the second quarter, up from only six in the first quarter. Everyone was up in arms. LRIs had *doubled*. He had to trudge down to administration that afternoon and let them know what respiratory care was going to do about these data. After he closed his office door, he began to rant about the injustice of it all. After all, it was probably the nurses' or doctors' fault. Why was RT being blamed? Shortly he calmed down. He tried to think carefully about the issue, but he was having trouble concentrating. He turned on his CD player and heard Roger Waters singing:

> I got to admit
> That I'm a little bit confused
> Sometimes it seems to me
> As if I'm just being used
> Got to stay awake,
> Got to try and shake
> Off this creeping malaise
> If I don't stand my own ground,
> How can I find my way out of this maze?
> —*Animals* by Pink Floyd

Suddenly, he started thinking about causes for why the number of infections seemed to have increased so much. He speculated that these infections might have been caused by changes in practice, for example poor compliance with hand washing, suctioning, or infection control policies. But the ICU had basically the same staff of RTs, RNs, and MDs that had been there for years, so it seemed unlikely that they would suddenly stop complying with policies. But what if they just had more patients and thus they should have more LRIs, he wondered? Then it occurred to him that maybe they had the same number of patients, but they stayed on the ventilator longer. So he decided to try to adjust the data so that they could be compared across different time periods when there were different numbers of patients and different numbers of ventilator days. He called up the decision support department and asked them to send him the total number of ventilator days for the last *two* quarters. The numbers turned out to be:

	1st Quarter	2nd Quarter
Number of LRIs	6	12
Number of ventilator days	295	734

He then divided the number of LRIs in each quarter by the number of ventilator days during each quarter. He then multiplied this number by 100, producing a rate of LRIs per one hundred ventilator days. He used the following formula:

$$\text{LRIs/100 ventilator days} = \left[\frac{\text{Total \# of LRIs}}{\text{Total \# of Ventilator Days}} \right] \times 100$$

It turns out that the numbers looked like this:

	1st Quarter	2nd Quarter
Number of LRIs/100 ventilator days	2.01	1.61

(Continues)

By now, Roger Waters was singing, "You better watch out, there may be dogs about." Joe sat there for a minute and pondered what he had just learned. Not only had the infection rate not gone *up*, it had actually gone *down*. He proceeded to make a nice graph, slapped it on his thumb drive, and headed for the meeting with administration, a broad grin on his face. He stopped by the bathroom on the way. After all, they *were* ventis.

Thus Joe discovered the practice of indexing, which in health care could be described as mathematical adjustments of data to make them comparable across different domains, for example time, populations, or organizations. Medication errors are indexed to the total number of doses given. Paid respiratory therapy hours are sometimes indexed to total numbers of respiratory care procedures (see below). If you are comparing the frequency of unhappy events, such as morbidities, you need to index them to the level of clinical activity such as numbers of patients or numbers of patient days. If you are analyzing costs, these too must be indexed to appropriate factors, such as admissions or discharges. In the example above, Joe multiplied the quotient by 100. This is simply a convention to make the number a little easier to get a grip on. For some reason, some of us can tell the difference between 2.01 and 1.61 more easily than we can tell the difference between 0.00201 and 0.00161. Go figure.

Benchmarking can be done internally, for example comparing your department's efficiency to other departments in the hospital. This is usually not a terribly useful exercise because the economics and practice models of the cost of respiratory care operations are not very comparable to these same dimensions in a radiology department or food service. There is also the practice of corporate benchmarking. Your hospital may be part of a corporation that owns other hospitals, in which case you may be assessed using benchmarking data from other hospitals inside the corporation. This can be very useful because you may have access to some pretty detailed cost data that you cannot get access to for departments that are not in your organization. This makes meaningful comparison a little easier. Or your hospital may subscribe to a commercial benchmarking database company. These businesses compile data from lots of hospitals, usually at the department level, and then develop comparative measures for analyzing your financial efficiencies. Occasionally they even have clinical process or outcomes measures, but usually the data available to you are limited to financial metrics. The quality of these services is highly variable, and they usually do not have very much respiratory data available. The AARC now has a benchmarking service available. For a very modest fee, compared to the cost of membership in some benchmarking organizations, you can submit your data online and then compare your department's performance with other RT departments.[iv]

Benchmarking companies can suffer from serious data quality problems. Not all the hospitals may count and represent their data in the same way. Clinical data are usually a little more suspect than financial. An example might be accidental extubation reporting. Some benchmarking companies gather and report the number of accidental extubations indexed to ventilator days. But not every hospital gathers its accidental extubation data the same way. Hospital A may have a voluntary paper reporting system. In other words, staff members are expected to self-report accidental extubations by finding the appropriate form, filling it out, and turning it in. These forms then have to be gathered, sorted, collated, counted, and finally reported to the benchmarking company. You can imagine (without a lot of effort) that there are lots of places for this reporting to break down. It is very possible that accidental extubations occur on the night shift, on the weekend, over the holidays, during very busy times, and/or during periods of short staffing. Quite probably, the staff may not have the inclination or the time to fill out said paperwork. Something as supposedly simple as not being able to find the appropriate forms can be a huge barrier to the staff's ability to complete such reports. Thus, not all of the events may get reported.

Conversely, Hospital B may have a clinical auditor who goes around to every ventilated patient every day, examines the medical record, and interviews the clinical staff for evidence of accidental extubations. This system produces much more accurate accidental extubation data. Hospital B is working harder and has a better system for identifying unhappy clinical events, but in the benchmarking system, Hospital A may look like they have a better system because their rates of accidental extubations are (falsely) low. Of course, nobody said life was supposed to be fair.

Better benchmarking companies work hard to ensure data quality, and they have periodic reviews of data gathering techniques and data quality with all their reporting hospitals. Regardless of the quality of the data you get from a benchmarking company, it is very inadvisable for you, as a director, to spend a lot of time in administration whining about the poor quality of the data. It is tantamount to career suicide to drag your feet and do nothing

---

[iv]http://www.aarc.org/resources/benchmarking/index.asp

when confronted with benchmarking data that suggests your department isn't doing very well. What you *should* do is tell administration you have concerns about the quality of the data while at the same time presenting your plans to work with the benchmarking company and reporting hospitals to improve the quality of their *data and what your plans are to improve your operation*, which after all is what administration really wants you to do.

Even if benchmarking data are not entirely accurate or quantitative, they may be *qualitative*. Maybe Taco Bellevue Hospital isn't as good as they look compared to you, but there may still be a lot you can learn from their RT department. You should spend a lot more time trying to learn from benchmarking data than you do trying to run away from it, or trying to 'splain it away. Circling the wagons or filling the moat will send a bad message that you aren't willing to learn. It is easy to slip into defensive mode. You work hard at your job and you have tried to design the best department possible. If you are a little arrogant (like me) it can be hard to admit that the dufus across town at that other hospital could possibly know more than you about running a department. As personally satisfying as this kind of thinking can be, it is dangerous. I think I am pretty good at what I do, but in every single aspect of running an RT department, I know directors who have better operations than I do. John Thompson, RRT, Tom Kallstrom, RRT, Rick Ford, RRT, Sue Ciariallo, RRT, and Scott Pettinichi, RRT come to mind (there are many others whom I hope won't feel offended because I did not mention their names).

A good thing to do with benchmarking data is to identify the hospitals that have operations comparable in scope and design to yours. Pick the two or three of these departments that have the best benchmarking data and go there and examine their operations. Talk to the staff, examine their systems, study their structure, and steal shamelessly from them the things that can make your operation better. Be sure to talk to the staff. Management has one view of reality and the staff has another view.

COST PER UNIT OF CARE

Immutable Truth #17: Not everything that counts can be counted, and not everything that can be counted counts.[v] As we proceed through the measurement

---

[v] OK, I admit it. I did not think this one up, although I wish I had. This has been attributed to Einstein. It is unclear to me whether he was the author or not. It is reported to have been a sign posted on his office wall. One of my favorite Einstein quotes: "Reality is merely an illusion, albeit a very persistent one."

chapter, I will propose many, many metrics. Not all of these measures are in existence, but I believe it is at least possible to measure all of these. I wish it weren't so, but we are nowhere near being able to measure all aspects of our operations. And the bitter truth is that some of it may never be measured, at least not in my lifetime. There is a conventional wisdom that goes something like this: if a phenomenon is real, it can be observed, if it can be observed, it can be measured. Before you start squirming in your seat about my obvious inconsistency here, let me head you off at the pass. I personally think consistency is somewhat overrated. At least from an intellectual perspective, we are forced every day, if we are careful observers, into regions of the mind that can only be accurately described by the term "cognitive dissonance." This is the ability to hold two completely opposing points of view at the same time and feel okay about it. Yes, I think all real phenomena can be observed and hence measured, and I think not everything that counts can be counted. I am down with this. Those of you who are troubled by this apparent inconsistency should build a bridge, and get over it.

Apparently, questions about the efficiency of respiratory therapy operations have been asked for a long time. From a recently unearthed ancient Greek dialogue, we learn that the ancient Greeks had RTs too. Who knew? In this papyrus scroll found in the trash can of a Coptic Egyptian monastery, Phaedrus is talking to Diogenes in the administrative conference room at the Rhodes Medical Center:

Phaedrus	*Gosh it seems like we have a lot of RTs around here. I wonder if we have too many? They sure seem to cost a lot.*
Diogenes	*Hhhhmmmm, I don't know how to define "too many," but I wonder if we have more than they have at Athens Community Hospital?*
Phaedrus	*Well, they have fewer beds than we do, so they probably wouldn't have as many RTs as we have anyway. Maybe my cousin Apollo can help us figure out if our RT department is lean and mean?*
Diogenes	*Maybe we should just calculate the number of RTs we have per occupied bed each day and then compare it to Athens?*

Phaedrus	*That might work, but we have way more pulmonary patients than the other hospital because of Pneumocrates, our world famous, hard charging pulmonologist, so we might need more RTs per occupied bed than that other hospital.*
Diogenes	*Yeah, I see your point. Great Zeus this is confusing. My candle is burning out.*
Phaedrus	*I am struggling too. My rhetoric seems to have failed me.*

Thus, Diogenes and Phaedrus are impaled on the horns of a common dilemma. They have access to *some* metrics. They have the technology. But turning data into information is more challenging. They don't know what to conclude from data they have access to. Diogenes and Phaedrus were focused, as many administrators and financial analysts are, on labor costs. But RT practice also consumes disposables and equipment—sometimes lots. Overly focusing on labor costs alone is somewhat myopic. And labor costs are mind-bogglingly hard to compare across healthcare systems because of the enormous variation in practice models. In some hospitals RTs do all the endotracheal tube suctioning, and in other hospitals nurses do most of it. In some places nurses do almost all simple oxygen therapy and pulse oximetry while other facilities have the RTs do almost all of these. Thus comparing labor or productivity metrics alone between hospitals does not adjust for these differences.

A better metric of financial performance is to calculate total RT costs per unit of care. This metric combines all the different costs in your operation—for example salary, supplies, equipment, education, training, etc.—and then indexes them to some level of activity that allows their comparison across various domains of time, population, and location. The challenge often lies in defining a unit of care. Many finance types think this ought to be *procedure counts* for an RT department. This is usually *not* a good idea. This is because of the following flawed assumption: A procedure is a procedure. Experience will soon teach you that this ain't necessarily so.[vi] What I mean is that different RT departments count things very differently.

[vi]I offer my apologies to my high school English teacher, Jim Gish, for the use of the word "ain't." To the purists among you, the use of the word "ain't" is troubling. But I like the word, as it is crisp and has a specific meaning that everyone clearly understands. E-mail, spam, netiquette, snafu, emoticon, newbie, and phat aren't real words either, but they seem to work well to me.

A simple example involves oxygen therapy. Many RT departments bill for oxygen therapy. Setting up and maintaining oxygen equipment is considered to be a "procedure." But how many oxygen procedures are there for 24 hours of continuous oxygen therapy? Some departments bill every 24 hours for oxygen therapy, others bill every 12 hours, and some bill every hour. Each billed procedure is included in the procedure count for purposes of indexing and calculating cost per procedure. Thus the department that bills every hour gets a procedure count of 24 for a day of oxygen therapy while another department that bills daily gets a procedure count of only 1. The two departments may be getting the same revenue overall for the oxygen therapy, and their labor costs may be similar. But if you divide their labor costs by 24 instead of 1, you get very different costs per procedure. Thus procedure counts are not very useful when it comes to using them for indexed measures of cost across different care models. They *can* be useful within a department to compare the efficiency of a system over time, but that is only if your billing system and methods for procedure count remain relatively constant over time, which often is not the case.

A better indexing variable for cost per unit of care is the relative value unit (RVU). This is essentially a unit of time. Why we don't just call them time units is beyond me. This is probably just an example of self-generated job security for *management engineers* who wanted to create an arcane and indecipherable language for writing reports that no one could understand. Thus a hospital would have to employ a *management engineer* just for their interpretive services.

Each billed procedure has an RVU attached to it, which represents the average amount of time it takes to perform this procedure. RVUs in some hospitals are represented in minutes, and others are represented in hours. Assume that a patient-ventilator system check takes 20 minutes. In a system where an RVU equals one hour, a patient-ventilator system check would have an RVU of 0.33, which equates to 20 minutes (one third of an hour equals 20 minutes). In a system where an RVU is equal to a minute, a patient-ventilator system check would equal 20 RVUs.

As noted, all billed procedures have an RVU attached. These are added up for all the billed procedures in a given budget period. The RVUs are then converted to FTEs, and this is how many clinical FTEs it should have taken your department to perform the clinical work you did. You should, by now, realize that building a very good billing system is vital. When building the billing system, be sure to spend the time to carefully evaluate the RVUs attached to each charge.

As I just pointed out, for the purposes of generating indexed cost per unit of care data, RVUs are better than procedures. Whereas some departments count 24 procedures for a day of oxygen therapy and others count only 1 procedure for a day of oxygen therapy, both departments should be taking about the same amount of time to set up oxygen equipment because oxygen therapy is largely standardized across the country. Thus if their billing system is properly designed, they will probably be reporting about the same RVU for oxygen therapy.

Regrettably, some departments do not have a system of RVUs that are attached to each billed charge. But even if your hospital has no formal RVU system, you could still develop your own. You could take your billed procedures each month and run them through an RVU grid using a simple spreadsheet function. This would yield total minutes of clinical care, which you could then use to track your own productivity by comparing this to total paid hours. These numbers will not be the same because you have plenty of paid hours that are not "clinical," including your own salary and that of your nonclinical employees.

The next best thing to using RVUs for measuring cost per unit of care is cost per patient day. This is simply the total cost of the RT operation divided by the number of patient days. The most accurate method for this metric is to use only patient days from patients who received some RT service. This is technically not difficult to do, but many hospital information systems do not have the infrastructure, nor the database querying talent, to produce such sophisticated slices of data. This is why data management and analytical skills are so essential to the development of a good department director; you may have to learn the querying and analytical skills to do these things yourself. Others will be luckier and have excellent decision support or finance departments that help with this kind of work.

If you cannot get patient days only for patients who had RT services, then just use patient days for all patients for the denominator. This is still generally better than resorting to procedures, which can be wildly different in different departments for essentially the same amount of work, owing to the variability in the design of billing systems, as stated above.

So now you are at the place of having indexed, cost per unit of care data. Then what? Is that your final answer? Sometimes it may be. You may not have access to any additional data that could help to make more meaningful analyses and comparisons across different time periods and different patient populations. But there are some additional things you can do to improve the comparability of data from different departments, hospitals, and time periods.

One important factor to consider when analyzing financial data is inflation. If your labor cost per unit of care went up 5% from one year to the next, it might be entirely caused by inflation in salaries as opposed to some change in the efficiency of your operation. This is also true for nonlabor costs, which are often subject to yearly price increases caused by inflation. The way to do this is to keep the costs constant in terms of the beginning year of comparison. The technique is relatively simple. You lay out your yearly costs in chronological order and divide them by one plus the inflation rate for each year, skipping the first year, and starting with the second historical year. Imagine that inflation is 6% per year over the five years of your data from 2000 to 2005. Leave the 2000 data alone. Divide the 2001 data by 1.06. Divide the 2002 data by 1.06, then divide that result by 1.06. Divide the 2003 data by 1.06, then again by 1.06, then again by 1.06, and so on, until you get to 2005. The resulting costs can be described as being "constant in year 2000 dollars." Table 4-2 shows an example of data on total respiratory therapy costs per RVU with and without adjustment for inflation. What looked like *increasing* respiratory therapy costs turned out to actually be *decreasing* after considering the effect of inflation, which is largely outside the control of the department director.

ADJUSTING FOR SEVERITY OF ILLNESS

One of the challenges of comparing data across different parts of the healthcare system is the inconvenient truth that patients have varying degrees of illness. Sicker patients typically take more time and energy and resources to care for. Applying a mechanical ventilator to an uncomplicated postoperative cardiac surgery patient is very different than applying a ventilator to a patient who is in status asthmaticus or who has adult respiratory distress syndrome. And yet systems that measure productivity through RVU counts would give both of these procedures the same number of RVUs.

One way to correct for this is to adjust data for severity of illness (SOI). This is also sometimes called risk adjustment, a very large topic about which much has been written.[2–9] Lisa Iezzoni describes the strengths and weaknesses of the many systems used for risk adjustment in her excellent book, which the interested student is encouraged to read.[10] Most severity measurement systems have one thing in common: They assign the patient a numerical severity score. How they go about this varies greatly from system to system. These scores are then used to adjust healthcare measures like cost.

Suppose you worked at Heavenly Gates Children's Hospital and your administrator approached you with some benchmarking data in the form of

Table 4-2.   Example of Adjusting for Inflation*

Before inflation adjustment	2002	2003	2004	2005
RT salary expense	$2,738,026	$2,964,686	$3,167,174	$3,293,861
Relative value units (RVUs)	45,672	49,089	51,033	50,091
Inflation rate		6%	6%	6%
RT salary expense per RVU	$59.95	$60.39	$62.06	$65.76

After inflation adjustment	2002	2003	2004	2005
Adjusted RT salary expense	$2,738,026	$2,796,874	$2,818,774	$2,765,589
Adjusted salary expense per RVU	$59.95	$56.98	$55.23	$55.21

Unadjusted change in expense per RVU from 2002 to 2005...................↑ 10%

Adjusted change in expense per RVU from 2002 to 2005.........................↓ 8%

*Note that after inflation adjustment, salary expense per RVU went from *increasing* during the historical period to *decreasing* during the historical period. The rate of inflation was assumed to be 6%.

the RT costs per RVU for the five hospitals in your corporation. It turns out that yours is the second most costly RT department in your organization, and something needs to be done about this. You are being asked to come up with a plan to address why you appear to be so costly compared to the other hospitals in the organization. The data you received are in Table 4-3.

It doesn't look good for the hometown team, and you are thinking about buffing up your resume when you have *a wave of crystallization*, a moment of insight, indeed a life saving mental maneuver. "Wait a minute," you think, "what if we are more costly because our patients are sicker?" This is, of course, one of the oldest tricks in the book for explaining away bad data and crummy performance. But maybe, just maybe, this time, it is true. You know for a fact that you have a lot more ventilated patients, and your pediatric cardiac surgery patients are very labor intensive to care for.

So you call the decision support department and ask them if there is any way to adjust these data from other hospitals for the severity of illness of their patient populations. Luckily, you get someone on the phone. It turns out they *can* adjust for severity of illness using the *case mix index*, which they have for every hospital for each year. They send you the numbers and tell you to divide the cost/RVU by the case mix index numbers. The last line in Table 4-3 shows you what happened to the ranking of the hospitals when the data were adjusted for severity of illness of their respective populations. You go from being the second most costly department to the second least costly department. You're so happy you can hardly count.

Case mix is a term that refers to the relative composition of your inpatient population. Tertiary referral hospitals usually have a much sicker population of patients than a suburban or rural community hospital. Case mix index is widely available. It is determined by comparing the relative mix of your patients to the average mix of all patients. Thus if your case mix index is 1.0, you have a population about equally as sick as the rest of the hospitals. If your case mix index is less than 1.0, your population is less sick than the group; and if your case mix index is greater than 1.0, your population is sicker than the group as a whole. Your finance department should be able to get your case mix index for you for any given period of time.

EXAMPLES OF METRICS

Tables 4-4, 4-5, 4-6, and 4-7 list various examples of types of measures you might consider in building a set of metrics for measuring department performance. Most directors spend most of their time measuring financial performance and productivity. This is usually because: (1) these are pretty important, and (2) these types of metrics are more widely available. Clinical quality is much more difficult to measure. So most departments don't do much to measure it. This has slowly begun to improve over the years, but good measures of clinical quality are still one of the least developed aspects of measuring RT department performance.

We instinctively think of clinical quality as making sure that we give therapies the right way, for example we are following the policies and procedures on how we should administer a given treatment. *The right treatment to the right patient at the right time* is one way to think of it. But unless you have

Table 4-3. The Power of Risk Adjustment*

		General Hospital	Our Lady of 142nd Street Hospital	St. Elsewhere Hospital	Heavenly Gates Children's Hospital	Taco Bellevue Hospital
The data that were given to you	Total procedures	63,713	296,100	107,622	76,984	146,518
	Total RVUs	2,162,271	10,982,787	4,303,581	5,938,908	6,802,593
	Total expense	$1,159,941	$4,928,591	$2,315,345	$3,598,913	$3,965,925
	Expense/RVU	$ 0.536	$ 0.449	$ 0.538	$ 0.572	$ 0.583
The data asked for	Case mix index (CMI)	0.766	1.473	1.042	1.706	1.125
The corrected data	Expense/RVU adjusted for CMI	$ 0.700	$ 0.305	$ 0.516	$ 0.336	$ 0.518

*RT department costs for 1 year in five different hospitals indexed to RVUs, adjusted for severity (risk). Expense/RVU adjusted for CMI is calculated by dividing (expense/RVU) by CMI. Note that Heavenly Gates Children's Hospital went from being the second *most costly* RT department to the second *least costly* RT department after adjusting for risk (severity of illness). This means that their increased expense can be explained by the increased severity of illness of their patient population relative to that of other hospitals.

Table 4-4. Metrics of Department Financial Performance[*]

Metric	Comment
Total expense per procedure	This is useful usually only for internal comparisons over time because there is lots and lots of variation in how procedures are counted between RT departments.
Total expense per RVU	This is a better measure, but not all departments have well designed RVU systems in place.
Total expense per patient day	Your RT expenses are spread out over the entire inpatient population. This is not sensitive at all to changes in the mix of different kinds of patients the hospital admits. If the proportion of patients with respiratory disease increases, your RT expenses ought to increase. But this metric does not adjust for any case mix changes.
Total expense per respiratory patient day	Better yet, this is the cost of the department spread out over only the days of patients receiving RT services. Respiratory patients can be identified as those receiving any billed RT charge.
Labor expense per procedure	Be sure to adjust these for salary inflation if comparing across time periods. Also if comparing between hospitals in different cities or regions, there are geographical adjustments for the cost of labor that can make these metrics more comparable for use between hospitals.
Labor expense per RVU	Another way of thinking of this is the labor cost per minute (or hour) of care administered.
Labor expense per patient day	This spreads your labor expense out over the entire inpatient population, but once again it is relatively insensitive to changes in case mix.

(Continues)

Table 4-4. Metrics of Department Financial Performance *(Continued)*

Metric	Comment
Labor expense per respiratory patient day	Some departments have very different scope of supplies bought by respiratory care. An example would be nitric oxide gas. In some hospitals it is paid for by the pharmacy and in some hospitals it is paid for by the RT department. Because it can cost a department in the millions of dollars for nitric oxide per year, it would not be reasonable to compare their supply expenses per unit of care to a department that did not pay the nitric oxide expenses.
Nonlabor expense per procedure	Nonlabor expenses represent all costs other than salaries, for example total expenses minus labor expenses. This includes supplies, equipment, maintenance, training, and administrative overhead costs.
Nonlabor expense per RVU	This can reflect the costliness of RT practice in terms of supplies purchased and used and practices that consume a lot of disposables.
Nonlabor expense per patient day	This also reflects the costliness of RT practice in terms of supplies purchased and used but spreads the cost out over all patient days.
Nonlabor expense per respiratory patient day	As stated above, this is more reflective of actual indexed RT nonlabor costs because it uses only RT patient days.

*All metrics are for department-level direct expenses of an RT department, although these would work for any hospital department.

Table 4-5. Metrics of Productivity

Metric	Comments
Volume adjusted versus actual FTEs	This metric is determined by adding all the RVUs reported for a given period, running them through an equation that converts them to the number of FTEs you should have used, which are then compared to the number you actually did use. This difference is then used for either your remedial instruction or exalted praise (don't count on it).
Paid hours per procedure Paid hours per RVU Paid hours per patient day Paid hours per respiratory patient day	The suggestion here is that the less time it takes to perform a procedure, the more efficient you are. While this *can* be true, it is not *always* true. Some procedures, if rushed through and done sloppily, can potentially cost you (and your patients) more later on, such as taping endotracheal tubes and chest physiotherapy.
Ratio of clinical to nonclinical hours	Nonclinical hours include those of any department member not directly doing billable clinical procedures. A higher ratio indicates that you are paying a lot of hours to managers, supervisors, coordinators, assistants, clerks, etc. This *may* indicate you have an inefficient operation.

Table 4-6. Metrics of Clinical Quality

Metric	Comments
Compliance with charting standards	The quality or completeness of charting can be an indirect representation of the quality of clinical care. Consistency and complete charting can reflect consistency in clinical practice. Usually represented as a percentage of things you want to be charted, such as:

(Continues)

Table 4-6.   Metrics of Clinical Quality *(Continued)*

Metric	Comments
Compliance with charting standards	• Was heart rate charted before and after treatments? • Were breath sounds charted before and after treatments? • Was the patient in the right position for the treatment? • Was the endotracheal tube position checked with each ventilator check?
Compliance with policy standards	If your policies are properly crafted, compliance with them indicates good quality care. You should be periodically measuring the degree to which your staff members comply with your policies. You might assume it is happening, but this assumption is usually about as reliable as preelection campaign promises. Examples include: • Are alarm limits properly set? • Are patients checked at the appropriate frequency? • Are patients properly monitored, for example is pulse oximetry or capnometry used on patients when it should be?
Compliance with protocol standards	If you have a protocol for the treatment of asthma, are you following it? Chances are pretty good that it is not always followed. Protocols are typically much more effective when compliance with the protocol is periodically monitored. Examples include: • Treatments may be given more or less often than indicated in the protocol. • Dosages vary from the protocol. • Was the patient assessed according to the protocol?

Table 4-6. Metrics of Clinical Quality *(Continued)*

Metric	Comments
Effectiveness of protocols	Having protocols to direct care is nice, but so is a back rub. The question is: Are your protocols working? Most of the inappropriate application of respiratory care interventions involves overtreatment. Thus measures of protocol effectiveness usually measure how much we are treating patients or how long it takes. Examples may include the following if this aspect of your care is guided by protocols: • Number of treatments per admission • Hours of oxygen therapy per patient • Length of mechanical ventilation • Extubation failures
Procedural quality	While a lot of respiratory therapy can, at times, be largely ineffective, some procedural interventions, if done poorly by respiratory therapists, can yield very bad outcomes: • Mechanical ventilation—Poor application of ventilation can result in ventilator-induced lung injury, which can be manifested by any of the following (not all VILI is avoidable). • Air leak rates including pneumothorax and pulmonary interstitial emphysema • Length of ventilation in days or hours • Chronic oxygen requirements (percentage of patients) • Airway management • Rates of accidental extubations (per 100 ventilator days) • Rates of extubation failure (percentage of all extubations that result in reintubation within 24 hours)

(Continues)

Table 4-6. Metrics of Clinical Quality *(Continued)*

Metric	*Comments*

Procedural quality	• Rates of accidental tracheostomy decannulation (per 100 tracheostomy days)
	
	• Others
	  • Changes in clinical scores. Many hospitals now use clinical scores such as an asthma score or a bronchiolitis score. A measure of procedural quality can be the percentage of patients who experience an improvement in scores after treatment.
	  • Lower respiratory tract infection rates. These are also variously called ventilator associated pneumonias (VAP). I don't like using the term pneumonia because there continues to be lots of debate about uncertainty in the diagnosis of pneumonia. These rates are usually indexed to ventilator days (100). They are related to a lot of factors other than RT procedural skill and diligence, but they can also be caused by poor management of endotracheal tubes, bad suctioning practice, and poor hand washing compliance.
	  • Readmission rates—If treatment of certain types of patients, such as those with asthma, emphysema, or bronchiolitis is done poorly or not often enough, it can result in the patients being readmitted to the hospital or return to the emergency department within a few days. Typically the standard is 48 hours, although some hospitals measure out to seven days.

Table 4-6. Metrics of Clinical Quality *(Continued)*

Metric	Comments
Procedural quality	• Asthma in particular has a unique set of measures that can help identify the quality of care all across the care continuum. If asthma is properly managed and patients are properly educated and are compliant with treatment and management principles both inside and outside the hospital, then future hospitalizations and emergency room visits ought to be significantly reduced.
Treatment efficacy	A great question to ask is how much of the therapy given by RTs is "appropriate," for example how much was clearly indicated according to evidence-based guidelines. Also how much was effective.

Table 4-7. Metrics of Business Operations

Metric	Comment
Billing accuracy	Billing accuracy is a very big deal. There have been some very prominent examples of practitioners and health delivery systems getting in a great deal of criminal trouble for producing inaccurate bills for patients, which amounts to fraud. It doesn't seem to matter much to the legal system whether you intended to produce an accurate bill or not. New guidelines related to compliance include the requirement that managers and hospitals attend very carefully to the accuracy of patient bills. Sadly, RT bills have been notoriously inaccurate. (Salyer JW. Improving the accuracy of a respiratory care billing system. *Advance for Respiratory Care Managers.*

(Continues)

Table 4-7. Metrics of Business Operations *(Continued)*

Metric	Comments
Billing accuracy	1993:3(1);44–47.) If you look good in an orange jump suit with stripes down the leg, just ignore your billing system.
Staff turnover	I estimate that it takes about 25 to 35 thousand dead presidents to train a newly graduated RT to the point where they can practice autonomously and safely in a state of the art hospital. Every time a staff position is turned over, it is costly. Some turnover is inevitable, but how much is acceptable is difficult to estimate. You should be tracking yours.
Internal staff satisfaction	Respiratory therapy staff satisfaction with the quality of the workplace is vital to develop engaged employees. Engagement can be thought of as the degree to which your staff members come to work wanting to help make things better and having the skill and energy to do so. Measuring it *and* managing it are essential to the long-term success of the department and the hospital.
Patient satisfaction	Of course, it is nice that your staff members are highly motivated and satisfied with the workplace, but this will not float your boat if you have problems with patient and family satisfaction. If your hospital doesn't ask specific questions about RT in the patient and family survey, you could always suggest to administration that they include some. Write them yourself.
External staff satisfaction	By this I mean the satisfaction of the other departments, services, and disciplines in the hospital with the quality of the interaction with your staff.

battalions of plain clothes observers skulking about observing RTs at the bedsides, it is somewhat difficult to measure the quality of the RT-patient interaction via direct observation. What you *can* measure more easily is the *result* of the RT-patient interaction. If the *result* of the RT-patient interaction is good, then it is reasonably safe to assume that the interaction was a good one. So what are the results of RT-patient interactions? To start with, patient response to treatment is a result of the interaction. This is reflected in improving signs and symptoms, improved clinical scores, or a reduced need for further treatment. But what if patients don't improve after treatment? Does this mean therapy is bad? Not always, but it could mean that the therapy was inappropriate, for example it should not have been given to begin with because it was not indicated for the treatment of the patient's condition. Or the treatment may have been indicated but simply didn't work, thus it was ineffective.

In spite of our vaunted technology and healthcare infrastructure, we do a great deal to and for patients that end up being of little value to them. This problem is much more prevalent than the general public, and many inside the healthcare industry, appreciate. Examples are legion. One of the most famous is the use of antibiotics in the treatment of otitis media in infants and children, a practice that has been repeatedly debunked as unnecessary in the vast majority of patients because of the fact that otitis media is overwhelmingly caused by viral infections for which antibiotics are useless.[11] Otitis media, it turns out, overwhelmingly resolves without antibiotics within two to three days.[12] The facts notwithstanding, antibiotics continue to be over prescribed in this population, likely contributing to the development of antibiotic resistant strains of bacteria.

Respiratory therapy examples are also legion, including the over use of chest physiotherapy, bronchodilators, continuous pulse oximetry, and oxygen therapy, to name only a few.[vii] These therapies are widely prescribed, often in patients for whom there is no evidence that they will be of benefit. One of the greatest forces in nature being inertia, when therapies are started,

---

[vii]A great resource for those interested in studying and improving the utilization of respiratory care is the American Association for Respiratory Care (www.aarc.org). They have an extensive bibliography related to the use of therapist driven protocols to improve utilization as well as lots of other tools to help you. While a lot of their resources are available to the public, some of the best are accessible only to AARC members. If you are not a member, shame on you because you are (1) limiting your effectiveness by not having all the tools available to you, (2) not supporting your professional field, and (3) obviously a dufus. No other single event or organization has done more to advance the quality of respiratory care and the professional lives of respiratory therapists than the AARC. Join now.

they tend to continue. Thus even when therapies are clearly of no benefit to patients, we continue to dutifully and precisely administer them. This phenomenon is caused, in part, by the *interventionist* culture of our clinicians (nurses, doctors, and RTs). When patients come under our care, we have to do *something*. Even though what we are doing doesn't appear to be having any benefit, we continue, comforted (often more so than the patients) in the fact that at least we are trying to do *something*.

By building clinical quality metrics around the utilization of appropriate and effective treatments, you will do a great deal to ensure and improve the quality of clinical care. What follows is a series of actual metrics of department performance taken from my own experience. I used all of these metrics at one time or another. Figure 4-1 is an example of a metric of the utilization of bronchodilators.[13] This figure describes the results of our study of the appropriateness of bronchodilator administration.

We simply sent out experienced RTs and asked them to give a treatment and then evaluate whether they thought the treatment was appropriate (should have been given to begin with) or effective (resulted in any apparent patient improvement). These data caused quite a stir when I presented them at the medical executive committee. It was one of the high points of my career at that time. Of course, that was during my "The Who period" when I was principally fueled by coffee, conflict, and continuous process improvement. These were arguably somewhat fluffy data because I did not define in the study what "appropriateness" and "effectiveness" criteria were in any detail. I simply left it to the judgment of the clinicians, who in this case were clinical supervisors, all of whom were skilled and experienced pediatric respiratory therapists (average experience was eight years).

Utilization of chest physiotherapy is also a useful metric. I list here two different methods of displaying utilization. In the first, Figure 4-2, the percentage of inappropriate chest physiotherapy that was ordered is compared to the amount of chest physiotherapy actually administered before and after the initiation of a protocol to guide the administration of the therapy.

You can see that physicians continued to order lots of inappropriate chest physiotherapy, but because of the wonderful intervention of the RTs, armed with a good CPT protocol, the percentage of the actual inappropriate treatments significantly dropped and remained low. We then wondered about the effect of this protocol on the total number of CPT treatments given. This is an example of data that needed to be indexed. If total treatments given had dropped, it

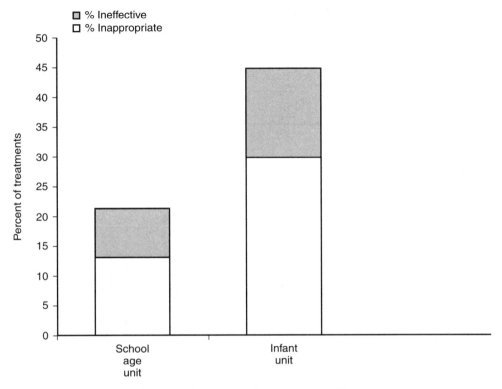

Figure 4-1. Measure of Appropriate Utilization of Bronchodilators
A typical utilization measure; the percent of all aerosolized bronchodilator treatments given that were deemed inappropriate or ineffective. In this case inappropriate indicates that the treatments probably never should have been given to begin with. Ineffective describes treatments that may have been indicated, but did not have the desired effect, i.e., relief of symptoms. This study was in pediatrics, thus the age of the patients.

might have been because we just had a slowdown in the number of patients. So we indexed total treatments to total patient days, which is shown in Figure 4-3.

As you can see, the protocol had a profound effect. We estimated that it reduced our labor expense by about $75,000 per year (in 1994 dollars).[14]

Another example of utilization measures is the utilization of arterial blood gases, which are notoriously over utilized (Figure 4-4).

I know of one pediatric hospital that did about 15 blood gases per ventilated patient per day in their PICU while another hospital did about four per day in their PICU. Both units had similar populations. You can see that resource consumption was very different in these two units. This is a classic

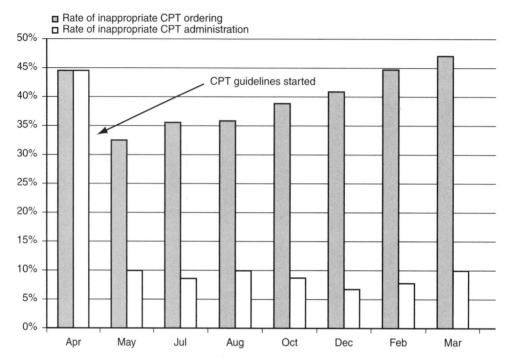

Figure 4-2. Impact of CPT Guidelines
Another measure of utilization: the percent of chest physiotherapy treatment ordered and given that were "inappropriate." Inappropriate in this case refers to whether or not the use of CPT complied with a therapist-driven protocol for CPT. Note that the rate at which physicians wrote inappropriate orders for CPT didn't really change. What changed was the intervention of RTs using a therapist-driven protocol that significantly reduced the rate of inappropriate administration. Changing physician behavior can be quite challenging.

example of unwarranted variation. I don't know what the right frequency of blood gases per ventilator day should be, but I know that differences of this magnitude demonstrate systems that are not well controlled. And blood gases are not benign. There are risks associated with both percutaneous and line drawn blood gas sampling. The data shown in Figure 4-4 were from an intensive care unit where ventilator care was being standardized over time and postoperative care process models were put into place. There was clearly something going on because you can see that there was a large and sustained decrease in the mean utilization of blood gases.

The incidence of lower respiratory tract infections (LRIs) has long been thought to be affected by the quality of hand hygiene and certain respiratory care practices, notably the frequency at which ventilator circuits are changed.

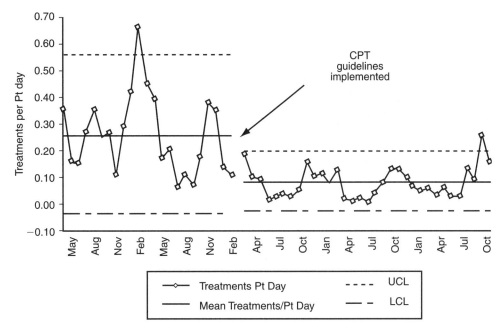

Figure 4-3. Measures of TDP Effectiveness in the Infant Med/Surg Unit
A measure of the effectiveness of a therapist-driven protocol (TDP), in this case for the administration of CPT. There were very large and sustained decreases in the number of treatments given. This form of chart is called a process control chart, and is a typical method of demonstrating whether a process has changed. UCL and LCL refer to upper and lower control limits. This are calculated limits of two standard deviations above and below the mean. The presumption is that in a normal system, 95% of data points will fall between the UCL and LCL.

We used this metric to test whether changes in our clinical practice had any effect on LRIs. Specifically we doubted that there was any relationship between the frequency of changing ventilator circuits and the incidence of LRIs. Figure 4-5 demonstrates that as we decreased the frequency at which we changed ventilator circuits from every 48 hours to weekly, there was no change in the LRI rates.[15]

Another example of a utilization metric as a clinical quality measure is the use of continuous pulse oximeters. Over use of continuous oximetry, especially outside the intensive care units, has many potentially undesirable effects. These include unnecessary costs, alarm desensitization, unnecessary blood gases, and possibly delayed discharge.[16] We wrote a clinical protocol for optimizing (reducing) the utilization of continuous pulse oximeters.[17]

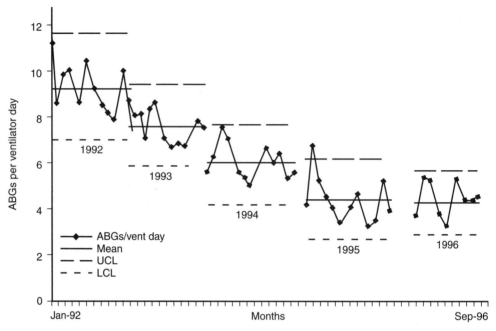

Figure 4-4. Utilization Measure of ABGs

The utilization of arterial blood gases (ABGs). This graph is another example of a process control chart. In this case, it is clear the process has been changing significantly each year for a period of several years. While not the direct result of a specific protocol, it was attributed to an increased awareness by physicians and RTs of the cost of care. Notice that the average number of ABGs for each month is indexed to the number of ventilator days. This removes the possibility that these reductions in blood gases are because of a reduction in ventilator days. Also note that the upper and lower control limits are recalculated for each subsequent year.

Figure 4-6 describes the effects of our protocol by comparing the same three month period between three different years.

Interestingly, this improvement in utilization was not sustained. It had originally been made possible when the respiratory therapists applied the protocol to all oximetry orders. Eventually the nurses took over this responsibility, and the gains realized early with the protocol were lost. The nurses, particularly nursing leadership, were not particularly engaged in administering the protocol. This is not to be construed as a criticism of the nurses. Little leadership was exhibited about this by the middle level nursing managers and so the staff nurses never got engaged in this process.

Manual ventilation of patients with handheld resuscitators is a frequently done procedure, especially in intensive care units. Yet not much is done about

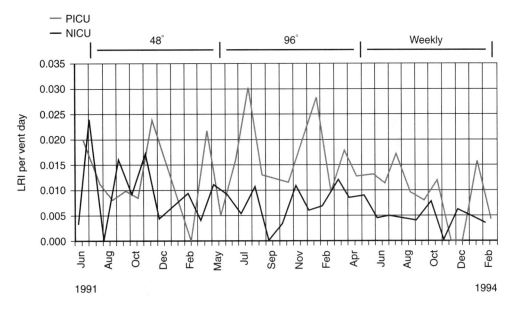

Figure 4-5. Ventilator Circuit Changing Frequency

Traditionally, ventilator circuits were changed every day. Slowly, this practice migrated to every other day. We showed that over a period of years, the frequency of ventilator circuit change did not appear to have any effect on the rate of lower respiratory tract infection (LRI). These LRIs are also a measure (at least indirectly) of RT quality of care. So this kind of comparison was particularly useful. (Salyer JW. The effect of 7 day circuit changes on lower respiratory tract infection rates in the NICU and PICU. *Respir Care* 1994;39:1109).

ensuring the competency of nurses and therapists who often do this procedure. Manual ventilation can be potentially risky because over distention of the lung can cause ventilator induced lung injury and air leak, especially in children. We set out to test the consistency of ventilation among and between different disciplines using different styles of resuscitators. Figure 4-7 shows the results of our study and was an important finding that led us to change our practice, doing away with flow-inflating bags because they produced much more variable ventilation.[18–19]

Serendipitously, we demonstrated that the quality of manual ventilation was better when done by RTs than when done by nurses. This would be a relatively simple ongoing measure of RT clinical quality. You could simply establish a minimum required manual ventilation consistency that you required of all staff members as a yearly competency.

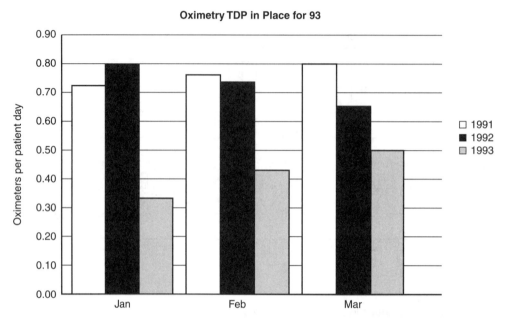

Figure 4-6. Utilization Measures: Oximetry
The Utilization of Continuous Pulse Oximetry. This chart demonstrates the effect of the implementation of a TDP on pulse oximeters in use. They are indexed to patient days and you will see that after the implementation in 1993, the utilization dropped significantly. (Salyer JW, Burton K, Keenan J. The effect of guidelines for the use of continuous pulse oximetry in a pediatric population. *Respir Care* 1994;39:1099).

Another important clinical function for RTs is patient education, the most notable of which is teaching asthma patients and their families to better manage their disease. It has been shown that asthma education can reduce the severity and frequency of attacks by helping patients do a better job at preventing attacks and identifying attacks earlier. We set out to test this and showed (Figure 4-8) that our asthma education program appeared to produce a very large reduction in hospital admissions and emergency room visits.

This study was done on 129 asthma inpatients who had asthma education compared to admitted asthmatics who did not have an educational intervention. This huge reduction in admission rates would have equated to a reduction in charges of approximately $333 thousand if applied to all admitted asthmatics for a year.

Business operations are often overlooked when metrics are developed. I have consistently insisted that we measure the accuracy of our billing operations.[20] Billing metrics need to touch every clinician, and in fact we typically did a sufficient amount of audits to ensure that we measured the accuracy of

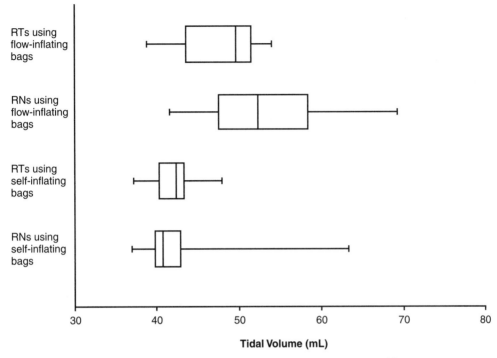

Figure 4-7. Distribution of Tidal Volume for Neonatal Patients Sorted by Bag Type and Discipline

The technical quality of the RTs is demonstrated in the chart of the distribution of tidal volumes between nurses and RTs when using two different styles of bags. Careful control and limitation of tidal volume delivered to neonates is a very important clinical and patient safety issue. The study was conducted to test the variability in tidal volumes between bag styles, but serendipitously revealed the difference in technical quality between disciplines. (Keenan J, Salyer JW, Ashby T, Withers J, Bee N. Ventilation variability using self-inflating and nonself-inflating resuscitation bags in a neonatal lung model. *Respir Care.* 1999;44:1253).

every clinician's billing. A sample of some results I once obtained is described in Figure 4-9.

Another example of business operations metrics is compliance with charting standards. Of course, charting quality is a surrogate for the quality of clinical care, but it is also a measure of the organizational risk with regard to documenting billed procedures. If your charting quality is poor you might not be able to prove that billed procedures were done. This is serious business, and unless you like embarrassment and lawsuits and lawyers and such, you might want to be sure that department billing is being clearly documented in the medical record. An example of this metric can be seen in Figure 4-10.

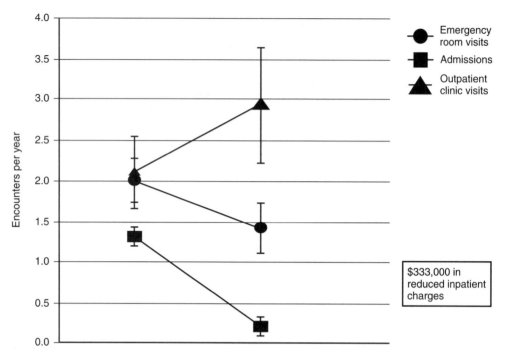

Figure 4-8. Effect of Asthma Education Program on Hospital Admissions and Emergency Room Visits

Measuring the impact of an asthma education program. The figure represents before and after rates of hospital admission, emergency room visits, and clinic visits of a group of 129 patients who entered the asthma education program at Heavenly Gates Children's Hospital. These data were very impressive as they showed that what happened was exactly what we wanted, i.e., less use of costly hospital and emergency room facilities and more use of the clinic. The intervention being tested was a very rigorous 2-hour asthma training program for patients and families, administered one-on-one by a respiratory therapist. Although the name of the hospital may sound goofy and whimsical, these are real data, which I compiled myself.

MEASURING PATIENT SAFETY

To discuss the measurement of patient safety we must first describe and define the phenomenon that has created the "patient safety movement." It is rare for a single publication to change the world. But that is what happened to the hospital world in 2000 when the Institute of Medicine published its exposé on the lamentable state of patient safety in health care, entitled *To Err Is Human: Building a Safer Health System*.[21] In this work, the authors claimed that as many as 100,000 Americans die each year from

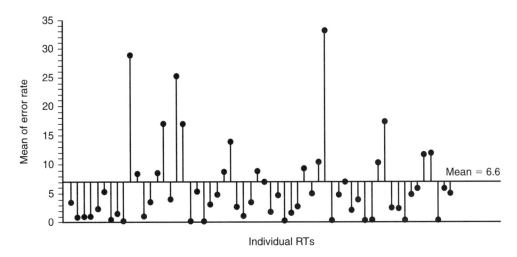

Figure 4-9. Billing Error Rates for all RTs Over a 1-Year Period
A measure of business operations: the accuracy of RT billing. Note that lots of RT managed to have perfect billing. This study was constructed so that the RTs were each audited repeatedly so that there was a sufficient amount of data on each staff member to make a fair judgment. The RTs who had high billing errors were counseled into a new awareness that their continued employment would depend greatly on improving their billing accuracy.

preventable medical errors in U.S. hospitals. Other authors have estimated that there are *225,000 deaths per year* in U.S. hospitals from iatrogenic causes.[22] In pediatric patients alone it is estimated that medical errors cost the system over $1 billion per year.[23] There also appears to be evidence that as many as 20–30% of patients get contraindicated care.[24] Thus was born the patient safety movement, which seems to have evolved a de facto definition: our corporate attempts to minimize mistakes and avoid harming or killing patients.

The scope of the problem becomes more easily understood when you consider the following list of causes of death per year in the United States:

- Motor vehicle deaths—44,000
- Breast cancer deaths—43,000
- AIDS deaths—17,000
- Murders—13,000
- Adverse drug deaths—7,000
- Total workplace deaths—6,000

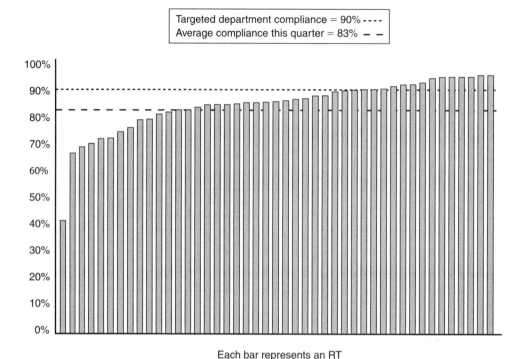

Each bar represents an RT

Figure 4-10. Individual and Departmental Compliance with Charting Standards
A measure of the quality of charting. Each department should have charting standards that, if complied with, will improve the quality of care and reduce organizational risk. This chart shows individual compliance with these standards and total departmental compliance. We do repeated audits over time so that we ensure that each staff member has a sufficient number of audits to be truly representative of the quality of their charting.

After the book was published, hospitals scrambled to respond. There was the initial round of denials and protestations. *Immutable Truth #18: The cycle of fear rules.* The cycle of fear has a profound influence on the governance of human affairs. It is innervated when its hapless victims are presented with unhappy news about shortcomings related to their performance (or the performance of their organizations). Figure 4-11 shows the basic functional structure of the cycle of fear.

Note that the cycle starts with fear. We have tremendous fear when things go wrong—fear of recrimination, blame, punishment, and having to work late. One of the visceral reactions caused by fear is denial. We deny the truth of the message. We try filtering the data, questioning its authenticity. Later,

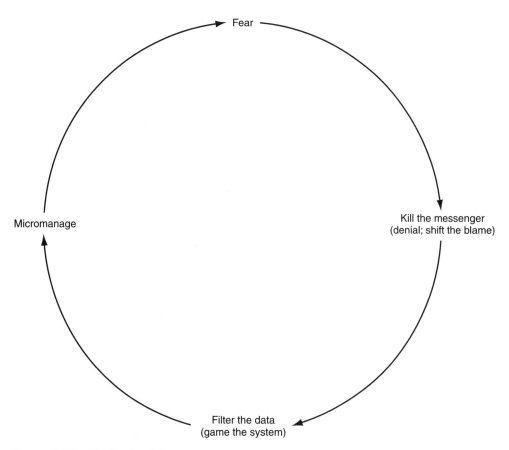

Figure 4-11. The Cycle of Fear
A ubiquitous governing law of nature that can be observed when people find out maybe things they are involved in or responsible for, aren't going so well—the meconium has hit the fan.

we move on to killing the messenger. We doubt the credibility of not only what is being said, but of who is saying it. Finally, we may move into micromanagement, for example trying hard to control everything. Fear causes distrust, so we can end up not trusting anyone, and we can begin to feel like we have to do it all to save ourselves. The descent caused by the cycle of fear can be steep and lead you to the edge of the abyss (a place I have been to so many times, all the bartenders know me by name). We can become paralyzed by the fear that may overcome us when we learn we have screwed up, when our plans have gone awry. As hard as it is to do, true leadership includes the ability to accept the imperfections of your leadership and embrace your mistakes and learn from them.[viii] Real learning often comes from pain. And the pain of facing our mistakes and shortcomings can often lead us to grow and develop and be more than we thought we could be.

The initial reaction of the healthcare industry to the claim that 100,000 Americans were being killed per year in hospitals was (in some places) less than admirable. There was a lot of denial and filtering of the data. Those of us who had done any work at all in measuring unwarranted variability in healthcare systems knew that the Institute of Medicine's estimate was probably low because it was only based on studies of what was in the medical record. Shocking as it might sound, sometimes bad things that happen to patients do not get put in the medical record.

But things have steadily improved. We have developed an entire field of endeavor called the patient safety movement. This function within the hospital helps us achieve the very first goal of the healthcare system, *primum non nocere* (Latin for "first, do no harm"). We may not be able to help patients, but we hope to the almighty that we don't harm them. Many hospitals now have patient safety officers, and some have patient safety departments. But the progress is slow, and many of the well known things hospitals could do to improve patient safety have not yet been widely implemented.[25]

In keeping with the principle that you cannot manage what you do not measure, most hospitals are working hard to build systems to measure patient safety as an initial and important foundation to building a safer system. But this is challenging. How do you measure the frequency of mistakes? How do you index mistake frequency? How can mistakes be classified? Are all our mistakes reported or captured by our error measurement systems? Most hospitals have systems for measuring errors that rely almost entirely on voluntary reporting of mistakes by the staff. Of course, many staff members do not feel safe in reporting errors due to fear of recrimination, punishment, loss of employment, and litigation. Forward thinking organizations are working hard to develop a blame-free culture in which clinicians are encouraged to report their mistakes so that the organization and the individual can learn from errors.

There is an old school and a new school regarding medical errors. The old school (which I was taught) says that "good clinicians" do not make serious mistakes. Of course this is ridiculous when you think carefully about it. Everyone makes mistakes with the exception, perhaps, of Jesus and your

---

[viii]While owning mistakes in the business, academic, personal, and professional worlds is quite admirable, the rules are different in politics where your enemies use your admission of mistakes as a cudgel to beat you to death with. While this may happen occasionally in business, it is ubiquitous in politics.

wife. But I believed it. Or at least I hoped it. But I soon learned otherwise. My mistakes as a clinician are legion. On the advice of my attorney (one A. Lewis Dewitt), I am declining to comment any further on this particular topic.

The folly of punishing staff members who make mistakes becomes apparent with the realization that all humans make mistakes. Eventually everyone in safety critical jobs like operating life support equipment or an aircraft will make a serious error. If you fire them for this, eventually everyone will be fired. Well probably not everyone because many grave errors are not reported and are in fact hidden.

As our industry has grown in stature, maturity, and wisdom, we are beginning to embrace the new school: *good clinicians report and learn from their mistakes.* But as a director–manager, you will eventually be faced with the temptation of slipping into the old school. When one of your staff members makes a serious mistake that injures or even contributes to the death of a patient, you will be tempted to punish him or her. Suspension, termination, reassignment, or strangulation will enter your mind. It takes some serious discipline to keep from initially over reacting this way. There are things you can do to help calm yourself. I prescribe one hour of listening to Diana Krall while gazing at Salvador Dali's *Dematerialization Near the Nose of Nero* and a glass (or two) of a respectably priced pinot noir.

Instead of the classical reaction, you have to dispassionately evaluate every mistake and analyze it from a systems perspective. The truth is that most mistakes in a complex system like healthcare delivery have multifactorial causes. They are rarely caused simply by someone screwing up, although this obviously does happen sometimes. Errors are often contributed to by the design of the healthcare systems people are working in. Some classic examples are overwork, sleep deprivation, and under staffing, lack of equipment standardization, inadequate policy development, poor patient monitoring, and poor alarm management. These can contribute to staff members making errors that are not entirely caused by a lapse or slip by the staff member. If you work too many hours too many days in a row, your judgment can become dulled. This phenomenon is well known in industries like the airlines and the railroad system. Sleep deprivation and disruption are also known to diminish cognitive and physical skills. And of course there is now a well known inverse relationship between inadequate staffing and the quality of care.[26–29] The interested reader who wants to dig deeply into the science of studying human errors is directed to the work of Lucian Leape[30] and James Reason.[31–32] Table 4-8 lists some common systemic causes of errors in respiratory care practice.

The measurement of patient safety is a very nascent field. Incident reporting systems are the first stop for many hospitals looking for a way to measure patient safety. Incident reporting systems are data repositories of self-reported errors or adverse events that are gathered and kept by the hospital. The organization uses the information for learning (hopefully) by doing deep analytical work around what causes these mistakes and what can be done to prevent them. But using the number or type of incident reports as a measure of patient safety can be a risky business. First, such systems rely on voluntary self-reporting of mistakes, or they rely on staff being willing to report others' mistakes. Both of these phenomena can be unreliable ways to get quantitative data on the number and types of errors. There is a strong reluctance of some staff members to report on others' mistakes. And of course there is an even stronger reluctance to rat ourselves out.

Many hospitals now use a system that conducts serious event reviews when mistakes are made. These are supposed to be meetings of all the disciplines involved in the care of a patient when an error occurred. They are typically run by a neutral party and are intended to be safe (e.g., no personal attacks or emotional outbursts will be permitted). They use root cause analysis techniques to try to determine what, if any, systemic design flaws may have contributed to this error. The idea is to learn not to judge, to learn why mistakes happened, and to build additional safety barriers into the healthcare systems. This requires a tacit admission on the part of the hospital that people lose it from time to time. They screw up. As pointed out earlier, if we tended to fire everyone who ever screwed up in a hospital, soon we would have few employees left.

Case Study 10: What, me worry?!?!

The baby on ECMO was not doing well at all. It was 0230 at Taco Bellevue Hospital, and the kid was going downhill. The attending physician, the nurse, the charge nurse, and two respiratory therapists were in the room. Hugh G. Lunger, RRT was the ECMO specialist, and he was feeling pretty stressed out. The patient was on a high frequency oscillator, had eight syringe pumps mounted on poles at the bedside, was on a pulse oximeter, cardiac monitor, end-tidal CO_2 monitor, and the ECMO pump. The room was crowded with machines, tubing, cables, IV poles, sensors, probes, chairs, tables, stands, people, parents, and of course, the patient. Hugh was trying to straighten up the area when he found an empty heparin syringe sitting on the ECMO pump. He got a sick feeling in his stomach because he didn't remember giving a dose of heparin anytime recently. With a sinking realization, he concluded that

he must have went to grab a saline flush syringe and inadvertently gave a bolus of heparin. He looked around to see if anyone had noticed. Apparently no
one had. For a few moments he thought about throwing out the syringe and
not telling anyone. He just couldn't bring himself to do it. He told the patient's
nurse and the attending physician about his mistake. Blood was drawn for
laboratory studies, which revealed very prolonged clotting times, which con-
firmed that too much heparin had been given. The patient had some bleeding
in the brain and some pulmonary hemorrhaging, but both of these had started
before Hugh had made his error. He filled out an incident report and wondered
what would happen to him. He went home and drank heavily.

The next day the RT department director looked up Hugh and asked
him how he was feeling about the incident and told him that there would be
a "serious event review" the next day. "Don't worry," he said, "we are just
going to explore what happened, why it happened, and what we can do to
prevent such an error in the future. I will be there and no one is going to beat
up on you, I promise." Hugh had a pretty restless night, resuming his heavy
drinking.

At the serious event review the following day, Hugh showed up and simply
recounted what happened. After much deliberation, it was learned that
the flush syringes and the heparin syringes were the same size and color.
They had labels on them that were the same size and color. You had to read
some pretty small print on the label to discern which syringe was which. They
further discovered that the syringes were arranged near one another in the
ECMO specialists' work space. It was decided that the error, while regrettable,
was probably bound to be made by someone eventually given the complicated
layout of the ECMO work space and the visual similarity between the different
medication syringes. The group decided to color code all heparin syringes
with a piece of pink tape wrapped around the barrel of the syringe.

After the meeting, Hugh took the director aside and said, "I was afraid you
were going to fire me."

"Why in the world would I want to do that? I just spent a lot of time and effort training you in how not to make medication errors. Now, had you recklessly
violated some known policy and been cavalier about this, I might have had a different opinion," replied the director as he headed out the door to his fifth meeting of the day. Hugh went home and poured the rest of his Jack Daniel's down
the drain.

Difficult as it is, there are things that you can and should measure with
regard to patient safety. You should go through your policy manual, identify the
policies and procedures that relate to patient safety, and set out to measure the

Table 4-8. Some Common Systemic Causes of Errors in the Delivery of Health Care

Insufficient equipment standardization	Too many different types of ventilators, monitors, ECMO machines, or any of a wide variety of other devices make it more difficult to train the staff and more difficult to maintain technical proficiency.
Poor equipment maintenance	Equipment that is not properly calibrated or maintained may not display accurate clinical measurements or may not deliver the therapeutic intervention as desired.
Inadequate training	This has repeatedly been shown to be a common cause of medical errors, including preventable ventilator related deaths.
Not enough equipment or supplies	An example might be an insufficient number of end-tidal CO_2 monitors to monitor all ventilated patients or not enough pulse oximeters or transcutaneous monitors.
Inadequate staffing	No one has yet scientifically established what safe levels of staffing are. But the nursing literature is full of examples of a relationship between poor staffing and unhappy outcomes of care.
Poorly designed work space	If the work space is cluttered and visually confusing, it might make the clinicians prone to slips or mishaps, for example grabbing the wrong medication or hooking up the tubing in the wrong way.
Incomplete or poor policy development	Alarm management is a great example. Exhaled minute alarms are available on the latest generation of ventilators, but my experience is that they are not often set properly. But if done so, they could alert the clinicians to large changes in minute ventilation. Precise requirements for safe alarm settings need to be described in policies. Another example is the number of people required at the bedside for risky procedures

Table 4-8. Some Common Systemic Causes of Errors in the Delivery of Health Care *(Continued)*

	like endotracheal tube retaping or changing tracheostomy tubes.
Slack enforcement of policies	Marvelously crafted policies bear little fruit if they are not enforced. To do this you must periodically measure the compliance of your staff with your policies.
Lack of competency assessment	Staff members can be put through all sorts of training, but this does not ensure that they have developed the skills they need. Skills (or competency) assessment is the only way to ensure this. Staff members should have to actually demonstrate important skills, either at the bedside or in a lab setting, during initial orientation and periodically thereafter.
Confusing labeling	One of my clinicians once brought me two virtually identically packaged drugs. They came in the same size and color container with the same size and color label. There was one slight difference: One was a tenfold stronger concentration than the other. But you had to read some pretty fine print to see this. Interestingly, these drugs were on the code cart and thus would be used under the most hectic and stressful conditions. We asked the manufacturer to make the labels different colors and the print larger. They were glad to help us out.
Jury rigging	Resist the temptation. Don't do it if at all possible. It is a recipe for disaster. The most famous examples are gas cylinder regulators that have had the pins knocked off to allow them to be put on gas cylinders for which they were not designed or labeled. Another is the Rube Goldberg setups I have seen for the administration of

(Continues)

Table 4-8. Some Common Systemic Causes of Errors in the Delivery of Health Care *(Continued)*

Jury rigging	helium into ventilator circuits for which they were not designed.
Poor communication	This is one of the most common threads seen in many disastrous clinical errors that I know about. Vital information was not passed on between shifts or between disciplines.

degree to which your staff are complying with these. A great example is the use of alarms on life support equipment. In this case, I refer to mechanical ventilators and patient monitoring systems. It is well known that bad management of alarms contributes to poor patient care, and in fact The Joint Commission reports that 80% of preventable ventilator related deaths are caused, all or in part, by mismanagement or malfunction of alarms. So your policies should describe pretty precisely how and when all alarms are to be set and used. Then you can simply do random, periodic audits of charting to see if alarm use as charted is in accordance with these policies. You can also do real time observational audits, for example have someone go from ventilator to ventilator and from monitor to monitor and measure the degree to which the ventilator and monitor alarms are set according to policy. This assumes that your policies have been designed to maximize patient safety as opposed to staff convenience.

Another good measure of patient safety is artificial airway security. How well are endotracheal tubes and tracheostomy tubes secured? Are they taped and tied properly? Are the taping and tying jobs performed according to the policy schedule? These can be audited by direct observation and/or through retrospective chart review. Of course the best measure here is rates of accidental extubation and/or tracheostomy tube dislodgement. Figure 4-12 shows accidental extubation (AE) data from an NICU. The data are summarized by quarter and indexed to ventilator days.

You can both track your own data and compare it to some national data. In this case the hospital in question belonged to a clinical benchmarking consortium that had data from nine other NICUs. The AE rate of 1.25 per 100 ventilator days is the average of all the reporting hospitals for all the data reported over five calendar quarters. But while averaging data sometimes makes it easier to display and understand, it can hide underlying

	NICU vent days	NICU AEs	NICU AEs per 100 vent days
3rd Quarter 2003	665	4	0.60
4th Quarter 2003	393	3	0.76
1st Quarter 2004	760	1	0.13
2nd Quarter 2004	781	0	0.00
3rd Quarter 2004	562	5	0.89
4th Quarter 2004	699	1	0.14
1st Quarter 2005	951	1	0.11
2nd Quarter 2005	767	4	0.52
		Mean	0.39

NICU AEs per 100 vent days
Benchmark NICU mean = 1.25 AEs/100 ventilator days

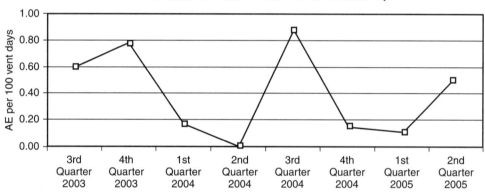

Figure 4-12. Accidental Extubation (AE) Data
Typical display of safety data. In this case rates of accidental extubation, which are indexed per 100 ventilator days. The benchmark in this case is the average AE rate for 14 reporting hospitals in a commercially available benchmarking consortium.

orders of variation. Figure 4-13 is the data from these 10 NICUs from which the mean of 1.25 was generated. Note the amount of variation between hospitals and the amount of variation within the hospital from quarter to quarter.

Particularly when evaluating clinical data you must remember that variation happens and often has natural and thus uncontrollable causes. More on this in a moment. The take home message is to avoid over reacting to individual data points, or even quarters, where data might look bad, especially in data as highly variable as accidental extubation data.

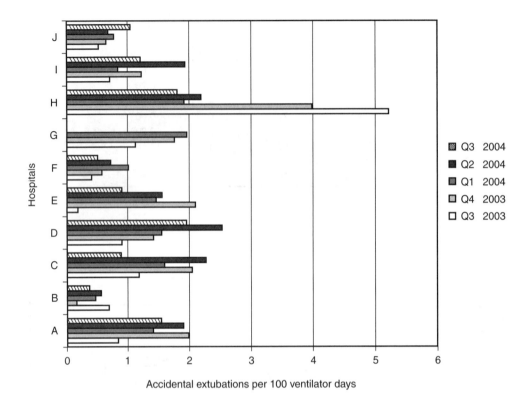

Figure 4-13. Neonatal Accidental Extubation Comparative Data from 10 Hospitals
Comparative data on neonatal accidental extubations. I have blinded the hospitals' names. These types of data normally have to be purchased via contract with a benchmarking company. In this case, these data are used with permission from Medical Management Planning, Inc., Los Angeles, CA.

PROCESS CONTROL CHARTS

When trying to measure the quality of your department's operations, you will eventually be forced to render a judgment. By this I mean you will look at some of your data and try to figure out whether it is good or bad. Benchmarking helps tremendously because you will have data from other departments or hospitals to help you make such judgments. But more often than not, you do not have external data to use to evaluate the quality of your own operation. There is a terrible lack of clinical and safety data on the national level to help you judge the quality of your operation. This is slowly changing, but there is a very long way to go until we have reliable data sufficiently detailed and comparable to help you judge the quality of your operation. Thus managers are forced to track their own data over time. At least this tells you if the quality of your operation is changing. But how much is it changing? Are the changes meaningful? Or are they just the result of normal variation like we see in our accidental extubation example above? Process control charts can help you answer these questions.[33] Process control charts are based on the mean and standard deviation of data from a given system. The assumption is that all systems have variation, but this variation occurs within inherent limits, which are described by combinations of the mean and standard deviation of the data from the system. All such charts have three basic components:

1. A centerline that is the mean of all data plotted
2. Upper and lower control limits that describe the inherent limits of normal variation in a system
3. Actual data plotted over time from the system being measured

The point of the control chart is to allow you to visually identify trends or data points that may indicate your system is operating outside the normal inherent limits. The statistical theory behind the process control chart indicates that about 95% of all data points should fall within two standard deviations above and below the centerline of the data. Thus the upper and lower control limits are calculated as follows:

$$\text{Upper Control Limit (UCL)} = M + 2 \times SD$$
$$\text{Lower Control Limit (LCL)} = M - 2 \times SD$$

where

$$M = \text{mean of all data plotted}$$

$$SD = \text{standard deviation of all data plotted}$$

When the chart is developed, which can very easily be done in any spreadsheet program, you should evaluate the data and look for any of the following findings that might indicate your data are outside the normal range of variation.

- One data point falling outside the control limits
- Six or more points in a row steadily increasing or decreasing
- Eight or more points in a row on one side of the centerline

Any of these can be indicative of concern that something other than natural causes of variation are occurring in the system you are measuring. A classic example is the plotting of quality control data from a blood gas laboratory. The laboratory staff will put a liquid with a known partial pressure of oxygen into the blood gas analyzer, in this case 100 mmHg. But the instrument is very unlikely to read exactly 100 mmHg. Instead it might read 99 mmHg. Repeat samples might read 112, 110, 92, 98, and so on. This is normal variation in the performance of a PO_2 electrode in a blood gas instrument. Over time, enough of the quality control data points are gathered to construct a process control chart. Then when regular quality control samples are run in the lab, they can be plotted on the process control chart. The occurrence of any of the findings listed above might alert the staff member who is running the blood gas instrument that the performance of the PO_2 electrode is outside the acceptable limits of inherent variation.

Figures 4-3 and 4-4 are both real life examples of process control charts. In both cases, the upper and lower control limits were calculated for different periods described on the charts. These periods correspond to interventions that were designed to improve the performance of the systems. In the case of utilization of chest physiotherapy, a clinical protocol was put into place, and you can see that the variation in the underlying system decreased considerably. In the case of the utilization of blood gases, we divided the data into calendar years for the sake of convenience. You can see that both control charts clearly indicate that the measurements of these clinical processes were clearly changing, indicating changes in the underlying processes. Fortunately, all these changes were desirable and indeed were the result of intentional interventions. Both of these charts were constructed using the standard charting functions in a spreadsheet program. There are also specialized statistical programs you can buy that produce process control charts.

REFERENCES

1. Hogberg D. Insurance Fraud. Let's not base policy on inflated statistics. *National Review Online.* June 15, 2004. http://www.nationalreview.com/comment/hogberg200406150914.asp.
2. Thomas JW, Longo DR. Application of severity measurement systems for hospital quality measurement. *Hosp Health Serv Adm.* Summer 1990;35(2):221–243.
3. Iezzoni LI. Assessing quality using administrative data. *Ann Intern Med.* October 15, 1997;127(8 Pt 2):666–674.
4. Hughes JS, Iezzoni LI, Daley J, Greenberg L. How severity measures rate hospitalized patients. *J Gen Intern Med.* May 1996;11(5):303–311.
5. Hariharan S, Zbar A. Risk scoring in perioperative and surgical intensive care patients: a review. *Curr Surg.* May-June 2006;63(3):226–236.
6. Herridge MS. Prognostication and intensive care unit outcome: the evolving role of scoring systems. *Cin Chest Med.* December 2003;24(4):751–762.

7. Apolone G. The state of research on multipurpose severity of illness scoring systems: are we on target? *Intensive Care Med.* December 2000;26(12):1727–1729.

8. Marik PE, Varon J. Severity scoring and outcome assessment. Computerized predictive models and scoring systems. *Crit Care Clin.* July 1999;15(3):633–646.

9. Orchard C. Measuring the effects of case mix on outcomes. *J Eval Clin Pract.* May 1996;2(2):111–121.

10. Iezzoni L, ed. *Risk Adjustment for Measuring Healthcare Outcomes.* Third edition. Health Administration Press; 2003.

11. Spiro DM, Tay KY, Arnold DH, Dziura JD, Baker MD, Shapiro ED. Wait-and-see prescription for the treatment of acute otitis media: a randomized controlled trial. *JAMA.* September 13, 2006;296(10):1235–1241.

12. Rosenfeld RM. Natural history of untreated otitis media. *Laryngoscope.* 2003;113:1645–1657.

13. Salyer JW, Lynch JL, Witte M. Preliminary report on the appropriateness of aerosol therapy in a pediatric population. *Respir Care.* 1992;37:1328.

14. Salyer JW, Burton KK, Poll K. Improving the utilization of CPT in a pediatric population. *Respir Care.* 1995;40:1160.

15. Salyer JW. The effect of 7 day circuit changes on lower respiratory tract infection rates in the NICU and PICU. *Respir Care.* 1994;39:1109.

16. Salyer JW. Neonatal and pediatric pulse oximetry. *Respir Care.* 2003;48(4):386–396.

17. Salyer JW, Burton K, Keenan J. The effect of guidelines for the use of continuous pulse oximetry in a pediatric population. *Respir Care.* 1994;39:1099.

18. Keenan J, Salyer JW, Ashby T, Withers J, Bee N. Manual ventilation technique variability in a pediatric lung model. *Respir Care.* 1999;44:1252.

19. Keenan J, Salyer JW, Ashby T, Withers J, Bee N. Ventilation variability using self-inflating and nonself-inflating resuscitation bags in a neonatal lung model. *Respir Care.* 1999;44:1253.

20. Salyer JW. Improving the accuracy of a respiratory care billing system. *Advance for Respiratory Care Managers.* 1993;3(1):44–47.

21. Kohn LT, Corrigan JM, Donaldson MS, eds. Committee on Quality of Health Care in America, Institute of Medicine. *To Err Is Human: Building a Safer Health System.* National Academies Press; 2000.

22. Starfield B. Is U.S. healthcare really the best in the world? *JAMA.* 2000;284(4);483–485.

23. Miller MR, Zhan C. Pediatric patient safety in hospitals: a national picture in 2000. *Pediatrics.* 2004;113:1741–1746.

24. Schuster M, McGlynn E. How good is the quality of health care in the United States? *Milbank Q.* 1998;76:517–563.

25. Longo DR, Hewett JE, Ge B, Schubert S. The long road to patient safety: a status report on patient safety systems. *JAMA.* 2005;294(22):2858–2865.

26. Cimiotti JP, Haas J, Saiman L, Larson EL. Impact of staffing on bloodstream infections in the neonatal intensive care unit. *Arch Pediatr Adolesc Med.* August 2006;160(8):832–836.

27. Tucker J, UK Neonatal Staffing Study Group. Patient volume, staffing, and workload in relation to risk-adjusted outcomes in a random stratified sample of UK neonatal intensive care units: a prospective evaluation. *Lancet.* 2002;359:99–107.

28. Bostick JE, Rantz MJ, Flesner MK, Riggs CJ. Systematic review of studies of staffing and quality in nursing homes. *J Am Med Dir Assoc.* 2006;7(6):366–376.

29. Seago JA, Williamson A, Atwood C. Longitudinal analyses of nurse staffing and patient outcomes: more about failure to rescue. *J Nurse Adm.* 2006;36(1):13–21.

30. Leape LL. A systems analysis approach to medical error. *J Eval Clin Pract.* 1997;3(3):213–222.

31. Reason JT. *Managing the Risks of Organizational Accidents.* Burlington, VT: Ashgate Publishing; 1997.

32. Reason JT. *Human Error.* New York, NY: Cambridge University Press; 1990.

33. Chamberlin WH, Lane KA, Kennedy JN, Bradley SD, Rice CL. Monitoring intensive care unit performance using statistical quality control charts. *Int J Clin Monit Comput.* 1993;10(3):155–161.

CHAPTER 5

Staffing Systems

It is never as bad as you think it is.

It is never as good as you think it is.

Few things generate more divergent opinions and passionate discourse in the staff room than a discussion of staffing. Within the context of this chapter, staffing can be thought of as the systems that are in place in the department to help ensure that you have the right number of people in the hospital at any given time (and that they are in the right place). If I have 10 people in the hospital doing clinical practice and I ask them about adequacy of staffing, I will get five different opinions. Once during a cycle of routine one-on-one meetings with my staff, I had a most interesting experience. On the same day, I met with two different therapists. In the course of these meetings I was told, "We are so habitually short staffed around here that it is sometimes dangerous and makes it really hard to do a good job" (therapist #1), and "My only gripe about this department is that there are often too many people here; staffing is pretty fat" (therapist #2). Welcome to my world.

As a director–manager, you will probably spend more time dealing with and worrying about staffing than any other single aspect of department operations. Hospital administrators are regularly blamed for being cold, heartless, calculating, bean counters for cutting staffing. I must say that in my 32 years of hospital work, spanning five states and seven hospitals, I have never actually seen a cut in staffing. By this I mean that I have never seen an involuntary reduction in force (otherwise known as layoffs). I have seen hiring freezes and limitations on overtime. But widespread layoffs in respiratory therapy or nursing, I just haven't seen. But I have spent most of my career in academic medical centers or nonprofit organizations. That is not to say that staffing isn't sometimes very thin. But this is almost always because we have been unable (as opposed to *unwilling*) to get more RTs in the building.

My experience tells me that the single greatest challenge in developing staffing systems is the highly volatile nature of the demand for RT services in most hospitals. In a typical 250 bed hospital, it is not uncommon to range from between 5 and 30 mechanical ventilators per day. On top of this is superimposed the seasonal variations that can contribute to large changes in the number of nonventilated patients receiving respiratory services in the hospital, such as asthma, bronchiolitis, or the influenza season. In the departments I have been in or studied, short staffing is almost always caused by some combination of (1) episodic absenteeism, (2) an aging work force, and (3) volatile and excessive demand. By episodic absenteeism I refer to the ubiquitous phenomenon of employees calling in sick for a single day. Far be it from me to suggest that they might possibly not be exactly entirely ill every single time they call in sick. But my blackened old cynical heart does indeed doubt it from time to time. It is hard to begrudge folks an occasional mental health day (as these episodes have come to be called by some), especially those who suffer the dual insults of working in a hospital *and* working nights. But these episodes of unnecessary absences are superimposed on necessary absences, for example staff members who are actually ill, such as those suffering from influenza or upper respiratory infections, or staff members who are out on medical leaves. When these cosmic forces all align with periods of high demand for services, things can get ugly in a New York minute. And of course, these forces do line up in just such a fashion, typically at the time when your department and hospital can least afford to have the RT department short staffed, yet again proving the old adage, "Whom the Gods would destroy, they first drive mad."

The RT workforce is aging. I personally find this outrageous and feel someone ought to do something about this. Any readers who have any ideas about what might be done are urged to contact me immediately. I will probably either be at the doctor's office, pharmacy, or at my water aerobics class. According to the American Association of Respiratory Care's 2005 Human Resource Study, the mean age of the RT workforce is now 45 years old. I have seen the effect of this in increasing amounts of short-term disability and medical leaves of absence. More staff members seem to be off work for a few weeks or a few months for health reasons. Knees, hips, shoulders, and backs seem to be the most frequent locus of dysfunction. This is probably due to the fact that next to nurses, RTs are the health professionals most often seen at the bedside.[1] This requires a lot of movement on the part of RTs. Moving parts tend to wear out.

There are other contributing factors to missed work in the RT workforce. As bedside personnel, RTs, like nurses, are exposed to every nasty despicable pathogen that our patients have the temerity to bring to the hospital with them. I have a theory that the clinical staff can be expected to miss more work than nonclinical staff from influenza and upper respiratory viral infections that they acquire from patients. Yet most hospital or department level absenteeism policies do not make allowance for this obvious fact and tend to want to hold all hospital staff to the same absenteeism standards. I can't prove my theory, but lack of proof has not stopped me from believing a wide range of speculative fiction before, so why should I start now? As far as I am concerned, Frodo and Bilbo live to this day in the undying lands.

Speaking of truth, the truth is that in my experience most departments and hospitals don't do much to manage absenteeism. They just put up with it. On a day-to-day basis, it is pretty much impossible to determine if that person calling in sick is really sick. So managers are forced to count absences and try to counsel employees when their rate of absences exceeds allowable thresholds. But what are the correct allowable thresholds? And do you count all absences against these thresholds or only those not accompanied by a physician's certification of illness? And if you count all absences against an employee, aren't you then punishing them for a legitimate illness? As far as I know, most illness is not a matter of choice by the victim.

Adding to the dilemma of attendance management is the mixed message mambo, meaning that hospitals are forced to send a mixed message to the staff regarding absenteeism. Many hospitals now have signs posted at the main entrances urging visitors with symptomatic influenza and upper respiratory tract infections to avoid coming into the building. Infection control nurses insist that staff members stay home if they are coughing and sneezing. On the other hand, managers and supervisors are counseling employees for excessive absenteeism and pounding their collective heads against the wall when they are short staffed due to illness.

MEASURING ABSENTEEISM

I have had some success at improving absenteeism. One of the most effective ways is through what I call the measure and report method.

Case Study 11: The Power of the Peer

It was raining hard in Frisco. Seth Sikelot, RRT just could not face the thought of going to work. He was bone tired. Normally he only worked two 12-hour shifts in a row and then had a day off before coming back for his third shift of the week. But he wanted that new iPod, so when a frantic supervisor called him asking him to do an extra shift on his day off, he agreed. Now he was staring right into the face of his fourth 12-hour shift of the week. It might not have been so bad, but he took his wife to the movies last night after he got home, so he really didn't get much sleep either. He didn't remember exactly how many times, but he knew he had called in sick a few times the last few months, but so did everyone else. "What the hell," he thought, as he picked up the phone and called in sick, saying "I am not feeling well." This was certainly true. Seth had a momentary, fleeting feeling of guilt, but it quickly passed. The supervisor who took the call hung up the phone and hung her head in misery. Seth was the third person to call in sick that shift.

The next week Seth strolled into work, grabbed a coffee, and headed for the report room. He passed the bulletin board and something caught his eye. He stopped to look. The board did not have its normal confusing appearance. It had been completely cleared of all the customary clutter. Instead there was one very large color graph (Figure 5-1).

To Seth's surprise, the graph seemed to show the sick leave information for the department with every single RT represented. No one's name was on the graph, but instead all the staff members were represented by a number. He asked the supervisor about the numbers and was told to check his mailbox. He discovered his double secret number was 27. He got a sinking feeling in his stomach. He had one of the worst attendance records in the department. And it turns out lots of people didn't miss any days. He went into the report room, and the department director was there, which was never a good sign. The director said, "I want everyone to review the attendance data I posted on the bulletin board." Seth had no idea anyone was measuring or analyzing attendance.

That night at home, he decided he had better get all of his material firmly compressed into one small container. Within six months he had one of the best attendance records in the department.

The measure and report method holds that if you measure performance of individuals within a group, you can change some behaviors by simply showing people how they compare to others. But this has to be done within the context of the culture of the group. For inexplicable reasons (to me), it is no longer acceptable to actually show different levels of performance of individuals in any public fashion. Things like school grades, job performance measurements, and attendance are now considered to be private. Many people feel that this kind of public revelation is degrading or humiliating. That would seem to me to only be true if you were on the low end of the performance scale. Nevertheless it is now not really acceptable to publicly identify low performers, even though in reality we all know who they are, and mostly so do they. A powerful alternative is to blind the data, for example show it in such a fashion that employees can see how they are doing

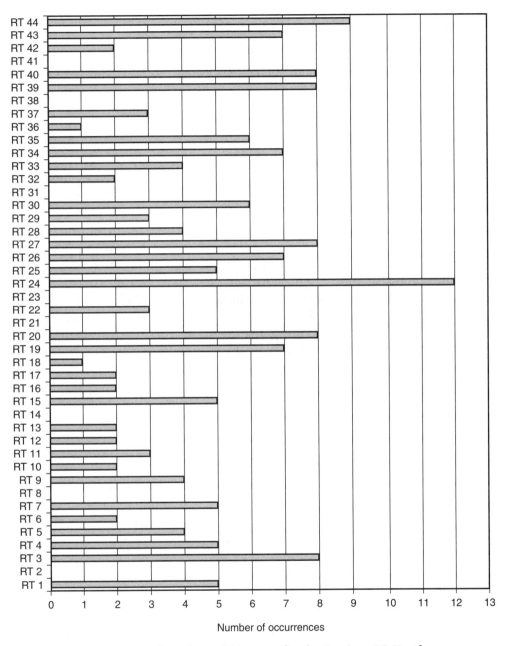

Figure 5-1. Occurrences of Unplanned Absences for the Previous 13 Months
Sick leave occurrences in the respiratory care department. This is an example of blinded reporting where each RT is assigned a number, known (theoretically) only by that RT.

compared to others, but they cannot see who the others are. Using this tool, we were able to reduce absenteeism by 23% in a department I worked in. We would periodically develop a graph like Figure 5-1 and display it in the department. We would also review the results with individuals during their performance review sessions. The improvement in attendance was impressive.

Figure 5-1 displays attendance in the form of counted "occurrences" of unplanned absence. An occurrence is defined as any missed shift (or part of a shift) or subsequent shifts that are not separated by a worked shift. Thus if you missed Monday and Tuesday, this would be counted as only one occurrence. Another method of measurement is to measure total missed hours and divide these by total scheduled hours for any work period. This produces an absenteeism rate or percentage. Both methods have their strengths and weaknesses. Counting occurrences is more proscriptive of the practice of frequent single missed shifts and is more forgiving of the staff member who might have had a bad influenza and missed two or three consecutive shifts. But it also might encourage a staff member to call in sick for two shifts in a row because this counts the same as calling in for one shift. The percentage of worked hours missed is simpler to track in some ways than occurrences, but it is not very good at measuring attendance in work groups that have different shift lengths. Missing one 8-hour shift is a smaller percentage of scheduled hours than missing one 12-hour shift.

I have seen departments that measure both occurrences and percentage of scheduled hours missed. They established acceptable thresholds of occurrences of unplanned absences (seven in a year) and percentage of hours missed (5%). If a staff member exceeds either level, they are counseled.

How much absenteeism is acceptable is a difficult threshold to determine. The Bureau of Labor Statistics measures this and reports an absenteeism rate of 4.1% in health care, which is the highest among industry sectors (see Figure 5-2).

My opinion, for what it is worth, is that acceptable absence levels ought to be established on the department level. Bedside clinicians can be expected to be sick more often than nonclinical staff because of their exposure to sick patients. My department threshold is set at 5%.

STAFFING SYSTEM

One of the most important functions of the leadership team is to establish appropriate levels of staffing. Practices here vary widely from hospital to hospital. Some departments have a fixed schedule, for example they use

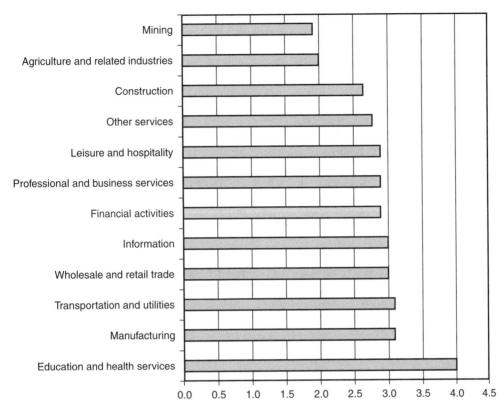

Figure 5-2. Absence Rate by Industry
Absenteeism by industry sector, from the Bureau of Labor Statistics, "Current Population Survey," 2005. (http://www.bls.gov/opub/ted/2006/feb/wk2/art02.htm) The rate reflects missed work hours divided by scheduled work hours.

historical patterns of demand for service to establish how many clinicians are needed. Thus every day they have more or less the same number of therapists in the building. This type of staffing system is pretty much fixed, for example it doesn't flex up or down with demand much. If there is a higher demand for services than the number of RTs scheduled, they just prioritize their work, pick up the pace of their work, and do the best they can. This usually results in increasing the time it takes to get a respiratory therapist to the bedside or to get new therapies started. The therapists also tend to shorten treatment times and skip absolutely unnecessary activities.

Some departments use a *flexed* staffing system. Flexed systems are clearly superior and are recommended by the Society for Critical Care Medicine.[2]

These can have several components, including a pool of per diem staff that can be added to the schedule on an as needed basis. They may be scheduled in advance but then not actually used in staffing if workloads do not require it. Other aspects of a flexible staffing program can include on-call systems where full- or part-time staff members sign up to work overtime, either full or partial shifts, in advance. They are only used if the workload requires it. Most of these systems pay an on-call premium to stay available for the shift, even if not called in at the beginning of the shift. This practice varies, but it is typically in $2.00 to $3.50 per hour range. In some pay models, these therapists would then get paid at a rate of 1.5 times their hourly rate if they are actually called in to the hospital to work. This is irrespective of whether or not they worked more than 40 hours in that week or 80 hours in that pay period in some systems, especially in workplaces governed by union contracts.

Also, some flexible staffing systems will send home regularly scheduled staff if the demand for service drops. Staff members can then decide to just have fewer hours worked on their paychecks or bring their hours up to their scheduled amount by using vacation or paid time off hours. Finally, these systems can be, and often are, supplemented by the practice of calling through the list of all employees on a shift-by-shift basis to see if anyone wants to work overtime.

Flexible staffing systems are probably the most efficient methods for trying to make sure there is the right number of RTs in the building, but there are many limitations. Usually the amplitude of the cycle of demand for services is greater than the amplitude of the cycle of available staff. In other words, the number of staff on-call may often not be enough to meet the spikes in demand. At the other end of the scale, demand for service can drop so low that you could possibly send almost the whole staff home. The problem with the extremes at both ends of this relationship between demand and availability of staff is the quickness with which conditions can change in hospitals. Consider this example of a 12-hour shift. You normally staff eight people, but it looks like you are only going to need four people for the shift, so you send four people home. Two hours into the shift, things start heating up and by the sixth hour you could have used all eight people. But by now you will not be able to get them back because they have all decided to go the beach and roast bratwursts. Or at the start of the shift you thought you needed six people, and you had six scheduled, so you did not bring the on-call therapist in to work, but by six hours into the shift, things have heated up and you wish you had brought them in.

Flexible staffing systems have to be carefully calibrated. If you hire enough staff to easily meet peak demand for services, you risk having lots of shifts during periods of low demand when you are sending a lot of staff members home without pay. They will then be forced to use up their paid time off to maintain their income. Clinical employees will do this for a while, usually because they like the time off to decompress from the stress of working in a hospital, but not for too long. Your employees will not long remain in a system where their income is not generally guaranteed. Some departments solve this problem by having a large part-time or per diem pool to flex the staff up during peak demand. Thus they keep the relative proportion of full- and part-time staff low so that there is less chance, during low demand periods, of having to send these people home without pay. Hospitals with a particularly specialized or advanced clinical practice model for respiratory therapists have difficulty using such a system because it takes a very long time to train such therapists, and they have to work with a predictable regularity to maintain their clinical skills.

One can get cynical about all this. As you gain experience in leadership you will watch your staff do amazing things. In spite of your best efforts, there will be shifts when staffing is very bad, for example the demand greatly exceeds the supply of staff. Somehow they will manage to plug the dike and get it all done, or at least get the vital stuff done, and apparently nothing bad will have happened, and you will breathe a sigh of relief. The casual observer might start to think that maybe staffing in general is too "fat." Because they appear to have gotten through this terribly short-staffed shift without any real trouble, maybe we could tighten up staffing in general. It sure would help the budget performance. But listen, my young Jedi: *Do not go down this path* because it leads to the dark side. Note that *apparently* nothing bad happened. *Immutable Truth #19: Directors–managers are often the last ones to know what is going on in their departments.* The truth is that there are sometimes unhappy things happening as a result of inadequate staffing; you just aren't hearing about them. Mistakes, lapses, and slips may occur that are not reported. Or they are caught and corrected by other RTs, nurses, or doctors before any damage is done, and you don't hear about these either. The culture in most hospitals has traditionally been *not* to report these things, unless they are terribly serious, because nobody wants to get anybody into trouble. The other danger is that if you have too many shifts where staffing is terribly short, people will get burned out. They will begin to lose coping skills and powers of concentration, and you risk creating serious disengagement of staff. We will talk more about disengagement later.

Managers and staff members have argued for a long time that inadequate staffing leads to poor quality of care. As obvious as this sounds, until recently, solid scientific evidence in support of this idea has been noticeably lacking. There is now a growing body of evidence linking staffing to clinical outcomes.[3-6] Most of this is in the nursing literature, but it conceptually translates well to respiratory therapy staffing. There is also evidence that the presence of respiratory therapists is related to improvements in patient outcomes as well.[7-18] The director–manager who is interested in demonstrating the value of having RTs around and trying to ensure that he or she has enough RTs on staff would do well to get steeped in this literature. Regrettably what the research on this subject lacks is the establishment of what constitutes safe staffing for either therapists or nurses. It is becoming clear that staffing and safe and effective practice are linked. It is not clear exactly how to establish what safe staffing levels are.

It is worth the time to do a slight review of what has transpired in the political arena regarding the establishment of safe staffing levels. As do a lot of things, the debate really began percolating in California where a strong political movement started to have the State establish standards for safe staffing levels.[19] A law was passed in 1999 requiring the State to establish minimally acceptable nursing to patient ratios and then to enforce these ratios in all California hospitals. In the initial round of discourse, the hospital association shamelessly proposed that the general medical surgical nursing staff to patient ratio be established at 1:10. In a shocking development, a nursing union initially proposed a ratio of 1:3.[20] Who could have predicted this? After much deliberation[i] and taking nearly 5 years, a general medical surgical nurse to patient staffing ratio was established of 1:5. There were also ratios established for intensive care, emergency department, and other areas of the hospital. Legislation has also been proposed at the federal level, mandating national staffing standards for nurses, but is still pending. The jury is still out on whether this law has had the desired effect on outcomes. I am sure it has improved the employment prospects of nurses in California. Whether or not it has been beneficial to hospitals as a whole, or to patient outcomes, remains to be seen. Early reports do not appear to indicate that any change in outcomes has been seen, but a lot of research remains to be done before this question can be answered.[21]

There are simply no good national standards on minimum acceptable staffing levels for respiratory therapists. Periodically urban myths

---

[i]It turns out that nearly everyone had an opinion in this volatile matter. The California Department of Health Services received 24,000 letters from various organizations and individuals during the public comment period. (Brook L, August K. State Health Department Releases Revised Nurse-to-Patient Ratios for Public Comment. California Department of Health Services, July 1, 2003.)

propagate that the JCAHO has established minimally acceptable RT staffing levels, but every time I look, they turn out to be only wishful thinking on someone's part. Even the AARC has never developed a specific, detailed recommendation that I can find. There are probably lots of reasons this hasn't happened, but two obvious ones emerge. Not surprisingly, they both have to do with variation. One is the large degree of variation from hospital to hospital in the severity of illness of patient populations. Hospitals vary in the communities and types of patients they serve. Some are in communities where prosperity and health abound, and as such they have a relatively low proportion of patients with complex, severe illnesses. Conversely, some hospitals are referral centers with lots of subspecialty care and thus have a population with a much higher proportion of patients with complex, severe illnesses than the general hospital community. The number of staff members required to care for the same number of patients at these two very different hospitals would indeed be, well, different. Thus staffing standards would be very difficult to develop that would be applicable at both types of hospitals.

The other large source of variation is RT practice models. Basically nurses and RTs have overlap in their respective scopes of clinical practice, and the amount of this overlap, or sharing of duties, very much affects the demand for RT services from hospital to hospital. So a hospital with a high degree of overlap in RT–nursing duties might require relatively fewer RTs than a hospital with a low degree of overlap. Of course this lower demand for RTs would probably be offset by a higher need for nurses. But let us not confuse this issue with logic and facts. We are discussing RT staffing, not nurse staffing.

One method of describing RT staffing is the ratio of RTs to ventilated patients. Typically these ratios range from 1:4 to 1:6, although this varies widely across dimensions of time and space. Speaking of the Twilight Zone, California has gotten a bad reputation for being the birthplace of strange. But this time, their leadership has turned out to be pretty good. The State's administrative code says the following about respiratory care staffing in the intensive care unit: "Sufficient respiratory therapists and/or respiratory therapy technicians to provide support for resuscitation and maintenance of the mechanical ventilators in a ratio of 1:4 or fewer on each shift."[ii]

Using this ratio as a quick and easy descriptor of the state of RT staffing is a popular tool because it is a relatively easy piece of data to lay your

[ii]California Code of Regulations, Title 22, Article 6, Section 70405.

hands on. But it can sometimes be very unrepresentative of the demand for RT services. Some ventilated patients require a lot more care than do other ventilated patients. In some hospitals, for every patient receiving mechanical ventilation there may be 5–10 other patients who are not on mechanical ventilators but are receiving RT services. One of the best pieces of work around studying respiratory care staffing was done by Mathews, Drumheller, and Carlow. They examined RT staffing patterns by querying national data repositories and conducting various surveys. They found that, in general, hospitals staff an ICU RT for about every 10.8 existing ICU beds.[22]

Because no national staffing standards exist that describe acceptable staffing levels, directors–managers must develop their own local standards. The key here is to develop logical standards and then do your best to live by them. There are some national resources that can help you. The AARC publishes a compendium of respiratory therapy procedures and the time it takes to do each procedure. The *Uniform Reporting Manual* is used by many directors–managers to construct a staffing protocol. The idea is simple. Near the end of one shift, the total estimated treatments and procedures for the coming shift are entered into a spreadsheet. The time units, sometimes called weights, are then multiplied by the volume of each procedure, which produces the total estimated amount of time it would take to complete all the anticipated work for the next shift. This total time is then converted to the number of people required by dividing the total estimated time to complete the scheduled work by how much time an RT can actually work each shift. Warning: The amount of clinical work an RT can do in 12 hours is actually *not* 12 hours. They must occasionally heed the call of nature, refuel, get coffee, and call home to see how the kids and/or the spousal unit are doing. Also, they must take and give reports, have an occasional break, and have time to check their stock performance or shop on the Internet. There is also travel time, time for rounds, and usually unplanned admissions and pesky things like internal transports. The real art of crafting a staffing program is not in counting procedures and time units. It is coming up with a reasonable estimate of the average amount of time an RT can actually produce clinical work in a given shift.

A constant criticism of staffing programs like these is that the time standards for given procedures are not representative. It is argued that patients (like the quality of television programming) are highly variable. Some patients require longer to treat than others. This is true, but it must be remembered that time standards for treatments and procedures should be developed as averages, recognizing that some patients take more time and *some take less.* Such a system of estimating staffing needs for pending shifts is far from perfect. If a staffing protocol is only done every 12 hours, which is typical, then any changes, admissions, or new RT orders are only going to be updated in the protocol every 12 hours. Things in a hospital can change much faster than that. But using such a staffing system is demonstrably better than not using any staffing protocol, which regrettably, is still widely practiced. Figure 5-3 is an example of such a protocol.

This spreadsheet calculates how many RTs are needed for each functional area using the estimated volume of procedures and weights or time standards. These time standards were developed internally such that they are unique for this hospital, so don't get all flummoxed about the actual weights. The spreadsheet also allows for some fudge factors, for example time needed for rounds and travel and so on. These are different in different parts of the building and on different nursing units. The issue to study here is the process by which volumes of procedures and time standards are used to predict staffing needs. Each weighting unit is approximately 20 minutes. Table 5-1 lists the definitions for each field in the spreadsheet.

The final product of the calculations is the total number of staff members needed. The supervisors then compare this number to the number scheduled and make adjustments, either calling in additional staff or sending unneeded staff home.

When staffing has to be adjusted downward, for example sending regularly scheduled staff home, care must be taken to administer this fairly. A system has to be in place to be sure to pass out these episodes equitably. Some people always want to go home if possible and others never want to go home unless they have to. Go figure. I am always happy to go home when I get the chance. Careful records must be kept of who got sent home voluntarily and involuntarily when the workload was low.

Adjusting the staffing upwards has its own challenges and is usually a teensy bit harder than adjusting staffing downward. When demand greatly exceeds the supply of RTs for any length of time, the staff is offered overtime either through prescheduled shifts when they are available to work overtime (on-call) or they are used just in time, for example staying over after their regular shift is complete. Typically, about 20–30% of the staff works about 70–80% of the available overtime. This is usually not by design, but because of the distribution of the normal patterns of human behavior in the department. In this case, some people just want or need more money and are willing to work overtime to get it.

PICU Interventions	Number	Weight	Staff
Ventilators	4	6.5	0.79
BPAP/CPAP/VPAP	2	5	0.30
Planned post OP admits	0	5	0.00
iNO/Special gases	0	0.45	0.00
Transcutaneous monit	0	1.2	0.00
ETCO$_2$	1	1.2	0.04
CONT Bronchodilat NEB	0	2	0.00
O$_2$-CONT aerosols	0	0.75	0.00
TX units (non-vent)	6	1	0.18
Rounds/travel	4	1	0.12
Weekday transports	0	4	0.00
PICU Total			1.4

NICU Interventions	Number	Weight	Staff
Ventilators	4	6.5	0.79
BPAP/CPAP/VPAP	0	4	0.00
Planned post OP admits	0	5	0.00
iNO/special gases	1	0.45	0.01
Transcutaneous monit	2	1.2	0.07
ETCO$_2$	2	1.2	0.07
CONT Bronchodilat NEB	0	2	0.00
O$_2$-CONT aerosols	0	0.75	0.00
TX units (non-vent)	0	1	0.00
Rounds/travel	4	1	0.12
Weekday transports	0	4	0.00
NICU Total			1.1

CICU Interventions	Number	Weight	Staff
Ventilators	5	6.5	0.98
BPAP/CPAP/VPAP	1	5	0.15
Planned post OP admits	0	5	0.00
iNO/Special gases	1	0.45	0.01
Transcutaneous monit	1	1.2	0.04
ETCO$_2$	4	1.2	0.15
CONT Bronchodilat NEB	0	2	0.00
O$_2$-CONT aerosols	1	0.75	0.02
TX units (non-vent)	0	1	0.00
Rounds/travel	5	1	0.15
Weekday transports	0	4	0.00
CICU Total			1.5

Acute Care	Number	Weight	Staff
Ventilators	3	6.5	0.59
BPAP/CPAP/VPAP	1	5	0.15
O$_2$-CONT aerosols	7	0.75	0.16
TX units (non-vent)	10	1	0.30
CONT Bronchodilat NEB	0	2	0.00
Rounds/travel	1	10	0.30
In-house transport per 15 min.	0	1	0.00
ACU Total			1.5
Grand Total			5.5

Monday–Friday		
Saturday–Sunday	X	

Figure 5-3. Staffing Protocol

An RT department staffing protocol. This spreadsheet is designed to calculate the number of RTs needed for a given shift. It is intended to be used by populating the various cells with the latest information available, typically about 2 hours before the start of the shift. The functional areas of the hospital described by the spreadsheet are PICU (pediatric intensive care unit), NICU (neonatal intensive care unit), CICU (cardiac intensive care unit), ACU (acute care unit). See table 5-1 for definitions of the various components of the spreadsheet.

Table 5-1. Staffing Protocol Labels and Definitions*

Label	Description
PICU interventions	This describes the unit of functional area. In this example it is a pediatric intensive care unit. It could be any function area of the hospital.
Ventilators	The number of ventilators in operation for that shift.
BPAP/CPAP/VPAP	The number of other ventilator assist devices in use, for example continuous positive airway pressure, bilevel pressure devices, whatever.
Planned post-op admits	If known in advance, these are planned post-operative admits that will likely be on ventilators after surgery. In this example these are pediatric cardiac surgery patients.
iNO/special gases	The number of patients receiving inhaled nitric oxide, heliox, subambient oxygen therapy, or any other weird, unusual, infrequent special gas therapies.
Transcutaneous monit	The number of patients on transcutaneous monitors.
ETCO$_2$	The number of patients on end-tidal carbon dioxide monitors.
Cont bronchodilat neb	The number of patients receiving continuous bronchodilator nebulizers.
O$_2$-cont aerosols	The number of patients receiving oxygen or cool mist or heated tracheostomy collars that are not on any other interventions listed here.
TX units (non-vent)	The number of 20 minute treatment units. These may be nebulizer treatments, chest physiotherapy treatments, cough-assist device treatments, or anything else you haven't already accounted for.
Rounds/travel	This is automatically populated by a calculation based on the number of ventilators in use and

(Continues)

Table 5-1. Staffing Protocol Labels and Definitions (Continued)

Label	Description
Rounds/travel	is intended to account for the time spent attending teaching or care planning rounds.
Weekday transports	If known in advance, this is the number of planned internal transports, for example CAT scan, MRI, cath lab, etc.
Weight	These are fixed values based on estimated average amount of time it takes for each of the interventions listed. Each unit of weight is 20 minutes. Thus for a ventilator the weight is 6.5. This value is multiplied by 20 minutes and thus there is 6.5 × 20 = 130 minutes per 12-hour shift allotted for a mechanical ventilator.
Staff	This is a calculated value indicating the number of staff needed. The formula is:

$$Staff = \frac{(number\ of\ treatment\ 3\ weight)}{33}$$

The number 33 is the approximate number of 20 minute treatment units a staff member can do in a 12-hour shift. It is based on the following assumptions:

Total minutes per shift		720
Nonproductive		
	Meals	30
	Breaks	30
	Report	30
	Productive	630
Divided by 20 minute units		÷ 20
Number of productive units possible		≈ 33

*Staffing protocol labels and definitions associated with Figure 5-3. All weights are based on average workload estimates for a 12-hour shift.

When staffing gets really short, you will be tempted to consider mandatory overtime. In most states, labor laws allow you to compel employees to work extra hours. Even some union contracts permit this. I have never given in to this temptation. As bad as staffing can be sometimes, consider how bad it might be if your ability to retain qualified staff suddenly takes a downturn as a result of disgruntlement[iii] related to the implementation of mandatory overtime, particularly if you are one of the few departments in your local labor market with such mandatory overtime. Mathews, Drumheller, and Carlow also studied the issue of the utilization of mandatory overtime in RT departments.[22] The study gives us some insight into the utilization of mandatory overtime. Of the RT departments surveyed (n = 30), only 47% had any policy allowing mandatory overtime. Interestingly, only 33% had any disciplinary sanctions in place if you refused to work mandatory overtime. Actual use of mandatory overtime apparently is very rare with only 23% of departments reporting using the policy monthly or more.

My main problem with mandatory overtime is it just won't work very well. By this I mean that I don't think it will really improve staffing much, but it may certainly put a serious dent in staff relations. The inefficiency of such a program is related to the two-sided coin of progress in telecommunications technology. I know what *I* would do as a staff member if I looked at my caller ID and saw that it was the hospital calling. I would not answer the phone. This is already what happens when we are calling around to try to get people to work voluntary overtime. They don't answer the phone when the hospital calls. Think how much worse it would be if they knew that I would compel them to come to work if they answered the phone.

The Joint Commission on Accreditation of Healthcare Organizations (JCAHO) has a standard that requires hospitals to conduct staffing effectiveness analysis (recommendation HR.1.30). This recommendation requires hospitals to periodically study the effectiveness of staffing and its impact on outcomes in at least two units. This was intended to focus on nursing units, and staffing effectiveness analysis is not mandated by the commission for RT departments, although hospitals may and certainly do choose to include RT departments in this program. I conduct staffing effectiveness analysis by comparing needed staff to actual staff for each shift. Needed, or what I call "predicted," staff is

---

[iii]The word "disgruntlement" intrigues me. Synonyms for this word include unhappiness and dissatisfaction, both of which have opposites: happiness and satisfaction. But disgruntlement does not appear to have an opposite. No one ever describes a happy staff member as one that is highly "gruntled." I have tried using "gruntled" in polite management circles, but I can't seem to get any traction with this.

calculated from the staffing protocol described in Figure 5-3 and Table 5-1. Actual staffing is recovered in our department from a department level database that we populate each shift. It contains the number of staff members who worked, the number of ventilators in operation, who called in sick, and where staff members were assigned in the hospital. Predicted versus actual staffing constitute my version of a staffing effective analysis, which can be seen in Figure 5-4.

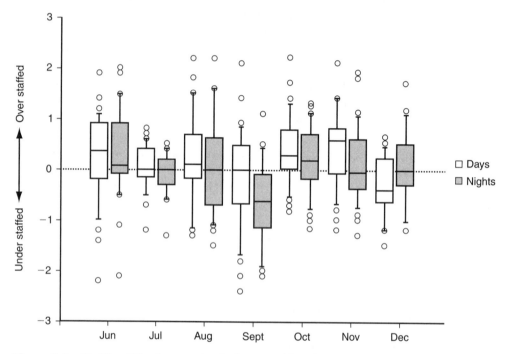

Figure 5-4. Staffing Effectiveness Analysis (Actual/Predicted Number of Staff)
The plots used here are referred to as box plots, or box and whisker plots. They are excellent ways to represent the distribution of a set of numbers. This plot represents the difference between actual staffing and predicted or desired staffing for each shift for 6 months. The upper and lower edges of the box represent the inter-quartile range, i.e., the 75th and 25th percentiles, while the line in the middle of the box represents the median or 50th percentile. The upper and lower whiskers represent the 90th and 10th percentiles. Don't confuse these with "error bars" in other types of plots. They do not represent error. The circles represent outliers above the 90th and below the 10th percentiles. Note that the inter-quartile range, which represents 75% of the data for each month is generally within one person of the desired staffing, which in this graph is represented by the zero line. In other words, in three quarters of shifts, staffing was within one person of the desired level. These data were in a department where baseline staffing was about 9 RTs so my analysis of these data indicate pretty good staffing, although there are individual shifts where staffing was considerably below (and above) desired levels. When you figure out a system to reduce this kind of staffing variation to zero, please give me a call or drop me an e-mail.

This graph demonstrates a truth about staffing. It varies as do the size of grains of sand and the luminosity of stars. To study the effectiveness of staffing you should look at it over time, as I do in this graph. You can see from the plots that the interquartile range, which describes 75% of the shifts, are all within ±1 person of the predicted (or desired) staffing. The circles that denote individual shifts above or below the 90th and 10th percentiles indicate that some shifts were certainly outside this range, but overall staffing was pretty good. As a measure of the performance of individual supervisors, I also plot these data by supervisor, using exactly the same plotting format. Note that I also analyze this for days versus nights. Box plots are powerful analytical tools. Unfortunately it takes statistical software to create them. There is a very complex and retro-engineered diabolical-type way to do them in Excel, but it ain't pretty.

SCHEDULING

Scheduling is distinctly different than staffing; it is the management function of creating and managing the schedule. The schedule, as an entity, has vast powers. It can create widespread joy and deep despair. It is hard to overstate the importance of how the schedule is created and how your staff perceives the fairness and efficiency of the scheduling process. Do not fall into the easy habit of ignoring the schedule. Like a junk yard dog who hasn't been fed in a while, it can reach up and bite you in the arse.

As a director–manager one of the first things you will have to decide is the length of your shifts. When I entered the field, sometime during the Jurassic period, everybody worked 8-hour shifts except the poor residents who seemed to work 72-hour shifts nonstop. They looked like it too. There have been many permutations of scheduling since then, including 4-hour shifts, 10-hour shifts, and the now famous 12-hour shift. As of 2005, the AARC Human Resources Survey reports that among hospital based RTs, 43.4% work 8-hour shifts and 33.2% work 12-hour shifts with the remainder working other various combinations. Among urban hospitals the prevalence of 12-hours shifts is much higher (72%). Most of the academic medical centers I have been in utilized 12-hour shifts, and the overwhelming majority of RTs that I have experience with prefer 12-hour shifts. The main advantage for the staff is less worked days per week, although each worked day is obviously longer. In congested urban areas, this is usually preferable because of the difficulty with commuting through bad traffic. One of the problems with 12-hour shifts is that there is no multiple of 12 hours that equals 40 hours, which is what constitutes full-time work in many hospitals. Some hospitals allow that 36 hours per week qualifies as full-time, and they pay benefits accordingly. Others use three 12-hour shifts in one week and three 12-hour shifts plus one 8-hour shift in the alternate week of the pay period, accepting that 4 hours will be paid in overtime, to qualify for full-time work. The length of shifts and the starting times of shifts also depend very much on the ebb and flow of work in the 24-hour cycle as well as the culture of the workforce. Whenever possible, schedules should be crafted to have the most people on board during the busiest times of the day.

The key to successful scheduling is being creative and flexible. Many departments are on an all 12-hour shift schedule while others utilize many and various combinations of 12-hour, 8-hour, and 4-hour shifts. Shift starting times sometimes vary too. The most common is obviously 0700 for both 8- and 12-hour shifts, but some departments utilize shifts that start at 1100 hours and run until 1900. Others have shift starting times between 0600 and 0730.

Self-scheduling is popular in some departments. This allows staff to self-select the days they want to work. When this selection process is complete, management makes adjustments attempting to even out the staffing across all shifts. In some scenarios, seniority is used to redistribute the staff to shifts they did not self-select with less senior staff being moved more often than more senior staff. Other departments use set schedules in which an individual always works the same days of the week. These types of positions are usually passed out according to seniority, although not always.

Working weekends is an unpleasant duty that also must be equitably distributed throughout the staff. There are a couple of schools of thought on this. First, some people believe that everyone on staff ought to work an equal amount of weekends. Typically this is every other weekend because there are two weekends in every pay period. The other camp believes that senior people ought to have to work fewer weekends than those with less seniority. In these types of systems you typically see senior people working one of three weekends and the least senior staff working two of three weekends. Then there are the unfortunate few, who, owing to the cruelties of fate and circumstance, finds themselves compelled to volunteer to work every weekend. God bless them.

My position regarding the use of seniority for scheduling purposes has undergone a metamorphosis over the years. For reasons inexplicable to me, when I was younger I did not favor placing a heavy weight on seniority when doling out the less desirable portions of the schedule. Now, having experienced the long passage of years, seniority seems more important to me.

Go figure. Actually I like to think that my position is a little more nuanced than just simply being motivated by blind self-interest. The longer I manage, the more valuable senior people have become to me. They bring what money can hardly buy—experience and judgment. They leaven the bread of the department. And typically hospital pay scales compress the salary advancement of the most senior people so there is little enough for them in terms of recognition for their years of experience. After about 15 years or so, many RTs are at or near the top of the pay scale. Usually human resource policies do not allow a person's salary to exceed the top of the pay scale. As an example, if the staff are getting a 4% raise, and a senior staff member is at the top of the scale, they might not get the 4% raise but instead get a lump sum of cash equal to 4% of their annual salary. This is nice, but later in the year when they work overtime, they will not be getting paid at the higher salary rate they would have if they had gotten the raise. Such systems inadvertently injure the salary progression of senior staff. Of course, the hospital has a reasonable business interest in keeping the growth in salaries manageable.

My current hospital does a great job of recognizing and rewarding senior people. Every quarter there is a beautifully catered service recognition breakfast for staff members who have been at the hospital for 15 years or more. Staff members are invited to come, and their manager comes too and makes brief personal remarks about what the employee brings to the organization. Luxurious gift baskets and handsome commemorative plaques are passed out. Notice: this is not my normal sarcastic shtick. I really *do* like these recognition breakfasts. The staff loves them too. I generally think we do not do enough to recognize the long service of our senior staff members.

Another potent form of abuse to which we subject our employees is the delight of working nights. While there may be the rare person who actually enjoys and even thrives on being awake all night, most sane people prefer to be asleep sometime between 2300 and 0700. This is why God made it dark at night. To attract and retain qualified night shift staff, most hospitals offer an incentive in the form of a pay premium or differential for working nights. Others choose to work nights because it fits the realities of their lifestyle, such as child care issues. Still others like nights because the suits aren't around. Other than the few who want to work nights, the rest of the night shift staff are diligently working, praying, fasting, and hoping to get off nights as soon as possible. This is because these folks know, either explicitly or implicitly, what the scientists are now beginning to prove. *Immutable Truth #20: Sleep deprivation, derangement, and disruption makes unhappy campers.* Nearly six million Americans work nights on a permanent or rotating basis.[23] As the science of sleep has developed, it has become clear to me that we have underestimated the impact of sleep difficulties on human performance and function.[24-30] Night shift work disrupts both sleep and waking because of the misalignment of circadian regulation and sleep–wake behavior. Diminished cognitive performance, memory loss, and other health issues have been described in night shift workers.[31,32] In about 5–10% of night shift workers, the sleep-wake disturbance is severe. Whenever I am adjudicating an employee performance issue involving a night shift staff member, I try to keep in mind the debilitating effects that nights have on work and home life. Whenever possible, I allow these factors to be considered as mitigation. If I could design a new staffing system from scratch with no limitations, I would build sleeping rooms for all night shift staff and arrange the system so they could periodically nap/sleep, which has been shown to improve performance.

There is no single best system for scheduling. One has to be crafted for the culture and circumstances of each individual hospital and department. Just remember to be as flexible and fair as you possibly can with the schedule. Failure to develop the schedule in an evenhanded and equitable manner can result in deep staff disgruntlement. In my opinion, scheduling in hospitals is one of the main causes of staff dissatisfaction and drives people out of the field (or keeps them from coming into health care). I have lost a number of highly trained and qualified clinical staff to other segments of the healthcare industry, for example home care or sleep laboratories, because they could get much better working schedules in those operations.

AGENCY STAFFING

There is a nationwide shortage of respiratory therapists. The history and causes of this shortage are very well described by Mathews, Drumheller, and Carlow.[22] The equation is quite simple. The demand for RTs is increasing while the supply has been stagnant or declining. In 1995 there were 100 applicants per year per respiratory therapy school. By 2001 this had dropped to 20. In 1995, advanced level schools graduated 4910 students, and by 2005 this had dropped to 3953. Combine this with the Bureau of Labor Statistics forecast that there will be a need for 5000 new RTs per year, and you can see the gap. The AARC Human Resources Study estimated that in 2005 there were 11,695 vacant RT full time equivalents (FTEs) out of 151,559 total RT FTEs, yielding a rate of 8% of all RT positions unfilled. About 6% of the general population hold more than one job while 29% of RTs report having more than one employer. Finally, hospitals report that 1% of RT positions are filled with supplemental or agency staffing.

This shortage is felt very acutely by some hospitals and departments. I took a director position once of a department with 42 FTEs that had 13 unfilled positions. For the first 14 months in that job, I had no qualified applications come across my desk. Circumstances like this drive directors to hire contract or agency staff. These RTs are employed and deployed by companies that provide you with temporary and allegedly trained and experienced staff on relatively short notice and for short periods of time when you have positions you cannot seem to fill and cannot do without. These types of RTs are sometimes called travelers because they tend to work in one hospital or city for a few months and then travel on to another city. Indeed these companies recruit RTs by offering them (among other things) the glamour of travel. They also pay them very well and give them generous housing allowances, which are usually not taxable. Directors pay a price for these staff members. The cost of these employees to the hospital ranges from $40–55 per hour depending on the region and the company. At first, this seems outrageous because it is almost double the average hourly rate of regular staff. But this can be misleading. The cost of an hour of RT labor is really much more than just the hourly rate. You must include benefits in determining the costs of an hour of labor. Benefits packages vary from hospital to hospital, but generally the cost of benefits is about 28–35% of the hourly salary. Thus you must multiply your hourly rate times approximately 1.3 to get the actual cost of your labor. By way of example, true labor costs per hour would be:

- Average hourly rate = $25.00 per hour
- True hourly labor costs = $25.00 × 1.3 = $32.50

Thus when comparing the cost of agency staff to your staff, be sure to use costs that are adjusted for benefits. And you must also factor in recruitment and training costs of hiring new regular staff. These can be substantial. The recruitment costs of hiring traveling RTs are already paid for in their hourly rate. The assumption is that they do not require very much training because they are supposed to be quite experienced, which is a good thing because paying $50 per hour to train them hardly makes much financial sense. But you will not be able to avoid doing some training and orientation of contract staff. Be sure to keep training and competency files on these staff members too because the JCAHO requires documentation of training and competency of contract staff.

My experience with contract staff has been uneven. Some are highly qualified and motivated. At other times, I have had contract staff members who either intentionally or unintentionally misrepresented their experience and training. And the enormous variability in the complexity of clinical practice between hospitals makes prehiring assessment of competency very difficult sometimes. An ability to work in one hospital may not translate into an ability to work in another hospital. I generally do not like using contract staff because they are typically not around long enough to establish relationships and trust with other RTs, nurses, and physicians. But I must admit that they have helped us through some very difficult times. Using contract staff is also a way to do back door recruiting. I have hired many contract staff members into permanent positions at the end of their contracts or shortly thereafter. Having them on contract first gives me a chance to evaluate them and gives them a chance to evaluate the department and the hospital. The caveat here is the company that provides you with contract staff may not be happy about you actively recruiting them. Some contracts have clauses that require you to pay a hefty placement fee if contract employees decide to take regular permanent staff positions after they have been with you as contract employees. Read the fine print. The fee may be worth it for a really gifted clinician, but be sure to evaluate what the contractual obligations are before you discuss a job with a contracted employee.

A heavy dependence for protracted periods on agency staff is usually a sign of deeper troubles. If you cannot recruit and retain staff in your department, it is time to start examining why this is so. Either your pay structure is not competitive or your working conditions are not good or both. I have seen this happen more than once when departments descended into a death spiral of poor working conditions, poor pay, lousy recruitment, and even worse retention. The responsibility for this always rests with leadership. I have seen many RT managers who like to blame conditions like these on administration. It is true that administrators make great boogey men and women, but the responsibility rests with department leadership. It is your job to make the case to administration and influence and convince them of what your department needs. Remember, administrators are real people too. And the overwhelming majority of all of them I have worked with responded positively when you present them with cogent, dispassionate, patient focused, data driven arguments. It is also very useful to enlist the support of your nursing and medical colleagues when confronting issues like these, for example what the hospital must do to recruit and retain competent RT staff.

In general, agency or temporary staff can make sense for short-term, episodic staffing needs. These can include replacement of staff members who are on medical leave or seasonal adjustments to staff. I also generally try to stick with a single company whose staff I have had experience with before.

REFERENCES

1. Kocher N, Chapman S, Dronsky M. Respiratory care practitioners in California: the center for the health professions. *UCSF.* July 2003.
2. Task force on Guidelines, Society for Critical Care Medicine. Guidelines for standards of care for patients with acute respiratory failure on mechanical ventilatory support. *Crit Care Med.* 1991;19(2):275–278.
3. Needleman J, Buerhaus P, Mattke S, Stewart M, Zelebvinsky K. Nurse-staffing levels and the quality of care in hospitals. *N Engl J Med.* 2002;346:1715–1722.
4. Cho SH, Ketefian S, Barkauskas VH, Smith DG. The effects of nurse staffing on adverse events, morbidity, mortality, and medical costs. *Nursing Research.* 2003;52:71–79.
5. Aiken LH, Clarke SP, Sloane DM, Sochalski J, Silber JH. Hospital nurse staffing and patient mortality, nurse burnout, and job dissatisfaction. *JAMA.* 2002;288:1987–1993.
6. Person SD, Allison JJ, Kiefe CI, Weaver MT, et al. Nurse staffing and mortality for Medicare patients with acute myocardial infarction. *Med Care.* 2004;42:4–12.
7. Shrake KL, Scaggs JE, England KR, et al. Benefits associated with a respiratory care assessment-treatment program: results of a pilot study. *Respir Care.* 1994;39:715–724.
8. Robertson RH, Hassan M. Staffing intensity, skill mix and mortality outcomes: the case of chronic obstructive lung disease. *Health Serv Manage Res.* 1999;12:258–268.
9. Orens DK, Kester L, Konrad DJ, Stoller JK. Changing patterns of inpatient respiratory care services over a decade at the Cleveland Clinic: challenges posed and proposed responses. *Respir Care.* 2005;50(8):1033–1039.
10. Burn SM, Marshall M, Burns JE, et al. Designing, testing, and results of an outcomes managed approach to patients requiring prolonged mechanical ventilation. *Am J Crit Care Med.* 1998;7:45–57.
11. Ely EW, Bennett PA, Bowton DL, et al. Large scale implementation of a respiratory therapist driven protocol for ventilator weaning. *Am J Respir Crit Care Med.* 1998;159:439–446.
12. Kollef MH, Shapiro SD, Silver P, et al. A randomized, controlled trial of protocol directed versus physician-directed weaning from mechanical ventilation. *Crit Care Med.* 1997;25:567–574.
13. Wood G, MacLeod B, Moffat S. Weaning from mechanical ventilation: physician directed versus a respiratory therapist directed protocol. *Respir Care.* 1995;40:219–224.

14. Horst HM, Mouro D, Hall-Jenssens RA, et al. Decrease in ventilation time with a standard weaning process. *Arch Surg.* 1998;133:483–488.
15. Stoller JK, Skibinski CI, Giles DK, et al. Physician ordered respiratory care vs physician ordered use of a respiratory therapy consult service: results of a prospective observational study. *Chest.* 1998;110:422–429.
16. Stoller JK, Mascha EJ, Kester L, et al. Randomized controlled trial of physician directed versus respiratory therapy consult service directed respiratory care to adult non-ICU inpatients. *Am J Respir Crit Care Med.* 1998;158:1068–1075.
17. Stoller JK, Haney D, Burkhardt J, et al. Physician ordered respiratory care versus physician ordered use of a respiratory therapy consult service: early experience at the Cleveland Clinic Foundation. *Respir Care.* 1993;38:1143–1154.
18. Kollef MH, Shapiro SD, Clinkscale D, et al. The effect of respiratory therapist initiated protocols on patient outcomes and resource utilization. *Chest.* 2000;117:467–475.
19. Rhone N. Debate over nurse staffing grows; health: implementation of minimum per-patient ratios is delayed as factions clash over defining adequate levels. *The Los Angeles Times.* April 5, 2001.
20. Doolan D. Keeping watch: California's staffing ratios. *Nurs Manage.* 2005;36(7):36–40.
21. Evans WN, Beomsoo K. Patient outcomes when hospitals experience a surge in admissions. *J Health Econ.* 2006;25(2):365–388.
22. Mathews P, Drumheller L, Carlow JJ. Respiratory care manpower issues. *Crit Care Med.* 2006; 34(suppl):S32-S45.
23. Czeisler CA, Walsh JK, Roth T. Modafinil for excessive sleepiness associated with shift-work sleep disorder. *N Engl J Med.* 2005;353:476–486.
24. Borges FN, Fischer FM. Twelve-hour night shifts of healthcare workers: a risk to the patients? *Chronobiol Int.* 2003;20(2):351–360.
25. Gold DR, et al. Rotating shift work, sleep, and accidents related to sleepiness in hospital nurses. *Am J Public Health.* 1992;82(7):1011–1014.
26. Gordon NP, et al. The prevalence and health impact of shift-work. *Am J Public Health.* 1986;76(10):1225–1228.
27. Parkes KR. Shiftwork, job type, and the work environment as joint predictors of health-related outcomes. *J Occup Health Psychol.* 1999;4(3):256–268.
28. Rosa RR. Extended workshifts and excessive fatigue. *J Sleep Res.* 1995;4(S2):51–56.
29. Gaba DM, Howard SK. Patient safety: fatigue among clinicians and the safety of patients. *N Engl J Med.* 2002;347(16):1249–1255.
30. Kurumatani N, et al. The effects of frequently rotating shift work on sleep and the family life of hospital nurses. *Ergonomics.* 1994;37(6):995–1007.
31. Rouch I, Pascal W, Ansiau D, Marquie JC. Shift-work experience, age and cognitive performance. *Ergonomics.* 2005;48(10):1282–1293.
32. Costa G. The impact of shift and night work on health. *Applied Ergonomics.* 1996;27:9–16.

CHAPTER 6

Billing Systems

And if you ask for a rise[i]

There's no surprise

They're giving none away

—Dark Side of the Moon by Pink Floyd

Respiratory therapy departments typically generate revenue—lots of it. In fact, much of the early growth of RT departments in hospitals happened because chief financial officers grew aware of the fact that more RTs on board usually resulted in more revenue. I am not saying this was all good, but it is the truth. We would like to think our success and growth was entirely because of our vast contributions to the welfare of patients. So sorry, but as delightful as this would be were it true, 'tis not. Don't get me wrong. RTs have long since proven their contributions to patient care as I documented in the last chapter. But the wise director–manager would do well to pay close attention to the revenue generating capabilities of the RT department. Of course, the clinical skills and technological wizardry of RTs are indispensable to hospital clinical operations, particularly in critical care. It is interesting to conduct a mental experiment. Ponder what would happen in your hospital tomorrow morning if none of the RTs showed up. Could patients still be placed on mechanical ventilators? Could blood gases be analyzed? Would pulmonary function testing get done? This goes back to one of my immutable truths. If a hospital could shut down your department, they should. What do they need you for anyway?

Well, one of the things they need you around for is generating revenue. Just like going to the dentist generates a bill, getting seen by an RT in the

---

[i]If you look up the lyrics to this classic on the Internet, the word is raise, not rise. But American pronunciation being what it is, when I try to sing it with raise instead of rise, it doesn't quite rhyme as nicely. So I am changing the lyric to rise. I hope David and Roger don't mind too much.

hospital almost always results in specific charges appearing on the patient's bill. Billing systems for RT departments vary enormously. Some are vast and mind bogglingly complex. Others are elegantly simple. I prefer simple. In this context, complexity refers to the number of different things that RTs charge for. The more cynical among us operate under the (false) assumption that their real value as employees of the hospital can be proven by the billing system and that the more varied and complex the charges that they bill for, the more they are beloved by administration. In their weaker moments they can be heard to say, "We wouldn't be here if we weren't generating revenue." In contradiction to this dark assertion I offer the following. When I worked for Kaiser Foundation Hospitals in California they did not bill patients. It was a true health maintenance organization (HMO) where members' employers paid a fee every month for each covered employee and then members could go to any Kaiser hospital. Because (Kaiser) the insurance company operated the (Kaiser) hospitals, it didn't bother billing itself. Thus the RT departments in these hospitals did not generate revenue and instead were simply naked cost centers. Yet these hospitals continued to have RT departments. And having worked at a few Kaiser hospitals, I can testify that they did not appear to have any more or less RTs than other non-Kaiser hospitals I have worked in. The Kaiser hospitals kept the RT departments around for a variety of reasons, none of which were at all related to generation of obscene profits.[ii]

Unnecessarily complex billing systems usually accomplish one useful thing. They manage to irritate the financial managers and business office staff of the hospital. This is because the more complex a system is the more prone it is to error and dysfunction. I know of RT billing systems that have been found to have huge undiscovered billing errors in them. By undiscovered, I mean that systematic errors were not identified for quite some time. Examples of these errors include double billing or billing for procedures that did not happen. When discovered, the hospital was forced to pay back insurance companies hundreds of thousands of dollars. There was no skullduggery involved, just shoddy design and poor execution. And of course there have been some very famous examples of criminal proceedings against health care organizations and individuals who have committed fraud by submitting fraudulent bills to the government payers, including a $35 million

---

[ii] I take it back. Profits are not and cannot be obscene. Profits result when the market is willing to pay more than the cost of producing goods or services. Of course, what you do with profits can be obscene. My only beef with profits is that I ain't getting enough of them myself. This is, of course, almost entirely my fault.

settlement between the University of Washington and the federal government for fraudulent billing practices and a $20 million settlement for the University of Pennsylvania.[1] In both of these cases, the problems were mostly related to billing for physician services, which most hospitals do not do. But there are plenty of problems with the rest of the billing universe too.[iii]

Listed below are various types of billing errors. Well, actually, not all of them are errors in a strict sense. Some of these are billing practices that have been identified as unethical or unnecessary. The following list is a compilation from my own experience, and there are many lists you can find on the Web sites of companies that will help patients challenge their hospital bills. These companies are very successful at getting patients' hospital bills reduced.

- Duplicate charges (i.e., more than one charge for the same item).
- Charges for services never rendered or at least not documented in the medical record.
- Separate charges for tests that together comprise a panel for which there should be a single charge.
- Charges for certain services that were performed by nurses or therapists, such as equipment monitoring, that should be included in the room charge.
- Charges for equipment monitoring services on occasions when the equipment in question was not in use.
- Separate charges for services and supplies that should be included in the charge for another item.
- Charges for items dated before the patient was admitted to the hospital or after the patient was discharged from the hospital.
- Charges for tests and services that had to be performed a second time because they were performed incorrectly the first time, because the results were lost or mislaid, or because of some other hospital mistake.
- Charges for unidentified items (miscellaneous charges).
- Charges for personal items, such as a toothbrush, a comb, or slippers, that the patient did not use.
- Charges for services that the patient refused.

[iii]In the first half of fiscal year 2006, the Office of Inspector General (OIG) reported expected recoveries of approximately $1.02 billion for discovered billing fraud and errors. During this period, 1540 individuals and entities were cited for fraud and abuse involving federal health care programs and/or their beneficiaries. There were 226 criminal actions against individuals or entities that engaged in crimes against departmental programs. In addition, there were 119 civil actions (http://oig.hhs.gov/publications/docs/press/2006/Semiannualspringrelease2006.pdf).

- Charges for routine supplies used by hospital staff, such as surgical gloves, coats, drapes, masks, urinals, bedpans, irrigation solutions, ice bags, IV tubing, pillows, towels, gauze, oxygen masks, oxygen supplies and syringes, blood pressure cuffs, heating pads, and thermometers and blah de blah blah blah, all of which should be covered in the room charge.
- Room charges that were incorrectly calculated, such as if the patient had a semiprivate room but was charged for a private room; the patient requested a semiprivate room but was placed in—and charged for—a private room because no semiprivate room was available; the patient was charged for a greater number of days in a specialized unit like intensive care or cardiac care than he or she actually spent there.
- Charges for operating room time; it's not uncommon for hospitals to bill for more time than was actually used.
- Up coding, which often occurs when hospitals shift the charge for a lower-cost service or medication to one that's more costly. For example, a doctor orders a generic drug, but the patient is charged for a pricier brand name.
- Charges for the day of discharge. Most insurance plans do not allow hospitals to charge for the day you leave the hospital. This is because the hospital will go ahead and bill the next patient who comes into the room, thus allowing double revenue for the room for that day.
- Charges that may have been scheduled but were later cancelled.
- Charges for physician services on the hospital bill when the doctor (such as an anesthesiologist or radiologist) bills for the same service.

A study by an insurer estimated that the average hospital bill contained almost $1400 in overcharges. The federal government estimates that 99% of hospital bills contain overcharges.[2]

I know of very little that has ever been published regarding the accuracy of respiratory care billing practices. I studied the accuracy of the RT billing system at a hospital where I once worked.[3] On the advice of my attorney (A.L. Dewitt), I am declining to name names. I initially discovered that the billing error rate was about 18%. We reviewed 45 randomly selected medical records of patients who received respiratory care. We examined their bills and compared the bills to what was documented in the medical record. We found two broad categories of errors: (1) procedures billed for that we could not find evidence of in the medical record and (2) procedures documented in the medical record for which no charge had been generated. There was a third type of error that we could not identify: billable procedures done for patients for which there was no charge posted and no entry charted in the medical record. Lots of errors occurred in both directions that resulted in underbilling and overbilling. When we extrapolated these error rates across the entire population of patients who received respiratory services, the net financial impact of correcting all these billing errors would have been an increase in revenue for the department of nearly $700,000 per year or about 7% of department revenue. The billing system in this department was operated separate from the clinicians. There were billing clerks that went in real time around the hospital every day and read the respiratory charting and then filled out a billing sheet for each patient based on what they read in the chart. These data were then entered into homegrown billing software.

Based on these findings and my deep-seated conviction that I would not look good in an orange jumpsuit with a stripe down the leg, I came to the conclusion that something must be done. We did three things. First we got a new billing system in which the clinical staff would be responsible for their own billing. This required the purchase of a $100,000 respiratory therapy department information system in which the staff did their own billing data entry during each shift. Second, we started conducting individual billing audits and fed this information back to the staff. We made billing error rates part of yearly performance appraisals. Third, we simplified the billing system as much as we could, reducing the number of different billing codes used. Within a year, the billing error rate for another sample of randomly selected medical records had dropped to 3%. I considered this still unacceptable, but I was very happy with our progress.

Part of what contributes to the frequency and types of billing errors are the sheer numbers of procedures and interventions billed for. Each different billable respiratory therapy procedure is typically referred to by a description (name) and code number. I know of departments that have as few as 50 different RT charge codes and others that have as many as 200 charge codes in spite of the fact that these departments were very similar in scope of practice.

Some charging systems include procedural charges (billing for what RTs do) as well as equipment and supply charges (billing for what RTs use). The latter is becoming less frequent because public and private payers are beginning to balk at paying for specific equipment charges, such as for respiratory monitors, which almost all patients have. They argue that these charges ought to be included in the room charge. As a result, some hospitals have changed their billing systems to reflect this philosophy and now bill only for procedures and not for supplies or equipment. As an example, in some departments there is no longer an equipment charge for a mechanical ventilator. Instead, there is a charge for mechanical ventilation, which includes the cost of the equipment, the labor costs and the supplies, plus, of course, the markup. More on this seemingly innocuous term later.

The list of all the different charges used by the RT department is typically called the chargemaster. To each charge there is also usually attached a price and a relative value unit (RVU), which I described in Chapter 4. RVUs are units of time and reflect the average amount of time it is expected that it would take an RT to complete this billable procedure. Table 6-1 lists a typical chargemaster and the associated RVUs.

Table 6-1.   Typical Charges for Respiratory Care Services at Taco Bellevue Medical Center

Cryptic charge code abbreviation	English translation	Frequency of charge	Relative value unit (minutes)
Airway clearance TX-initial	The initial assessment and treatment with any alternative airway clearance technique including autogenic drainage, assisted cough, PEP mask, external chest wall oscillation	Once per patient at initial treatment	45
Airway clearance TX-subsq	Subsequent assessment and treatment with any alternative airway clearance technique including autogenic drainage, assisted cough, PEP mask, external chest wall oscillation	Per subsequent treatment	25
BIPAP/CPAP initial	Initial assessment and treatment using bi-level positive airway pressure or continuous positive airway pressure	Once per patient at initial setup	130

Table 6-1. Typical Charges for Respiratory Care Services at Taco Bellevue Medical Center *(Continued)*

Cryptic charge code abbreviation	*English translation*	*Frequency of charge*	*Relative value unit (minutes)*
BIPAP/CPAP subsq shift	Subsequent patient– equipment system assessment/adjustment of bilevel positive airway pressure or continuous positive airway pressure	Each subsequent shift	90
Bronchial brushing	Obtaining bronchial brushing samples from intubated pa-tients using closed sheath bronchial brush systems	Per procedure	45
CBG draw	Percutaneous capillary blood gas sampling	Per procedure	20
ABG draw	Percutaneous arterial blood gas sampling	Per procedure	15
Cont neb initial	Initial assessment and setup of continuous aerosol for the administration of inhaled medications	Once per patient at initial setup	40
Cont neb subsq	Subsequent patient– equipment systems assessments/adjustments	Per subsequent shift	35
CPR	Cardio-pulmonary resuscitation	Per 15-minute increment	15
CPT comprehensive initial	Initial assessment and treat-ment with chest physiother-apy and postural drainage; includes all lobes and all positions	Once per patient at initial treatment	45

(Continues)

Table 6-1. Typical Charges for Respiratory Care Services at Taco Bellevue Medical Center *(Continued)*

Cryptic charge code abbreviation	English translation	Frequency of charge	Relative value unit (minutes)
CPT comprehensive subsq	Subsequent assessment and treatment with chest physiotherapy and postural drainage to all lobes and all positions	Per subsequent treatment	30
CPT initial	Initial assessment and treatment with limited chest physiotherapy and postural drainage; only selected lung lobes and positions used	Once per patient at initial treatment	30
CPT subsq	Subsequent assessment and treatment with limited chest physiotherapy and postural drainage; only selected lung lobes and positions used	Per subsequent treatment	20
EKG	Electrocardiography	Per procedure	45
ETT retape	Retaping endotracheal or nasotracheal tubes	Per procedure	15
Extubation	Removal of endotracheal or nasotracheal tube	Per procedure	20
Heliox init	Initial assessment and setup of equipment for the administration of HeO_2 gas mixtures either via mechanical ventilator or other gas delivery apparatus	Once per patient at initial setup	120

Table 6-1. Typical Charges for Respiratory Care Services at Taco Bellevue Medical Center *(Continued)*

Cryptic charge code abbreviation	*English translation*	*Frequency of charge*	*Relative value unit (minutes)*
Heliox subsq	Subsequent assessment and adjustment of equipment for the administration of HeO_2 gas mixtures either via mechanical ventilator or other gas delivery apparatus	Per subsequent shift	60
Indirect calorimetry	Determination of basal metabolic rate using indirect calorimetry	Per procedure	120
Infant pneumogram	Multichannel recordings of physiologic variables to identify and quantify the presence of infant apnea	Per procedure	120
In-house transport	Transport of ventilated patients in-house for diagnostic and treatment purposes; charged in 15 minute increments	Per 15-minute increment	15
Intubation assist	Assisting with the insertion of endotracheal or nasotracheal tubes	Per procedure	45
Manual ventilation	Positive pressure ventilation with manual resuscitator	Per 15-minute increment	15
MDI TX-init	Initial assessment and treatment with inhaled medication via metered dose inhaler	Once per patient at initial treatment	20

(Continues)

Table 6-1. Typical Charges for Respiratory Care Services at Taco Bellevue Medical Center *(Continued)*

Cryptic charge code abbreviation	*English translation*	*Frequency of charge*	*Relative value unit (minutes)*
MDI TX-subsq	Subsequent assessment and treatment with inhaled medication via metered dose inhaler	Per subsequent treatment	12
Mech ventilation init	Initial assessment and setup of conventional mechanical ventilators	Once per patient at initial setup	130
Mech ventilation subsq	Subsequent patient ventilator system assessment/ adjustment	Per subsequent shift	110
Nebulizer tx-init	Initial assessment and treatment with inhaled medication via handheld nebulizer	Once per patient at initial treatment	25
Nebulizer tx-subsq	Subsequent assessment and treatment with inhaled medication via handheld nebulizer	Per subsequent treatment	20
Nitric oxide initial	Initial assessment and setup of equipment for delivery of $_iNO$	Once per patient at initial setup	60
Nitric oxide subsq shift	Subsequent patient–equipment systems assessment/adjustment	Per subsequent shift	10

Table 6-1. Typical Charges for Respiratory Care Services at Taco Bellevue Medical Center *(Continued)*

Cryptic charge code abbreviation	English translation	Frequency of charge	Relative value unit (minutes)
O$_2$ initial	Initial assessment, setup and treatment with continuous oxygen	Once per patient at initial setup	20
O$_2$ subsq shift	Subsequent patient–equipment assessment/adjustment of continuous oxygen therapy	Per subsequent shift	20
Resp monit, noninvas-init	Initial assessment and setup of devices for continuous monitoring of the respiratory system including pulse oximetry, capnography, or transcutaneous carbon dioxide monitoring	Once per patient at initial setup	30
Resp monit, noninvas-subsq	Initial assessment and setup of devices for continuous monitoring of the respiratory system including pulse oximetry, capnography, or transcutaneous carbon dioxide monitoring	Per subsequent shift	20
Trach care	Care of the tracheostomy tube and stoma site, including cleaning, skin care, and changing ties	Per procedure	15
Trach change	Removal of existing tracheostomy tube and insertion of new tube	Per procedure	30

(Continues)

**Table 6-1. Typical Charges for Respiratory Care Services at Taco
Bellevue Medical Center** *(Continued)*

Cryptic charge code abbreviation	*English translation*	*Frequency of charge*	*Relative value unit (minutes)*
Ventilator HFOV init	Assessment and setup of high frequency oscillatory ventilator	Once per patient at initial setup	130
Ventilator HFOV subsq shift	Subsequent patient ventilator system assessment/adjustment	Per subsequent shift	110

These charge frequencies and relative value units are based on a 12-hour shift billing program. Each RT bills for their procedures during each shift. The relative value units are stated in minutes and are completely homegrown, that is, developed internally based on a panel of staff RTs and supervisors. The cryptic charge code descriptors are taken right out of a hospital billing system. I left them in their current form so you could see that abbreviations and terminology are usually very local in flavor and sometimes more difficult to interpret than Klingon.

Table 6-2 is another example of a chargemaster, in this case from a group of RT departments that were trying to make a chargemaster that would work across a number of departments for comparing productivity. Note that neither list contains any price information.

PRICING

Prices for RT services vary enormously between hospitals. I know of charges for mechanical ventilation as low as $250 and as high as $1200 per day. There is no national repository of RT prices across the country. But there are some clues as to the magnitude of the variance. Ohio has a law requiring that hospitals publish lists of their most commonly used charges. Thus you can work the Web and find out the prices of selected RT charges at hospitals in Ohio. I spent a bit of time doing this (not much). I came up with the following ranges of prices from a group of nine hospitals in the Buckeye State.

Table 6-2. Sample Charge List for Respiratory Care Procedures from the Acme Benchmarking Service

Charge description	Frequency of charge	RVU (in minutes)
Blood gas analysis	Per procedure	10
Intensive chest physiotherapy	Per procedure	40
Bilateral chest physiotherapy	Per procedure	20
PEP therapy	Per procedure	15
IPV treatment	Per procedure	25
High frequency chest wall oscillation	Per procedure	20
Cough assist	Per procedure	25
Intermittent positive pressure breathing	Per procedure	20
Metered dose inhaler	Per procedure	15
Small volume nebulizer	Per procedure	15
Sputum induction	Per procedure	30
Treatment aerosol special	Per procedure	45
Continuous drug aerosol	Per day	60
Standard mechanical ventilation	Per day	180
Noninvasive positive pressure ventilation	Per day	120
External negative pressure ventilation	Per day	180
Oscillator/jet ventilation	Per day	200
Bronchoscopy	Per procedure	120
Bedside spirometry tests	Per test	15

(Continues)

Table 6-2. Sample Charge List for Respiratory Care Procedures from the Acme Benchmarking Service *(Continued)*

Charge description	Frequency of charge	RVU (in minutes)
PEAK flow, FVC and NIF, incentive spirometry	Per test	15
E_TCO_2 monitoring and T_cCO_2 monitoring	Per day	30
Oximetry spot check	Per test	5
Oximetry continuous	Per day	20
Nitric oxide	Per day	45
Oxygen	Per day	45
Specialty gases	Per day	60
Surfactant administration	Per procedure	30
Therapist assist	Per 15 minutes	15

This example is taken from a benchmarking group. It represents sort of average relative value units developed by representatives from several hospitals. In this case, the charging program was based on daily charges as opposed to charges per shift.

Procedure	Price range (minimum to maximum)
• Arterial blood gases	$43–$224
• Mechanical ventilation per day	$125–$990
• Aerosolized medication treatment	$31–$127
• Pulse oximetry	$30 per day–$74 per hour

I have also seen data from propriety services that compare the subscribing hospital's pricing to other subscribers' prices. I am not at liberty to list the prices, but ranges of this magnitude are not uncommon, indeed there are many that are much larger. What could account for such a range of prices for procedures that are very similar at hospitals in the same geographic region? The practice of "cost shifting" explains a great deal of this variation. This practice has the costs of running the hospital distributed throughout the revenue generating departments through the practice of marking up prices for certain procedures.

Blood gases are a great example. A blood gas analysis is one of the least expensive of all laboratory tests. It has been a while since I have managed a blood gas lab, but I estimate that the supplies, reagents for a test, and depreciation expense of the analyzer probably cost no more than $8 to $10 per study. Because the procedure from start to finish takes less than 15 minutes, the labor costs are probably no more than one fourth of an hour of RT salary, which, including benefits, is about $30 or about $7.50 per quarter hour. So now we are up to about $20 in actual costs for a blood gas (I am estimating high here, I think it is probably less). The rest of the price is markup or the increase above cost that is added to pay for other operating expenses that cannot be billed. The hospital management novitiate might be shocked by the amount of markup that goes on in establishing RT prices. Frankly, sometimes I am shocked too, but you must remember that this markup is paying for biomedical services, linen distribution, management overhead, supplies, training resources, risk managers, payroll, accounts payable, paint, trashcans, computers, floor wax, paper clips, toilet paper, and a thousand other things that it takes to run a hospital. Do not be confused by thinking there is any systematic approach to setting RT prices between hospitals. The amount of cost shifting and the way nonrevenue departments spread their costs out in revenue generating departments varies tremendously from hospital to hospital. Thus there is an enormous variation in prices. Were we to look across the entire country, the price ranges for similar procedures would be even more breathtaking. Another major contributor to the tremendous variation in price setting is the tremendous variation in reimbursement. Some procedures are paid for by payers pretty much without question. Thus the temptation is to raise the price of these procedures to offset the costs of other procedures and interventions that are not well reimbursed by payers (if at all). That is why I did not list any prices in Tables 6-1 and 6-2. You might be tempted to think that you are over- or undercharging for certain procedures based on any pricing information that I might list. This would be illusory.

However, an apparent lack of price consistency between hospitals does not absolve you of responsibility from trying to establish some rational price setting system within your own department.

Case Study 12: Mr. Markup Comes to Visit

It was raining hard in Frisco. Rose Reviknew, RRT was working on the billing system she had inherited when she took over as RT department director at Our Lady of Perpetual Billing Medical Center. The business office had called and said that the insurance companies were auditing a lot of respiratory therapy bills and were complaining that there seemed to be no rhyme or reason to how RT prices were set. It turns out that the prices for RT procedures had been created 9 years ago and then automatically increased by a certain percentage each year since then. Rose decided that setting prices should follow a basic formula as much as possible. The price of a procedure had four basic components: (1) cost of equipment used, (2) cost of supplies consumed, (3) labor costs, and (4) Mr. Markup. Rose decided to start with the daily charge for mechanical ventilation.

1. The cost of equipment used
   A) This is sometimes also called depreciation expense. The actual dollars used to buy the equipment were spent in the year it was purchased. But for accounting purposes, we would like to post the expense of buying the device across its useful life. It can easily be calculated by taking the original capital cost of the equipment and then dividing that by the estimated number of times it will be used over the life of the device.
   B) Rose's new ventilators cost $30,000 each and have a useful life of 5 years. Of course, Rose knew that all the ventilators would not be used every day of those 5 years, so she had to estimate the percentage of the time they would be used.
   C) She calculated ventilator usage using historical billing records for ventilators and the number of ventilators historically in her fleet. Her department typically billed for 6000 ventilator days in a year, and they had 25 ventilators. Thus if all ventilators were in use every day, there would have been 25 × 365 = 9125 days of mechanical ventilation billed for in a year. Because only 6000 were billed for, she assumed that her ventilators were utilized about 66% of the time (6000 of 9125).
   D) In a 5-year period there are 5 × 365 days or 1825 days. She estimated the ventilator was in use 66% of these days or 1205 days.
   E) To calculate the depreciation expense each time the ventilator was used, she divided the acquisition cost of $30,000 by 1205 days, which was about $25. Thus the cost of acquiring a $30,000 ventilator, spread out over each time it will be used, was about $25 per ventilator day. She used this to establish the depreciation expense component of the price.

2. The cost of supplies consumed
   A) Rose decided that the supplies consumed in applying a mechanical ventilator included the ventilator circuit, the humidifier chamber, and the water used. These had to be estimated for the average ventilator application.
   B) She knew that the average length of ventilation at Our Lady of Perpetual Billing Medical Center was about 5 days. Because ventilator circuits were changed weekly, most patients used only one ventilator circuit and humidifier chamber. She looked up the following costs: circuit cost = $15, humidifier chamber = $12, water = $40 (for 5 days). Thus the total supplies cost for her typical ventilator application was about $67. She divided this by her average length of ventilation, 5 days. Thus daily supply costs were $67 divided by 5 = $13.
   C) Then came Mr. Markup. It turns out that he is a very large guy. He likes to throw his weight around. Rose called the budgeting office and asked what the hospital policy was about markup. They said they typically mark up supplies and labor costs about three- to fivefold for the purposes of setting prices. Rose's momma didn't raise no fool, thus Rose chose the higher number. Using a fivefold markup, she set the supply cost component of the price for a mechanical ventilator at $65 per day.

3. Labor costs
   A) To calculate labor costs, Rose determined her labor costs per minute and multiplied this times the RVU for a ventilator charge. Then she remembered to include her close and personal friend, Mr. Markup.
   B) Labor costs per minute can be determined by using your average hourly rate for RTs and an estimator for benefits costs. The average hourly rate for RTs is simply the total RT salary dollars for any given period divided by total hours paid in that period. This includes overtime costs. Rose used all salary costs of both management and staff because all these costs were part of the costs of providing mechanical ventilation, if, of course, you assume that managers have something to do with the quality of care.
   C) Rose knew it was a convention to use about a 30% markup for benefits costs. She determined that her average hourly rate for RTs was $24. She got this number from the budgeting department. She multiplied $24 × 1.30 to adjust for a benefits expense of 30%. She got an hourly labor cost of $31.20, which equates to about $0.52 per minute in RT labor costs.
   D) Mr. Markup then came to visit again. Using the standard fivefold markup, labor costs per minute would be $0.52 × 5 = $2.60. Now she determined

> the number of minutes associated with a day of mechanical ventilation. This is where her RVU came in. Using the RVU of 180 minutes for a day of mechanical ventilation, the daily total marked up labor cost would be $2.60 × 180 = $468.
>
> E) She added it all up. The labor component was $468, supplies were $65, and equipment depreciation expense was $25, totaling $558. She set the price for a day of mechanical ventilation at $558. One down and only 75 more charge codes to go. Rose got up, put some music on the CD player, and ate some chocolate covered espresso beans.

Let me point out some caveats in this example. First, I would never set prices in an isolated fashion like this but would instead get a team of staff and supervisors together to make sure that all our assumptions were sane. Second, I have gone through this process and come up with some prices that were very different than the current prices. There is one thing the business office will require of any price revisions: revenue neutrality. Simply put, folks, get mean when you mess with the green. They usually require that any revisions have no overall net effect on the total RT revenue generated. Thus you will be required to make further, sometimes illogical, adjustments to prices in addition to the systematic approach listed above. I usually maintain revenue neutrality by spreading them out proportionally across all charge prices. If my new pricing ended up reducing RT revenue by 4%, I would simply increase all prices by 4%.

There is usually a yearly adjustment in respiratory procedure prices. This adjustment has, at least so far in my career, always been upward. The prices are adjusted to accommodate the hospital's increased operating expenses for the coming year. The hospital's operating expenses go up every year because you and your staff all get raises every year, and the cost of supplies and equipment the hospital buys also goes up. The business office typically calculates the price adjustment needed. Throughout my career this yearly price increase has almost always been two to three times larger than the general inflation rate except for a brief period in the mid- to late 1990s when health care inflation slowed a bit.

Each year you may also be asked to estimate procedural volumes for the coming year. This means that you will be expected, like Dorothy, to find a crystal ball and gaze into it and predict the future. Don't be nervous. Good managers predict the future every day. This is called forecasting. Fortunately most people above you in the food chain aren't a whole lot better at it than you are, so you can usually survive if your forecasts turn out to be spectacularly wrong, which mine have sometimes been.

Predicting volumes of billed procedures for respiratory therapy usually involves consideration of several factors.

1. Facilities growth—If the hospital is expanding its bed capacity, you may assume that you are going to have more inpatients. As an example, if you were adding 100 new inpatient beds, you could come up with an expected increase in RT volumes. One way to do this would be to determine the average number of RT procedures billed per inpatient bed per year from your existing beds and then use this to model expected procedures with 100 new inpatient beds. This assumes that your new beds are as fully occupied as your existing beds.
2. Service line growth—It may be that the hospital is expanding a given service line. There may be three new pulmonologists coming to your organization or locale and thus you might expect a growth in pulmonary patients. Other examples of service line growth could be the closure of competitive hospitals or medical practice groups that might change referral patterns and bring you more patients. Also the hospital may add or expand service lines that are expected to increase the respiratory therapy procedures, such as a cardiac surgery line or a neonatal intensive care unit. These need to be carefully considered when modeling volumes for the future.
3. Changes in care models—Be careful to consider any practice changes that you are implementing or planning to implement. If you are about to put a protocol in place to reduce the number of chest physiotherapy treatments, be sure to include this in your forecasts and predictions for the volume of billable procedures for the coming year. In most budgeting and productivity measurement systems, your hospital's system for measuring department performance will be built, in part, around your procedural volume predictions.

There are usually people in the business office or the finance department that have market data and have some ideas about what might happen to referral patterns in your market and thus could help you consider the factors listed above.

BILLING PROCESSES

How the bill is generated varies greatly across RT departments. The following is a discussion of models that I have seen.

Paper Systems

By paper systems I mean billing programs where pieces of paper are generated that contain billing information for patients. Some systems generate a separate form for each patient, and others have documents that can contain information for multiple patients. One model has RTs filling out these forms and then having them be entered into the hospital billing computer system by clerks. Figure 6-1 is an example of a billing sheet, in this case one that can be used for multiple patients.

As always, at every hand off there are potential sources of error. One famous error that I know of involved such a billing sheet. The therapist intended to charge for two nitric oxide charges. But instead of writing the customary "2," he put two hash marks on the billing sheet, intending each hash mark to be interpreted as a single charge. The hash marks looked something like this "II," which looked hauntingly like the number "11." Because Murphy's Law is as ubiquitous as gravity, these hash marks were interpreted by the billing clerk as "11." Owing to the high price for nitric oxide, this error amounted to about $60,000 in overbilling for one day for one patient. Fortunately, the department in question had a person whose responsibility it was to look at charges each week and scan for unusual amounts, and thus this error was caught and corrected before it was posted on the patient's bill, probably preventing a heart attack, which of course could have also been billed for.

Another paper system I know of has all the charge codes printed on every respiratory therapy charting form. As the RT staff charts clinical care, they also write numbers on the billing section of the flow sheets and charting forms. All forms are in duplicate, so at the end of the shift the RTs bring copies of all their charting to the department where the supervisors make a quick review of what is indicated for the billing and make corrections for any mistakes they find. Then billing clerks later enter the data into the hospital billing system. This system does contribute somewhat to deforestation.

Paper systems are obviously a little more labor intense because someone, either the clinicians or the billing clerks, has to first find and fill out the paper forms and then enter the billing information into the hospital's billing system. I prefer to have clinicians enter their own billing data because it causes them to get more invested in the process, and no one knows better than they do exactly what they billed for. And it allows for individual auditing of each RT's billing accuracy, which is an essential part of improving the accuracy of any billing system. This is only possible if relatively simple

| RT Name | | | Date | | | | | | Respiratory Care Charge Sheet | | |

CDM	Description	Freq.	CDM	Count	CDM	Count	CDM	Count	CDM	Count	CDM	Count
01387	Airway Clearance TX Initial	once	01387		01387		01387		01387		01387	
01379	Airway Clearance TX Subsq	each	01379		01379		01379		01379		01379	
89218	BIPAP/CPAP Initial	per s/u	89218		89218		89218		89218		89218	
89531	BIPAP/CPAP Subsq Shift	per shift	89531		89531		89531		89531		89531	
06360	CBG DRAW	each	06360		06360		06360		06360		06360	
40609	Cont Neb Initial	per s/u	40609		40609		40609		40609		40609	
40708	Cont Neb Subsq	per shift	40708		40708		40708		40708		40708	
09018	CPT Comp. Initial	once	09018		09018		09018		09018		09018	
09026	CPT Comp. Subsq	each	09026		09026		09026		09026		09026	
09034	CPT Initial	once	09034		09034		09034		09034		09034	
09042	CPT Subsq	each	09042		09042		09042		09042		09042	
06394	EKG	each	06394		06394		06394		06394		06394	
00751	ETT Retape	each	00751		00751		00751		00751		00751	
83898	Heliox Initial	per s/u	83898		83898		83898		83898		83898	
70804	Heliox Subsq Shift	per shift	70804		70804		70804		70804		70804	
04456	Manual Ventilation	per 15"	04456		04456		04456		04456		04456	
09067	MDI TX Initial	once	09067		09067		09067		09067		09067	
01544	MDI TX Subsq	per visit	01544		01544		01544		01544		01544	
01312	Neb TX Initial	once	01312		01312		01312		01312		01312	
01353	Neb TX Subsq	each	01353		01353		01353		01353		01353	
00959	Nitric Oxide Initial	first 24 hr	00959		00959		00959		00959		00959	
00967	Nitric Oxide Subsq Shift	per shift	00967		00967		00967		00967		00967	
83807	Nitrogen Initial	per s/u	83807		83807		83807		83807		83807	
70705	Nitrogen Subsq Shift	per shift	70705		70705		70705		70705		70705	
03235	02/Aero Initial	per s/u	03235		03235		03235		03235		03235	
03243	02/Aero Subsq Shift	per shift	03243		03243		03243		03243		03243	
89564	Resp Monit, Noninvas-Initial	per s/u	89564		89564		89564		89564		89564	
89556	Resp Monit, Noninvas-Subsq	per shift	89556		89556		89556		89556		89556	
80001	Rounds	per shift	80001		80001		80001		80001		80001	
00355	SX ETT/Oral/NP	each	00355		00355		00355		00355		00355	
00553	Trach Care	each	00553		00553		00553		00553		00553	
00660	Trach Change	each	00660		00660		00660		00660		00660	
40500	Vent Convent Initial	per s/u	40500		40500		40500		40500		40500	
09075	Vent Convent Subsq Shift	per shift	09075		09075		09075		09075		09075	
89820	Vent HFOV Initial	per s/u	89820		89820		89820		89820		89820	
89838	Vent HFOV Subsq Shift	per shift	89838		89838		89838		89838		89838	
	Other											
	Other											
	Write in Other											
33224	Airway Clearance Initial OP	once										
07954	Bedside Airflow Measure	each										
40005	Bronchial Brushing	each										
71109	Clinic PT Assess-OP	each										
09851	CPR	per 15"										
09059	Discharge Plan/Ed	per 15"										
00165	Extubation	each										
40104	Intubation	each										
82122	Neb Pari W/Filter (Tobi)	each										
33216	Trach Tube	each										
81793	Valve, Passy-Muir	each										
89812	Vent, MRI	per hour										
40534	Infant Pneumogram	each										
24009	Indirect Calorimetry	each										

Bottom of each count-column block: Patient ___ / DOB ___ / Medical Record# ___

Figure 6-1. Respiratory Care Charge Sheet

Sample of a paper billing sheet that allows billing data to be compiled on multiple patients. CDM is an abbreviation for charge description master and refers to the number that is entered into the hospital billing system. The RTs carry the billing sheets around with them and then turn them in at the end of each shift. The data are entered into the billing system by equipment techs who double as billing clerks.

billing software is used because training all the clinicians on a complex computer interface can be a potent form of self-abuse.

Computerized or Automated Systems

One type of computerized or automated billing system has the RTs doing their charting in a computer program, and billing is automatically generated by what was charted in the software. Such systems remove a large number of potential errors, but they are expensive and difficult to implement. In my experience, those departments that have actually implemented such systems end up being very happy with them. There are also some hybrid systems around where the charting is done in an electronic format, but billing is not automatically generated from charting. Instead there is a facility in the software for therapists to pull up a billing list and select what should be billed for each patient. Obviously automated billing systems are the best systems for reducing billing errors associated with poor documentation or erroneous data entry.

You will have to carefully study the computer infrastructure in your hospital and the cultures of the clinical staff and business office to determine the best design for your own billing system. You may already have an excellent billing system, but you cannot know this if you do not periodically study its accuracy.

CPT CODES

Unfortunately, no review of departmental billing systems is complete until CPT codes have been discussed. CPT is an acronym for Current Procedural Terminology. The purpose of the coding system is to provide uniform language that accurately describes medical, surgical, and diagnostic services. A CPT code is a five digit numeric code that is used to describe medical, surgical, radiology, laboratory, anesthesiology, and evaluation management services of physicians, hospitals, and other health care providers. There are approximately 7800 CPT codes. Two digit modifiers may be appended when appropriate to clarify or modify the description of the procedure. The CPT codes were first developed by the American Medical Association and have been adopted by the federal government for use in the Medicare and Medicaid payment coding system. This system, the Healthcare Common Procedure Coding System (HCPCS) is now required by the Medicare and Medicaid systems for anyone submitting claims to these payers (and some private payers).

In the interest of not reinventing the wheel, I will quote extensively here from the U.S. Department of Health and Human Services Web site.

Each year, in the United States, health care insurers process over 5 billion claims for payment. For Medicare and other health insurance programs to ensure that these claims are processed in an orderly and consistent manner, standardized coding systems are essential. The HCPCS Level II Code Set is one of the standard code sets used for this purpose. The HCPCS is divided into two principal subsystems, referred to as level I and level II of the HCPCS. Level I of the HCPCS is comprised of CPT (Current Procedural Terminology), a numeric coding system maintained by the American Medical Association (AMA). The CPT is a uniform coding system consisting of descriptive terms and identifying codes that are used primarily to identify medical services and procedures furnished by physicians and other health care professionals. These health care professionals use the CPT to identify services and procedures for which they bill public or private health insurance programs. Decisions regarding the addition, deletion, or revision of CPT codes are made by the AMA. The CPT codes are republished and updated annually by the AMA. Level I of the HCPCS, the CPT codes, does not include codes needed to separately report medical items or services that are regularly billed by suppliers other than physicians.

Level II of the HCPCS is a standardized coding system that is used primarily to identify products, supplies, and services not included in the CPT codes, such as ambulance services and durable medical equipment, prosthetics, orthotics, and supplies (DMEPOS) when used outside a physician's office. Because Medicare and other insurers cover a variety of services, supplies, and equipment that are not identified by CPT codes, the level II HCPCS codes were established for submitting claims for these items. The development and use of level II of the HCPCS began in the 1980's.

The rules for assigning the appropriate CPT code are complex, and much of the so-called fraud in health care may well be the result of inadvertent misuse of these codes. The reason this matters to respiratory therapy directors is that each billable respiratory therapy charge code should have an associated CPT code. There are CPT manuals and computer programs that can help you assign a CPT code for each of your billable procedures.

REFERENCES

1. Chan SP. $35 million settlement announced in UW billing case. *Seattle Times*. May 1, 2004.
2. Rosenthal E. Confusion and error are rife in hospital billing practices. *New York Times*. January 27, 1993.
3. Salyer JW. Improving the accuracy of a respiratory care billing system. *Advance for Respiratory Care Managers*. 1993;3(1):44–47.

CHAPTER 7

Budgeting

Budget: An orderly system for living beyond your means.

Budgeting in hospital departments has two distinct parts: the capital budget and the operating budget. Although these two are members of the same family, they are also like estranged brothers who fought over a woman 30 years ago and haven't spoken since. They do not talk with one another. The capital budget is used to purchase movable or fixed assets that increase the assets of the company. To simplify this definition, it is usually defined in hospitals as equipment that costs more than a certain amount, often $1000. The capital budget is not used to purchase supplies or other products that are consumable. The operating budget is used to pay for everything else. Money from the capital budget should not be used to pay operating expense, and money from the operating budget should not be used to purchase capital equipment. Why, you may ask, aren't these monies supposed to be comingled? Businesses are supposed to operate under a set of rules governing how expenses, profits, and taxes are recorded, counted, sorted, sifted, and otherwise reported to the government and shareholders. These rules are referred to as GAAP (generally accepted accounting principles).[i] Of course, owing to the public scandals associated with companies like Enron, we know that some companies (and some former accounting firms) sometimes stray from the GAAP pathway.

Operating budget money is more readily available to you. You generally just order stuff or sign invoices and operating money gets spent. This will tempt you to try to find ways to spend operating money to get much needed capital equipment. There are work-arounds, such as using a lease–buy agreement where monthly lease payments (from the operating budget) go toward the eventual purchase of capital equipment. This does not technically violate GAAP, and some hospitals do this, but most hospital accounting and

---

[i] The "modern" system of double-entry accounting was actually first carefully described by Luca Pacioli, an Italian monk, in the 15th century, but it may have been used as early as the 12th century.

budgeting offices will catch you and call your boss and then you will be in somebody's office trying to explain things. This is generally to be avoided.[ii] The reason they sometimes object is that using lease–buy methodology to obtain capital equipment allows you to avoid the rigors of the capital budgeting process, which is supposed to be a filter to make sure that only really needed capital equipment comes into the hospital.

Besides irritating you to the point of distraction, the budgets serve very important purposes. They give you a barometer of the financial performance of your department. They can help you plan the future and study the past. Because money has an inherent natural power (that some find intoxicating), it has powerful influences in hospital operations, and some of the best developed sources of data in hospitals are records of financial transactions.

You will be expected to create a capital and operating budget and to present and defend these budgets to the hospital financial illuminati. When your budgets are approved, however mangled they emerge from the process, you will then be expected to manage to these budgets. The natural temptation is to practice avoidance therapy. Ignoring the budget can be very rewarding in the short-term but usually has unhappy long-term consequences. If you are having trouble managing to your budget, don't wait until the administrators call you about this, demanding an explanation. Be proactive. Develop and present a plan for dealing with budgetary problems before they call you to make you develop and present a plan for dealing with budgetary problems. No one expects budget performance to be without difficulties all the time. Most administrators I worked for understood this and were patient. But administrators do expect you to actively deal with your budget issues.

Department heads have historically not gotten a lot of good training in budget development. It is often something you sort of learn as you go along. If you are not really comfortable with numbers or with confrontations that can arise while trying to get your budget approved, you will be tempted to let others do this. By this I mean that some hospitals don't expect a lot of budgeting expertise from their directors. Most hospitals have well developed budgeting departments that will be happy to write your budget

---

[ii]Generally I operate under the principle that it is better to ask for forgiveness than permission. The former is sometimes a little easier to get than the latter. And of course, by the time you ask for the former, you have already committed the deed in question and the genie is out of the bottle. However, you can only survive using this principle under a couple of conditions. First, what you are doing without permission better have a very compelling argument to support it and you better not use this defense too often. The judge will get tired of hearing it.

for you. In this case you must be assertive about being the creator of your department's budget. Sometimes budgeting officers tend to keep their cards pretty close to their vests and may try to keep some of the secrets of the budgeting priesthood, well, secret. Budgeting, especially calculation of staffing needs, is usually full of ratios and coefficients, some of which are rather complex. The tendency is to skip over how these ratios and coefficients are calculated and how they affect the development of your budget. Avoid this. Persuade your budgeting department to teach you all the subtleties of how your budget is created. If you do not learn and master these tools, you are not representing your staff and your patients to the best of your ability. This is where the mastery of spreadsheet skills are essential. It is possible to write and manage a budget without spreadsheet skills, but it will take you much longer than it ought to. You simply must learn moderately advanced spreadsheet skills to be really good at budgeting, or at least to be competitively fast at doing it.

CAPITAL BUDGETING

As a respiratory therapy director you will be constantly confronted with new technology. I once had a doctor call me a "gadgeteer." She did not mean it as a compliment, but I chose to take it that way. Respiratory therapy practice is heavily dependent on technology. You acquire most of this technology by writing masterfully crafted capital budgets. But health care technology is marketed very much like cars. The basic function of a car is to get you from here to there. Of course, there is a rich diversity of styles and features in cars, including a somewhat large range of prices. But all cars still fundamentally are designed to get you down to the 7-Eleven to get a gallon of milk and get you back, although admittedly a DeLorean will do this with a lot more style than a '78 Cutlass. A lot of health care technology is the same way. It has basic functions that haven't changed much over the years but has become festooned with fabulous features. I devote an entire chapter to the issue of evaluating technology later in this book. Here we will simply focus on what you do after you have decided that the technology you are assessing performs the way the manufacturer says it does and that it will be of value to your patients and makes financial sense.

For the purposes of discussing a capital acquisition in an RT department, I will focus on the example of purchasing mechanical ventilators. Almost all respiratory department heads will eventually come to the place where they have to think about expanding or replacing some or all of the ventilator fleet.

One of the first things you realize in this process is that there are many *stake-holders*. These are individuals who have a stake or interest in a particular process in human organizations. Stakeholders in the acquisition of new ventilator technology include respiratory therapists, physicians, nurses, clinical engineers, and financial managers. But the budgeting responsibility for acquiring ventilators has to reside in a single budget and this is usually the RT budget.

The capital budgeting process in hospitals is typically a 3–4 month cycle each year. You will be given a deadline to submit capital budget requests. The memos bugging you about the capital budget will typically start arriving about 3 months before the deadline. But to really make a good capital purchasing decision, you will have to have been working on this for some time. My leadership team once spent 18 months in an evaluative project to choose and acquire new mechanical ventilators.

The process of budgeting for capital equipment can be broadly described as the following process. This list is an idealized conceptual model. The phases of this process sometimes overlap and sometimes don't happen in exactly this order. But a really finely tuned capital budgeting process ought to have all these components. I ought to know. I have made many mistakes in acquiring equipment in the past, and these lessons have been dearly bought.

1. Request for proposal
2. Product selection
3. Price negotiation
4. Terms and conditions
5. The final decision

Request for Proposal (RFP)

This is the part of the process where you inform vendors of your possible interest in acquiring their products. They typically respond by arranging demonstrations and developing quotes, which is essentially their first attempt at establishing prices. This assumes some preliminary work has been done and you have a working knowledge of the market of the products you are considering acquiring. You select the manufacturers you are interested in evaluating and tell them you are considering buying ventilators. If your process is formalized you would do this in writing by sending them an RFP. Your finance department probably has some boilerplate RFP forms for you to use.

Product Selection

Product selection is where I believe we have historically not done a very good job as an industry. I will elaborate on this at length in the next chapter. Here I will simply say that this ought to be a very rigorous project and take a considerable length of time and involve product testing. If you do not do a good job of product selection, you may very well be sorry.

Case Study 13: Acquiring the Amazing Acme Pulse Oximeter

Heavenly Gates Children's Hospital had decided to acquire new pulse oximeters for the neonatal intensive care unit. They already had Acme pulse oximeters at every bedside, but they were stand-alone oximeters and took up space at the bedside. The care environment had become increasingly cluttered as technologies had been added to the clinical arsenal, and by now the immediate bedside was a cluttered mess. Acme engineers had a solution. They had developed a pulse oximeter module that went into a slot on the multiparameter bedside cardio-respiratory monitoring system with the saturation readings being displayed on the cardiac monitoring screen.

The respiratory care director, Albert Olskuel, RRT heard about this new technology and called the vendor for a demo. The Acme sales staff set up a great demo for Al and a handful of respiratory therapists, and they were all impressed. Everyone liked the performance of the 4000 Acme pulse oximeters the hospital already had, and the sales staff ensured the RT director that this was exactly the same oximeter, just fitted in a different box. Al submitted a capital budget request for 35 of the new pulse oximeter modules (total cost $125,000), and to his everlasting amazement, they were all approved.

Within two weeks of installation Al started hearing grumbling about the inconsistency of the performance of the new Acme devices. He initially chalked this up to normal grousing and unfamiliarity with the new devices. But the volume and frequency of the complaints grew. Finally, one morning, the chief of the neonatology division called Al and asked him to come to the unit and look at a patient. The chief had placed one of the new Acme pulse oximeters on the left hand and another on the left foot of the same patient. One was reading 92% and the other was reading 22%. They had identical wave forms. Al felt a knot in his stomach. He immediately had the entire fleet of Acme oximeter modules pulled from service, but not before getting hard copies of the recordings from this patient. Al also gathered anecdotal reports from many clinicians of similar troubles. When he called the Acme engineers and sales staff they insisted it must have been either a misapplication of the oximeter, a bad sensor, or something about the patient that made the oximeter reading perform so poorly. Acme claimed they had installed these devices in other neonatal intensive care units and Heavenly Gates was the only hospital having these kinds of problems.

So Al called some other neonatal units that had recently converted to the Acme oximeter. It did not take him long to discover another large unit where they had documented similar troubles with this product. He asked the director of that department to write him a letter outlining the troubles they were having.

He then set up a meeting with the leadership of Acme and also invited his boss and the hospital CFO. At this meeting Acme again denied there was anything wrong with their product, also claiming they knew of no other hospitals that were having these kinds of problems. At this point Al produced and projected the letter he had received from the other hospital that was having troubles with the Acme pulse oximeter.

A stony silence ensued, followed by a pregnant pause and a great deal of squirming. Before the meeting ended, Acme had agreed to a complete refund. Al and the hospital had dodged a bullet.

But imagine how much easier things would have been for Al if he had done his due diligence and called around and asked about the Acme pulse oximeter before he bought it or if he had done a rigorous clinical trial. He assumed the device would work based on the performance of other products from the same company. This is a risky assumption.

You may think this is a silly example and that this could not have happened. This is a true story. And there are many other true stories of RT directors buying equipment in a relative vacuum without adequate testing or input. I know of a purchase of nearly 100 mechanical ventilators that were sent back to the manufacturer because of an inadequate decision-making process prior to purchase. I know of another case of ventilators being purchased for a neonatal ICU without adequate testing or physician input, resulting in the medical staff refusing to use them. I also know of ventilators being purchased in a vacuum by an RT director–manager without any RT staff input. When they arrived the staff just simply would not use them, and they collected dust in the corner of the equipment room.

Al was able to obtain a refund from the manufacturer, but he was very, very lucky. You might not be so lucky.

Price Negotiation

Product selection and price negotiation really need to be happening at the same time. If you allow vendors to know that you have already decided to buy their product before you really start hard-nosed price negotiation, you have lost a lot of negotiating power. During the process of selecting products you need to be playing the vendors back and forth off of one another. Get quotes early in the process and then compare them. I have historically shown quotes from one vendor to another. For reasons that no one has ever adequately explained to me, some vendors think there is something wrong with this. The conversation goes something like this, "I will give you a lower price but you really can't tell anyone else about this." Obviously one of their concerns is that other hospitals will find out about your lower price and then demand it from the vendor also.

One important tool for you to use in negotiating pricing is to know what others are paying. There are a number of ways to do this. You can use your own network of contacts in other RT departments. There is tremendous value in establishing connections with other directors and managers so that this information can be shared. Sometimes this is done formally through memberships in hospital associations and consortia or informally through meetings and conferences.[iii] Another way to learn about pricing is through commercial services that your hospital may subscribe to, such as MD Buyline (www.mdbuyline.com). This Web-based software allows you to input what you are thinking about buying and returns detailed information on what other hospitals have paid. This works because member hospitals input their capital purchase data.

Another tool for pricing is participation in group purchasing organizations (GPOs). Your hospital participates by combining its purchasing power with many other hospitals to negotiate prices on a wide range of products. Some GPOs are financed by administrative fees paid by the vendors, and some are funded by fees paid by the hospitals. The large potential volume of purchases gives these buying organizations power to negotiate prices. Your hospital probably belongs to one of these buying groups and as such you can get access to price lists guaranteed by the contract. But be aware that you are not obligated to pay the contract price if you can negotiate a lower price. The manufacturer is obligated to charge no more than the contract price.

[iii]Some examples of associations, consortia, or meetings where RT directors network very effectively are University Healthcare Consortium, Children's Health Corporation of America, the International Respiratory Congress of the AARC, the Summer Forum of the AARC, The Focus Conference, and various state respiratory society meetings. If you are not regularly attending your state and national RT meetings, you are not giving yourself all the opportunities to learn and be a better director–manager.

Pricing in the acquisition of capital equipment like a ventilator is not as large a decision driver as it might be in the purchase of other RT products like disposables. The useful life of a ventilator is somewhere between 5 and 10 years depending on the pace of technological advances. Spreading the capital acquisition costs over a period as long as this helps give you a perspective on the small magnitude of the long-term impact of these costs. Also the market for ventilators is pretty competitive, and every time I have purchased ventilators, the different manufacturers have ended up bidding prices that are pretty close to one another when comparing ventilators with similar features. To me, terms and conditions are more important than pricing. Of course the most important consideration is the utility and performance of the device.

Terms and Conditions

When you purchase capital equipment, you will enter into a sales agreement (also sometimes called a procurement agreement), which is a form of a contract. Appendix D is an example of a procurement agreement. This procurement agreement will have terms and conditions (T&C). These are intended to clarify exactly what you expect of the manufacturer before, during, and after the purchase, and conversely what the manufacturer expects from you with regard to payment and other details. I have been in hospitals where almost no attention was paid to terms and conditions, and I have worked in hospitals where a lot of effort went into the negotiation of terms and conditions. Sometimes the purchasing department imposes on you what may at the time seem to be unnecessary and petty requirements in the terms and conditions. But I have learned that it is a good idea to be as detailed as you can manage in the T&C. When you are negotiating, do not be afraid to propose and push and plead and persuade. Sometimes we don't get what we want simply because we are, inexplicably, reticent to ask for it.

When you are developing terms and conditions consider including the following items:

- Shipping costs—These can be considerable and should not be overlooked in quotations and sales agreements.
- Details of delivery—This should include when equipment will be delivered, as well as where and by whom equipment will be uncrated and assembled. For a large purchase this can be a very big deal. As an example, when purchasing 28 new ventilators, I had to carefully consider

where we would receive these devices, where they could be uncrated and assembled (in the receiving department after hours), and where we would store them until we could complete training and implementation activities.

- Conditions of payment—I typically include only a partial payment up front with the remainder to be paid upon clinical acceptance, for example after the devices are assembled, tested, and used for a while to ensure the quality of their performance. This typically takes about 2–3 months.
- Training—Training is a very big deal and should be spelled out in detail. For devices like ventilators, I suggest two rounds of postsales training. The first round should occur immediately upon receipt and should be mandatory for all clinical staff members before they apply the devices to patients. The manufacturer is obligated to provide all this training. However, in particularly large departments, it is not unreasonable for the manufacturer to train some of the clinical staff to help with training. The second round of training should come 1–3 months following the rollout of the new ventilators. This will be focused on training for more advanced features of the device. Ventilators now have so many features that it is not really possible to train the staff adequately on the whole range of functions initially. I would let the staff get very comfortable with the basic operations of the ventilator before I did widespread training on advanced features. Be sure to spell out what you expect from the manufacturer for this postsales training.
- Warranties—Aim high. Try to negotiate extended warranties as part of the sales agreements, especially if the technology is relatively new. All the bugs may not yet be worked out. Review warranty language carefully and make sure you understand its limitations. Ensure that peripherals like cables and sensors are included in the warranty. Manufacturers may be reluctant to do this. Keep pushing them.
- Legal mumbo jumbo—These will include issues like *indemnification, insurance, remedies, force majeure* and other words that give you a headache. *Indemnification* in this context refers to the manufacturer's attempts to insert language that will shield them from liability claims if their products are defective and this results in injury to patients. I have had gas companies try to include language that would shield them from damages if they fill the tanks with the wrong gas. They claimed it was the hospital's responsibility to make sure the oxygen tank had oxygen in it. *Insurance* refers to requiring that the manufacturer carries

sufficient liability insurance to pay for any damages resulting from product defects. A customary required minimum is $1 million/$3 million in coverage, meaning $1 million per claim and aggregate coverage of $3 million, although most large manufacturers carry much more than this. By way of comparison, a 250 bed hospital might carry about $40 million dollars in coverage (for which they pay about $1 million dollars in premiums per year). *Remedies* are details of what will happen if either party doesn't meet all the obligations of the procurement agreement. The hospital's legal counsel or contracting specialist should review all the terms and conditions of sales agreements you are considering entering into. Be sure to clearly understand who is empowered in your organization to sign such a sales agreement. In some hospitals it will be the department director–manager but in others it will be the purchasing or materials director. *Force majeure* refers to natural disasters or other "Acts of God", which usually frees one or both parties from liability or obligation when circumstances beyond the control of the parties, prevents one or both from fulfilling their obligations under the contract.

Filling Out Forms and Making a Decision

The final decision about funding your capital budget request will be made by some committee somewhere based on a combination of the clinical and financial implications of your proposal, the quality of your proposal/presentation, how grumpy the committee members are feeling that day, and other mysterious and inexplicable cosmic forces. You will be expected to make evidence-based arguments for any new clinical equipment that you want. This is usually done first in the form of a written capital budget request. Appendix D includes an example of a typical template you might be expected to fill out. I realize that you probably loathe paperwork and find it, correctly so, to be a useless nuisance and obstacle to the routine discharge of your responsibilities. So do I. But in the case of a capital budget request, a form like this can help you organize your thoughts and arguments for why the hospital should invest in your proposal.

Helpful hints here are to focus on the patient safety aspects of new equipment or programs that you want to fund. This is a hot topic nowadays. Of course it is helpful if your idea actually has a snowball's chance in hell of really improving patient safety. See the next chapter on evaluating new technology. If you are proposing a programmatic change, such as funding an asthma education capability or program, be sure to include a solid bibliography on the topic of the effect of asthma education on clinical and financial outcomes. If you aren't familiar with the literature on asthma education, why in the world are you proposing it to begin with? You had better be the reigning expert in your facility on the extant clinical, laboratory, and health services research related to any capital budget requests you make. If there is no extant research in support of what you are proposing, you probably shouldn't be proposing it anyway. His willingness to fund unproven alleged technological advances is one factor that contributes to the continuing double digit inflation in health care costs every year.[1] This has been called "technology creep."

A decision as complex and costly as replacing or expanding a fleet of ventilators has many contributing factors and can be overwhelming. There are systematic approaches to making such a large decision. One of the best resources you can use to help you is the approach proposed by my mentor and former boss, Rob Chatburn. His paper entitled "Decision Analysis on Large Capital Purchases,"[2] demonstrates a rigorous and systematic approach to making such a complex decision. This approach can be used on any large capital purchase. There is a Web-based software version of this approach available at a Web site called VentWorld.[iv]

As I pointed out earlier, the decision to approve or deny your capital budget request will almost certainly reside somewhere in some committee. Most hospitals have a capital budgeting committee. My experience is that these committees have a chairperson, and in the end, that is the person that makes the final decisions, usually with the help of a trusted advisor or two. Some committees have a more formalized process where each capital budget request is scored by each committee member and then these scores are averaged and the resulting average scores for each request are ranked. The committee then approves the requests from highest to lowest ranked until they run out of money. This system seems to me to be the most fair as long as there is cross representational membership on this committee. Here's a helpful hint. Use your vast powers of corporate navigation to get on this committee. Then there will be at least one person on the committee that you know for sure will vote for your capital budget requests. How do you get on committees? The best way is just to ask either your boss or the committee chair or

---

[iv]VentWorld describes itself as "the Internet's premier source of ventilator product and supplier information, news, discussion, education, tools, and vent resources for the respiratory and critical care community!" The Web site is operated by Amethyst Research LLC, which is a company that sells computer and Web-based resources for acquiring and operating mechanical ventilators (http://www.ventworld.com/equipment/pdtAnnounce.asp).

both. Of course they will know that your interest in this committee is entirely self-serving, but you might get lucky.

In some circumstances you may only be asked (permitted) to submit a written request to the committee, and in other systems you may get the chance to make a presentation to the committee to defend your submission. If you only submit a written request, be sure to find out who the committee members are and contact the key decision makers to make your case in person. *Immutable Truth #21: Generally speaking, most folks don't read much, if any, of the stuff you send to them.* I really hate to be the one who bursts your bubble, who shatters the myth, who creates in you a lasting disillusionment, but it is simply and honestly true that the higher up you go in the food chain, the less likely you are to read a lot of what is sent to you. In the age of practically instantaneous transmission of textual information and the ease with which such text is created, executives and administrators (and directors–managers) are often overwhelmed with the volume of material that they receive. This is why the *executive summary* was created. Use this tool. Make a few important bullet points that will contain breathlessly cogent and compelling arguments that will get an executive's attention. Then include the more mundane details (such as actual evidence to support your arguments) in the body of your proposal. You are much more likely to get their attention long enough to win them over using this technique. I have personally and painfully made this mistake in the past. I have sent written arguments up the ladder to support my capital budget requests. These arguments were heavily referenced to compelling, controlled scientific literature, as well as being flawlessly concocted (if you ask me). The only possible explanation for why my budget requests were not approved—they just didn't read my submission. Because my proposal was about 25 pages long, this is almost certainly true. I am not saying you shouldn't submit your budget proposal with a lot of supporting documentation. But unless you follow up with one-on-one, eye-to-eye, or at least phone-to-phone connections with those decision makers, your proposal will probably not be funded until there is ice skating on the lake of fire.

However, there is a caveat here. Every once in a while you run into some thorough, analytical, logical, gifted, and totally irritating administrator who goes through your submissions with a fine tooth comb. So be sure to have all your T's crossed and your I's dotted, just in case.

There are some financial analytical tools that may be required of you when you submit a capital budget request. Basically, the finance department wants to know two things. First, how long will it take to recoup their capital investment?

Respiratory therapy particularly enjoys the benefit of being able to bill for their services. Thus the finance department may have an expectation that this new equipment you want to buy will generate revenue and they can anticipate a time when their initial capital investment is returned. This is called the payback period. Second, they want to know that this is the best investment for their money. In a real business the main purpose of the business is to maximize profits. A company (your hospital) could invest in your proposal or they could take the money you are asking for and invest it in other relatively secure wealth generating instruments like the bond market in which they can count on a known return on investment over the years. Thus they will want to calculate the amount of growth in the capital money you are requesting if they simply invested it in these other types of investments. They will compare this to the present value of the future cash flow that will be generated from your request minus the present value of the money they will invest in your request to get you started. This is called the net present value (NPV) of your project and includes an analysis of the future cost of money. In his seminal book, *A Brief History of Time* (which I highly recommend), Stephen Hawking points out a great truth about publishing. He noted that the sales of a book are inversely proportional to the number of equations in the book. But hey, I was born to have adventure, so here is the equation for NPV:

$$\mathrm{NPV} = \sum_{t=0}^{n} \frac{C_t}{(1+r)^t} = \sum_{t=1}^{n} \frac{C_t}{(1+r)^t} - C_0$$

Where:

t = The time of the cash flow
n = The total time of the project
r = The discount rate
C_t = The net cash flow (the amount of cash) at that point in time
C_0 = The capital outlay at the beginning of the investment time (t = 0)

Beyond the obvious and elegant beauty of this cool looking equation with stylish Greek symbols and exponents, you might be asking yourself why I included it. If by chance you are one of the few, the proud, who like equations, here is something for you to sink your teeth into. The principal feature of the equation is the discount rate (*r*). This is how much the money you are investing would have earned per period (typically per year) had it been invested in something else other than your project, or thought of another way, what is the future cost of the money. If the money is borrowed, this is the interest rate that must be paid in the future to get this money now. To really get a grip on this equation, you have to do what I suggested earlier in this book—get an MBA.

But here is some additional conceptual visualization that might help. Another way to look at this equation is:

$$NPV = Initial\ Investment + \frac{First\ Year\ Cash\ Flow}{(1+r)^t}$$

$$+ \ldots \frac{Final\ Year\ Cash\ Flow}{(1+r)^n}$$

The initial investment is actually a negative number because you initially had an outlay of cash. To this is added the yearly cash flows adjusted for the discount rate to adjust for how much the money will be worth in current dollars. So you can see how, if the initial outlay is large and the cash flows are small or the discount rate is high, the NPV might be less than zero.

Because the finance department will usually actually do this work, you don't really need to be able to do this equation,[v] but you do need to be able to interpret its output. Like the proverbial "p" value of inferential statistics, this is something that can cause you grief if you don't at least understand the results of the mathematical treatment. This might help:

- If the NPV > 0, the project is profitable and ought to be funded
- If the NPV ≤ 0, the project is a loss and should not be funded

Obviously, decisions to fund clinical equipment requests are complex and driven by more than just the finances of the request. But this is often how the financial managers of the project will view the economics of your proposal. A common mistake is failure to account for all costs in a capital budget proposal. Some types of capital budget acquisitions end up costing you operating expenses. An example would be a new ventilator that has a disposable flow sensor. Other examples might be the acquisition of pulse oximeters, which will almost certainly generate operational costs associated with the sensors. Frequently a capital budget request is funded but directors–managers fail to increase the operating budget for the additional costs

---

[v]There is an NPV function in Microsoft Excel.

associated with the approved capital budget. One way to avoid this is to use a good payback analysis.

The payback period is conceptually simple. When will you recoup your initial investment of cash if you buy the equipment you are proposing? But there are a lot of technical details here. The cash flows from the equipment in the future must be adjusted to keep them in current dollars so comparisons can be made. Consider this. The SUV you bought last year for $30,000 would have been a very different financial transaction if you had bought it ten years ago for $30,000. This is because ten years ago 30,000 dead presidents was a very different amount of money. This is also true for cash flows in the future. They must be adjusted (discounted) to keep them in current dollars. Appendix D-3 shows a customary method of calculating the payback period for a capital purchase. It takes into account the acquisition costs of the equipment, the operating costs of various types, the future cash flows, and the discounted future value of the cash flows the equipment would generate.

Note the detailed analysis of all the potential "noncapital" costs associated with your capital budget request. What are not listed here are the potential costs from your information technology department (IT). If your equipment needs to be interfaced with the hospital's local area network, there will be costs associated with this and these should be included in your modeling. Because almost all clinical capital equipment costs in hospitals now have the capacity to be interfaced with the hospital's information systems, you should probably have someone from IT review all your capital equipment proposals. If you don't, you may end up getting capital equipment funded and purchased and not be able to use it because your IT department doesn't have the human resources it needs to get the network interfaces for your equipment working.

RENTING VERSUS OWNING

There is an entire industry devoted to renting you the respiratory therapy equipment you need and even plenty you don't need (if you are not careful). They will rent you oximeters, ventilators, capnometers, BiPAP machines, transcutaneous gas monitors, and pretty much anything else you can convince them you will use regularly enough for them to invest the capital to buy and then rent to you. Rental companies can be lifesavers. They can also be leeches that suck off a great deal of money from your operation. Renting is a nice tool for meeting episodic spikes in demand for clinical equipment that exceeds your capacity. But you can find yourself constantly renting the same devices month after month. If this is true, you need to consider biting the bullet and acquiring more capital clinical equipment to meet this need and reducing your operating expense. Note that rental costs are an operating expense and as such can be something that becomes difficult for you to manage.

There are a wide variety of pricing schemes involved in renting equipment. The best systems involve metered equipment. Many companies will leave equipment on site all the time and only bill for it when it is used. You know when it was used because it is equipped with a time meter which ticks inexorably, like a cab meter in Las Vegas, but only when the equipment is turned on. Go for this plan, but be sure to train your staff to turn off rental equipment that is not in use. Of course they will also rent you stuff by the month, but often you don't use it that much and such a plan is not very fiscally sound. You need to have a good system for managing rental equipment. In the case of ventilators, what often happens goes like this:

- You are short of ventilators so you call and rent some.
- They come into the building and get put on patients.
- Then the angel of healing flies over the intensive care units, and many patients are extubated, and ventilator usage drops.
- According to the immutable truth of Murphy's Law, the patients on rental ventilators will not get extubated. And in the corollary, these patients will remain on the ventilator for several hundred days.
- Thus you will be paying for rentals when you have your very own, perfectly good, paid for ventilators sitting around.
- Speaking of immutable truths, these rental ventilators will not get replaced on patients unless you go and direct someone to do it or you train your supervisory staff to pay attention to this and make sure it happens. Switching out a ventilator is bothersome and can be risky, and it obviously should only be done on stable patients.

OPERATING BUDGETS

Capital budgeting is something you have to enjoy/endure only a few months of every year. But creating and managing an *operating* budget is a joy that stays with you year round like Christmas lights that you decide to leave up after the holidays because you will just have to put them back up in 10 or 11 months if you take them down in January. The more care you take in crafting your operating budget, the less heartache you will have in the long run. Creating and managing an operating budget is hard work. In fact a lot of managers have trouble doing it right. It is pretty typical for hospitals to have periodic difficulties with finances because of poor control of budgeting.[3]

To begin you must learn the terminology of budgeting. You might assume that the language of budgeting is the same language as the Magna Carta and the Declaration of Independence, but you would be wrong. It is unique and very special. Table 7-1 lists some translations of frequently used terms that might help you.

I tend to think of budgeting in basically two broad categories, although they are obviously linked: (1) spending accounts budgeting and (2) staff budgeting. Spending accounts are categories like medical supplies, salary dollars, office supplies, gases, etc. Staff budgeting is the process of calculating how many positions you need, how many you used, the difference between the two, and what in the world you are going to do about it. The nomenclature of management requires people to be renamed. Instead they are full time equivalents or FTEs. An FTE is really a calculator or a way to standardize how we count hours worked. If you worked 8 hours a day, 5 days a week for all 52 weeks, you were the perfect employee; you would have worked 2080 hours. This is the calculator for FTEs in a year. A great example to remember

Table 7-1. Operating Budget Terminology

Term	Definition and other witty comments
Actual budget	Actual budget is what was actually spent in a given expense account.
Fixed budget	Fixed budget is what you should have spent in a given expense account. This is customarily the total amount you should have spent for the year divided by 12 (budgeting in hospitals is almost universally done in monthly epochs). There is sometimes some seasonal adjustments in these categories based on historical trends for given times of the year.
Flexed budget	This is also sometimes called the volume-adjusted budget. It is an adjustment to the fixed budget based on the activity of your department for that month. If you were busier, you should have spent more money. Thus flexed budgets for busier times are higher. This is good. But they are also lower during slower times. This may not be so good if you don't have a way to adjust your staffing down during slower times. This adjustment is usually based on the amount of reported work that is done for the reporting period, which is usually derived from what was billed.

(Continues)

Table 7-1. Operating Budget Terminology *(Continued)*

Term	Definition and other witty comments
Variance	Variance can be good or bad. Good or favorable variance is when your actual amount of spending in any budget category was less than your budgeted amount. Bad or unfavorable variance is when it was more. When unfavorable variance exceeds certain thresholds, you will be required to explain why this happened and what you intend to do about correcting it. This is pretty much what they are paying you for.
Traditional budgeting	This is the most prevalent form of budgeting used in hospitals. It assumes that you do not have to build your budget from scratch. The hospital tacitly agrees that your current level of approved spending has already been justified and that the only detailed budgeting work required for next year is your justification of any additional or new spending you are proposing above existing levels of spending.
Zero-based budgeting	The converse of traditional budgeting, this requires a complete rebuild and justification of every budget category every year.
Full-time equivalent	Full-time equivalent, or FTE, is how we count people. And remember, we count people because people count. In the calculus of hospitals, a person is not a person. If a person works 2080 hours in a calendar year, *then* a person becomes a full-time equivalent. If this same poor fool only works 1040 hours in a year, he would be considered 0.5 of an FTE. Don't worry though because this does not mean that we think he is only half the man he used to be. No, no, it just means that in calculating staff costs we have to find a way to standardize the description of worked hours.
Position	A position is also called a job. These can be full-time, part-time, per diem, permanent, or temporary. If you have 10 people in your department and you want to have 11, you create a new position. This is not a real creative act, in a strict technical sense, although actually pulling it off can seem miraculous sometimes.
Direct expense	This is any expense that is posted to your budget that you actually have some control over.

Table 7-1. Operating Budget Terminology *(Continued)*

Term	*Definition and other witty comments*
Indirect expense	This is any expense that is posted to your budget that you do not actually have some control over. These are cleverly re-named by some accountants as allocations, accruals, trans-fers, whatever. They are conceptually the costs of running the hospital that are transferred from nonrevenue generating departments. Examples include the cost of utilities, the cost of the clinical engineering department, or the costs of the payroll department. This is done to share the pain and link expense with revenue. Sadly you have no control over these expenses, and they seriously affect your bottom line (profits), or in the case of nonprofit hospitals, margin.
Variable hours	Variable hours are the paid hours related to work that varies depending on the business of the hospital. Typically clinical RT work is always variable hours.
Nonvariable hours	The hours of employees who come to work whether it is busy or slow are called nonvariable hours. Their total worked hours are generally not affected by how busy the hospital is. If you are a manager, your hours are almost certainly all nonvariable hours because you come to work every day no matter the volume of patients (at least your boss thinks you're coming in every day).
Posting	Posting is the act of entering a debit or credit into the gen-eral ledger. This is how expenses get assigned to your ex-pense account.
Accrual	Accrual is the accumulation of a benefit over time. For example, paid time off is accrued as is seniority.
FOB	In the United States freight on board (FOB) refers to when the title for goods passes from the seller to the buyer. "FOB shipping point" means that the title transfers from seller to buyer at the origination point of shipping, and thus the buyer pays shipping costs. "FOB destination" means the title trans-fers when the goods reach their destination, and thus the seller is responsible to pay for shipping. Make sure you get FOB destination.

about FTE calculation is that it takes 4.2 FTEs to staff one RT around the clock 365 days per year. Here is how that calculation works:

$$\frac{365\ days}{1\ year} \times \frac{24\ hours}{1\ day} \times \frac{1\ FTE}{2080\ hours} = 4.2\ FTE's$$

Of course the world is seldom quite this perfect. This calculation does not take into account vacation, sick leave, and other vagaries. We will discuss this more shortly.

Budgeting for spending accounts in hospitals usually follows the traditional method where your current budgeted level of spending is considered to be automatically justified by the very fact that it already has been spent. Thus what you must work on justifying is any increase in spending you may be proposing for the coming budget cycle. Spending accounts are normally adjusted upward each year automatically by an agreed on inflation factor. "Agreed on" is a slight euphemism here because it won't really matter much whether you agree on this inflation factor or not. Someone else, notably the CFO or budgeting director, will agree on the inflation factor and you will have been rather unceremoniously informed of this factor. The inflation factor is supposed to take into account the yearly increase in the cost of the supplies you buy.

The new budgeting cycle will start a few months before the end of the current fiscal or calendar year. Some hospitals use a calendar year and some use a fiscal year, which is a convention whereby the year end for financial purposes does not fall at the same time as the year end of the calendar. This mostly came from retailers who are very busy indeed at the end of the calendar year with the intense feeding frenzy of conspicuous consumption attendant with the deeply religious nature of the celebration of Christmas. Who wants to spend November and December trying to hammer out a budget for next year when there is all that football to watch, turkey to eat, and parties to attend? It also came from the academic world where the expenditures are closely associated with the cycle of the academic year.

To budget for the coming year, you will have to figure out what you have and will spend by the end of this year. Unfortunately you start planning the budget long before the actual end of the fiscal year. Therefore you will have to engage in one of my favorite things, forecasting, which (understandably) is also called conjecture and guessing in my thesaurus. While easy to do on paper, at least from a budgetary point of view, forecasting can be somewhat risky in its prosecution. Consider the following remarkable predictions:[4]

- Radio has no future. Heavier-than-air flying machines are impossible. X-rays will prove to be a hoax. (Lord Kelvin, English scientist, 1899)
- Everything that can be invented has been invented. (Charles H. Duell, Office of Patents, 1899)
- There will never be a bigger plane built. (A Boeing engineer after the first flight of the 247, a twin engine plane that carried ten people)
- There is no reason anyone would want a computer in their home. (Ken Olson, president of Digital Equipment Corp., 1977)
- Ours has been the first, and doubtless to be the last, to visit this profit-less locality. (Lt. Joseph Ives after visiting the Grand Canyon in 1861)
- There is not the slightest indication that nuclear energy will ever be obtainable. It would mean that the atom would have to be shattered at will. (Albert Einstein, 1932)
- We don't like their sound. Groups of guitars are on the way out. (Decca executive, 1962, after turning down the Beatles)
- Who wants to hear actors talk? (H.M. Warner, Warner Brothers, 1927)
- It will be years—not in my time—before a woman will become Prime Minister. (Margaret Thatcher, 1974)
- With over 50 foreign cars already on sale here, the Japanese auto industry isn't likely to carve out a big slice of the U.S. market. (*Business Week,* August 2, 1968)
- Computers may weigh no more than 1.5 tons. (*Popular Mechanics,* 1949)
- The bomb will never go off. I speak as an expert in explosives. (Admiral William Leahy, U.S. Atomic Bomb Project)
- I'm just glad it'll be Clark Gable who's falling on his face and not Gary Cooper. (Gary Cooper after turning down the lead role in *Gone with the Wind*)
- We don't need you. You haven't got through college yet. (Hewlett Packard excuse to Steve Jobs, who founded Apple Computers instead)
- I think there's a world market for about five computers. (Thomas J. Watson, chairman of the board of IBM)
- Airplanes are interesting toys, but they are of no military value whatsoever. (Marshall Ferdinand Fock, Professor of Strategy, Ecole Superieure de Guerre)
- Stocks have reached a permanently high plateau. (Irving Fisher, Professor of Economics, Yale University, 1929)
- No matter what happens, the U.S. Navy is not going to be caught napping. (U.S. Secretary of Navy, December 4, 1941)

I bring all this up for its obvious humorous value and as a cautionary tale about the utility of predictions. The more time you spend developing your predictions the greater chance they have of approximating reality. But in the highly dynamic and sometimes volatile nature of the hospital business, predicting can sometimes be pretty inaccurate, and you should take care not to base your success or failure entirely on the accuracy of a prediction.

Forecasting spending accounts starts with just forecasting the remainder of the year. Consider the example of the hospital that has a fiscal year that ends in December. Sometime in August or September you will probably be asked to start budgeting. At that time you have financial data probably through August. To estimate spending for the entire calendar year you will have to use a technique called "annualization." Here you take the data you have for 8 months and project it out to 12 months, assuming the last 4 months will be about the same as the first 8 months. Most of the time this is okay, but sometimes patient volumes or the mix of patients can change pretty drastically, and this can greatly affect your budget predictions. There is no cure for this, but the disease can be treated to minimize the symptoms. Patient mix is an important aspect of the cost drivers in a hospital. Some types of patients cost a lot more than others, and cost estimations can be profoundly affected by relatively subtle changes in this mix. An example might be patients who receive inhaled nitric oxide, a pulmonary vasodilator. A single patient can use $12 thousand worth of nitric oxide in 96 hours. It doesn't take too many of these patients to skew your budget for the expense of nitric oxide.

The best way to minimize the effect of unpredictable variation is to get all the historical data you can. It is useful to look back at least three years to see if there is any recognizable seasonal variation that can help with the accuracy of your prediction. Five years would be even better.

The formula for annualizing any account is simple:

$$A = \left[\frac{YTD}{M}\right] \times 12$$

Where:
A   = Annualized spending (forecast)
YTD = Year to date spending in a given account
M   = Number of months in the year to date

When you have made this simple mathematical estimate of the annual spending for an account, you must then put on your thinking cap and ponder if there is anything on the horizon that might change spending for this account for the remainder of the year or into the next year. Some factors that might contribute to spending in the coming year include (but are not limited to):

- New stuff—New procedures or technology that might be coming soon or have already been included in the capital budget. An example might be a doctor who advocates the use of Heliox therapy. Heliox is very expensive, as is inhaled nitric oxide, Ribaviran, ECMO, certain kinds of high-flow nasal cannula circuits, and lots of other stuff. Keep your ear tuned to potential changes in the utilization of costly interventions. Ask around. Check with key medical staff members about what might be brewing. Also new technology might be on the horizon and coming like a battleship at flank speed. You can stay abreast of these changes by attending conferences and symposia, as I mentioned earlier.
- Changes in the physician referral patterns—New physicians may come to your area or current ones may leave. Some specialties generate a lot of business for the respiratory therapy department, like pulmonary, neonatology, cardiac surgery, internal medicine, etc. Keep an ear open for any changes that might increase the referral of respiratory patients to the hospital. Ditto for changes that might decrease these types of patients.
- Changes in the supply chain—Perhaps new vendors are entering the market or existing ones are leaving. Prices might change. This happens a lot in the rental business. Also changes in contracting can affect your supply costs. If you have been in a group purchasing organization (GPO) or supply contract of some type for a few years, the contract may be up for renewal, and prices might increase.

No one can accurately predict all of this stuff, but keeping these things in mind and doing some investigation and research can help you make better budgeting predictions.

Immutable Truth #22: There is wisdom in the counsel of many. One of the best ways to develop a sound budget is to not do it with the door to your office closed. I believe in open book management. There are departments where hardly anyone but the director–manager ever sees the budget. This generally ain't good. Your staff should periodically see the performance of the budget. I periodically show the actual budget reports to the staff. This can be done at staff meetings or at various department council meetings. I would be careful in distributing printed copies simply because it is sensitive information and papers tend to have mysterious abilities to travel to remote and unwanted locations. Here is one example of how I did operating budgeting at one hospital:

1. Schedule a leadership team meeting, usually an off-site, all day affair.
2. Arrange for projection equipment and computer resources.
3. Create a budget spreadsheet with all the accounts annualized and next year's projected spending all linked up with formulae so that the bottom line would reflect any change in any given account (see Figure 7-1).
4. Project the spreadsheet and go through the budget a line at a time.
5. Encourage everyone to participate. If some folks stayed quiet, I would go around the room and "poll the jury" for every suggested change to the budget.

Another technique for cost control and effective budgeting is the use of accounts payable detail. This is sometimes called the AP detail report and contains information on everything spent in all the accounts for your department. You can get this report from your budgeting department. Sort the information by dollar amount from highest to lowest. Then start at the top of the list and analyze where you are spending the most money. This will help you focus on where you might have a chance to reduce expenses.

To budget for salary expenses, I like to use what I call a position control chart. An example of one can be seen in Figure 7-2.

This spreadsheet helps you account for basic salary expenses. In addition, I have constructed this analysis to account for some expenses that are often not carefully considered, including shift differential, the cost of benefits, and the cost of replacement. When your staff takes advantage of the paid time off they have accrued, you may well have to replace them and pay others to work in their place either using overtime, per diem staff, or agency staff. This additional cost of replacement is often not budgeted for. This spreadsheet takes into account each individual's rate of paid time off (PTO) accrual. It assumes that clinical staff members have to be replaced about 75% of the time. This will vary from hospital to hospital. For nonclinical staff it assumes no replacement. Notice that the position control chart can be used to calculate both salary expenses and the number of FTEs you will need to plan for in your budget. So you can see how these two spreadsheets, Figures 7-2 and 7-3, can be used to construct a reasonable budget. Only one thing is missing: the cost of overtime. Very few departments are able to function without utilizing some overtime. The simplest way to budget for this is to simply look at the 3- to 5-year history of total overtime hours paid, and use this to estimate overtime hours for next year. In the case of budgeting hours, there is no real need to account for inflation, just simply budget the average number of hours you have used over the last few years.

EXPENSES

ACCOUNT DESCRIPTION	LAST YR ACTUAL A	YR TO DATE ACTUAL B	CURRENT YR END FORECAST C	CURRENT YR END BUDGETED D	NEXT YR BUDGETED E
OXYGEN AND OTHER GASES	$82,800	$65,457	$87,276	$87,868	$87,276
MINOR MEDICAL EQUIPMENT	$17,447	$14,409	$19,212	$15,450	$19,212
MEDICAL SUPPLIES	$533,358	$425,601	$567,468	$557,000	$567,468
OFFICE-COMPUTER-PRINTING SUPPLIES	$20,552	$17,049	$22,732	$21,785	$22,732
BIOMEDICAL SERVICES	$59,992	$46,253	$61,671	$60,500	$61,671
PHYSICIAN ADMINISTRATIVE	$65,650	$52,368	$69,824	$69,589	$69,824
OTHER PURCHASED SERVICES	$24,482	$18,657	$24,876	$25,950	$24,876
EQUIPMENT RENTALS	$83,636	$68,952	$91,936	$90,000	$91,936
OTHER MISCELLANEOUS EXPENSES	$12,416	$13,922	$18,563	$12,500	$18,563
TRAVEL/CONFERENCE	$9,512	$8,122	$10,829	$9,750	$10,829
TOTAL PROJECTED CURRENT YEAR EXPENSE			$974,387		
TOTAL BUDGETED CURRENT YEAR EXPENSE				$950,392	
TOTAL NEXT YEAR'S BUDGETED EXPENSE					$974,387
% INCREASE THIS YEAR'S BUDGETED TO NEXT YEAR'S BUDGET					3%

Figure 7-1. Operating Budget Planning Spreadsheet

An example of an operating budget planning spreadsheet. Actual spending year to date is used to "annualize" (forecast) spending for the remainder of the year. In this example, you are in the 9th month of the year. Hence the formula for the year end forecast is [(B/9) × 12]. Next year's budgeted amount is simply this year's forecasted spending. Typically, you are given a maximum percentage increase from budget to budget which you cannot exceed. In this example the budget-to-budget difference is 3%. If you use a spreadsheet with the formula set up properly, you can then adjust amounts for individual accounts and immediately see the effect on the bottom line.

Name	Budgeted FTE	Budgeted Paid Hours	Hourly Rate	Base Salary	Job Title	Shift Worked	Shift Differential	Base Salary + Shift Differential	Benefits Adjuster	Total Compensation	PTO Accrual Rates	PTO Earned (Hrs)	Replacement %
James, L	1.00	2080	$18.00	$37,440	Secretary	Days	$0	$37,440	1.243	$46,538	0.1308	272	0%
Johnson, M	1.00	2080	$42.00	$87,360	Director	Days	$0	$87,360	1.243	$108,588	0.1308	272	0%
Russel, B	1.00	2080	$38.00	$79,040	Manager	Days	$0	$79,040	1.243	$98,247	0.1308	272	0%
Wilkins, L	0.90	1872	$27.00	$50,544	Staff RT	Days	$0	$50,544	1.243	$62,826	0.1116	209	75%
Wade, D	0.90	1872	$27.00	$50,544	Staff RT	Days	$0	$50,544	1.243	$62,826	0.1116	209	75%
Unseld, W	0.90	1872	$27.00	$50,544	Staff RT	Days	$0	$50,544	1.243	$62,826	0.1116	209	75%
Thomas, I	0.90	1872	$27.00	$50,544	Staff RT	Days	$0	$50,544	1.243	$62,826	0.1116	209	75%
Stockton, J	0.60	1248	$27.00	$33,696	Staff RT	Days	$0	$33,696	1.243	$41,884	0.1116	139	75%
Sloan, J	0.60	1248	$27.00	$33,696	Staff RT	Days	$0	$33,696	1.243	$41,884	0.1116	139	75%
Sikma, J	0.90	1872	$27.00	$50,544	Staff RT	Days	$0	$50,544	1.243	$62,826	0.1116	209	75%
Robinson, D	0.90	1872	$27.00	$50,544	Staff RT	Days	$0	$50,544	1.243	$62,826	0.1116	209	75%
Oneil, S	0.90	1872	$27.00	$50,544	Staff RT	Days	$0	$50,544	1.243	$62,826	0.1116	209	75%
Nash, S	0.75	1560	$27.00	$42,120	Staff RT	Days	$0	$42,120	1.243	$52,355	0.1116	174	75%
Malone, K	0.60	1248	$27.00	$33,696	Staff RT	Days	$0	$33,696	1.243	$41,884	0.1116	139	75%
Jordan, M	0.90	1872	$27.00	$50,544	Staff RT	Days	$0	$50,544	1.243	$62,826	0.1116	209	75%
Johnson, M	0.60	1248	$27.00	$33,696	Staff RT	Days	$0	$33,696	1.243	$41,884	0.1116	139	75%
James, L	0.90	1872	$27.00	$50,544	Staff RT	Days	$0	$50,544	1.243	$62,826	0.1116	209	75%
Irving, J	0.75	1560	$27.00	$42,120	Staff RT	Days	$0	$42,120	1.243	$52,355	0.1116	174	75%
Havlicek, J	0.90	1872	$27.00	$50,544	Staff RT	Nights	$2	$50,546	1.243	$62,829	0.1116	209	75%
Lambier, B	0.75	1560	$27.00	$42,120	Staff RT	Nights	$2	$42,122	1.243	$52,358	0.1116	174	75%
Frazier, W	0.90	1872	$27.00	$50,544	Staff RT	Nights	$2	$50,546	1.243	$62,829	0.1116	209	75%
Schayes, D	0.90	1872	$27.00	$50,544	Staff RT	Nights	$2	$50,546	1.243	$62,829	0.1116	209	75%
Ewing, P	0.90	1872	$27.00	$50,544	Staff RT	Nights	$2	$50,546	1.243	$62,829	0.1116	209	75%
Duncan, T	0.60	1248	$27.00	$33,696	Staff RT	Nights	$2	$33,698	1.243	$41,887	0.1116	139	75%
Archibald, N	0.90	1872	$27.00	$50,544	Staff RT	Nights	$2	$50,546	1.243	$62,829	0.1116	209	75%
Bird, L	0.90	1872	$27.00	$50,544	Staff RT	Nights	$2	$50,546	1.243	$62,829	0.1116	209	75%

Name	FTE	Hours	Hourly	Salary	Role	Shift	Diff	Salary	Factor	Salary+Benefits	Accrual	PTO Hrs	Repl %
Salyer, J	0.90	1872	$27.00	$50,544	Staff RT	Nights	$2	$50,546	1.243	$62,829	0.1116	209	75%
Chamberlin, W	0.60	1248	$27.00	$33,696	Staff RT	Nights	$2	$33,698	1.243	$41,887	0.1116	139	75%
Bryant, K	0.75	1560	$27.00	$42,120	Staff RT	Nights	$2	$42,122	1.243	$52,358	0.1116	174	75%
Barkley, C	0.90	1872	$27.00	$50,544	Staff RT	Nights	$2	$50,546	1.243	$62,829	0.1116	209	75%
Abdul-Jabar, K	0.90	1872	$27.00	$50,544	Staff RT	Nights	$2	$50,546	1.243	$62,829	0.1116	209	75%
Vacant	0.90	1872	$27.00	$50,544	Staff RT	Nights	$2	$50,546	1.243	$62,829	0.1116	209	75%
Vacant	0.90	1872	$27.00	$50,544	Staff RT	Nights	$2	$50,546	1.243	$62,829	0.1116	209	75%
Walton, B	0.90	1872	$34.00	$63,648	Supervisor	Days	$0	$63,648	1.243	$79,114	0.1231	230	100%
Monroe, E	0.90	1872	$34.00	$63,648	Supervisor	Nights	$2	$63,650	1.243	$79,117	0.1231	230	100%
Gervin, G	0.90	1872	$34.00	$63,648	Supervisor	Days	$0	$63,648	1.243	$79,114	0.1231	230	100%
Homachek, J	0.90	1872	$34.00	$63,648	Supervisor	Nights	$2	$63,650	1.243	$79,117	0.1231	230	100%

Total Budgeted FTEs	31.2		Total Salary Dollars	$1,840,002
Currently Filled	29.4		Total Salary Dollars+Benefits	$2,287,122
Average Hourly Rate	$28.22			
FTEs for PTO Replacement	2.6		Total PTO Hours Earned	7448
Total Necessary FTEs	33.8		Converted to FTEs	3.6
			Average Replacement %	72%
			FTEs Needed	
			For Replacement	2.6

Figure 7-2. Position Control Chart

Sample of a position control chart. This spreadsheet helps you keep track of your positions, whether or not they are filled, and the total salary costs of running the department (excluding overtime). Notice that it includes an estimate of the number of FTEs required to replace staff who are taking earned time off. The accrual rates for paid time off (PTO) in this example includes total accrual for vacation, sick days, and holidays. Replacement rates are estimates of the percent of a position's time off that must be replaced by another staff member while they are gone.

FIXED VERSUS FLEXIBLE BUDGETING

When you have estimated the expenses in various budget categories for the coming year, they are divided by 12 and thus you have budgeted monthly expenses. Because these expenses are the same every month, this is typically called a fixed budget. Sadly, the ebb and flow and daily life in hospitals is hardly ever this constant. Some months are busier than others—way busier. Thus a fixed budget might not work so well for all months. Enter the flexed budget, which is also sometimes called the volume adjusted budget. The flexed budgeting process takes your fixed budgeting amounts and adjusts them up or down based on the relative change in activity from the original budget. "Activity" in this context refers to some measure of how busy the hospital is. Hospital activity is usually measured by occupied bed days. But this doesn't always work so well for respiratory therapy departments because your hospital might at times be mostly full of patients who don't require a lot of respiratory care. Or your hospital can be running at relatively low occupancy, and yet a large proportion of the patients may have a high demand for respiratory services. Some hospitals use occupied bed days anyway to describe how busy the hospital is when flexing the respiratory budget. I have also seen intensive care bed days used because some respiratory departments heavily concentrate their activities in the intensive care units.

Conceptually, flexed or volume adjusted budgeting works this way. You take the fixed budgeted amounts for a given month. This includes the volumes of procedures you anticipated doing and the actual volumes and amounts of money spent in various accounts. If you did a lot more procedures than you originally budgeted for, your expense accounts are flexed or adjusted up to account for this increased level of activity because you will surely have spent more money to deliver these additional procedures. Thus you would be allowed to have spent more money. The converse is true during times when your workload was slower than anticipated.

Not all hospitals use flexed budgeting. I have no real sense of how many do. I have seen it both ways. If your hospital does use flexed budgeting, you would serve yourself and your staff very well indeed to learn the intricacies of how the flexed numbers are created. Flexed budgeting formulae can be mind-numbingly complicated. You must try your hardest to understand how the finance department develops your numbers.

Whatever budgeting system is used, you will get a monthly report describing your budget performance. It typically includes your performance against your budget for the given month and year to date. Figure 7-3 is a

ACME REGIONAL MEDICAL CENTER

MONTHLY STATISTICAL REPORT

DEPARTMENT: Respiratory
MONTH/YEAR: May—76

REVENUE	May Budget	May Actual	May Variance	May Variance %	YTD Budget	YTD Actual	YTD Variance	YTD Variance %
INPATIENT REVENUE	$1,469,040	$1,163,550	($305,490)	(21)	$11,364,150	$10,393,428	($970,723)	(10)
OUTPATIENT REVENUE	$7,575	$9,733	$2,158	28	$59,135	$63,395	$4,260	8
GROSS PATIENT REVENUE	$1,476,616	$1,173,283	($303,332)	(21)	$11,423,286	$10,456,823	($966,462)	(10)
EXPENSES								
MANAGEMENT & SUPERVISORY SALARY	$35,462	$41,232	($5,770)	(16)	$224,123	$229,215	($5,092)	(2)
CLINICAL STAFF SALARY	$144,268	$127,406	$16,862	12	$1,345,380	$1,151,866	$193,514	14
CONTRACT/AGENCY SALARY	$0	$85,808	($85,808)		$0	$683,705	($683,705)	
EMPLOYEE BENEFITS EXPENSE	$44,353	$48,862	($4,509)	(10)	$413,958	$374,203	$39,755	10
MEDICAL GASES	$2,685	$2,226	$458	17	$32,745	$63,230	($30,485)	(93)
MINOR EQUIPMENT	$1,957	$3,272	($1,314)	(67)	$15,656	$12,716	$2,940	19
MEDICAL SUPPLIES	$23,063	$55,439	($32,376)	(140)	$281,255	$380,629	($99,374)	(35)
OFFICE AND OTHER SUPPLIES	$449	$1,057	($608)	(135)	$3,518	$9,798	($6,280)	(179)
BIOMEDICAL REPAIR & MAINT	$4,569	$3,609	$960	21	$37,800	$42,956	($5,156)	(14)
EQUIPMENT RENTALS	$11,910	$4,070	$7,840	66	$95,273	$54,332	$40,941	43
OTHER MISCELLANEOUS EXPENSE	$399	$1,603	($1,204)	(302)	$3,127	$10,699	($7,572)	(242)
EDUCATION/TRAVEL/CONFERENCE	$581	$239	$342	59	$4,554	$3,133	$1,422	31
TOTAL EXPENSES	$269,697	$374,823	($105,127)	(39)	$2,457,390	$3,016,482	($559,092)	(23)
FTEs								
MANAGEMENT & SUPERVISORY STAFF	6.2	6.4	(0.2)	(3)	6.2	6.5	−0.3	(5)
CLINICAL STAFF	29.3	27.7	1.6	6	40.0	35.9	4.2	10
CONTRACT/AGENCY SALARY	0.0	5.8	(5.8)		0.0	9.1	−9.1	
TOTAL FTEs	35.5	39.9	(4.4)	(12)	46.2	51.5	(5.3)	(11)

Figure 7-3. Typical Monthly Financial Report

Example of a typical monthly financial report. This particular month was not a good one for the Director of Respiratory Therapy at Acme Regional Medical Center. Notice all the numbers in parentheses. This is a standard way of notating "unfavorable" variance. In fact, it appears that 1976 has been a bad year altogether for this department, because they are seriously over budget on expenses and under budget on revenues. This combination tends to make administrators a little testy.

typical example of a monthly financial report. I made this one up to demonstrate how *lousy* budget performance would look. You would not want to see too many months in a row like this. I have absolutely no comment whatsoever whether this actually represents my budget performance in some other lifetime.

If you are significantly over budget in any of your accounts for a given month you will probably be asked to write a variance report. This may be called other things in different hospitals, but it is intended to be your explanation for how and why you were over budget, and what your plans are for correcting the budget performance in the near future. There are two bad things you can do about poor budget performance: (1) ignore it and hope it goes away, and (2) panic. While panicking can be fun in the short run, it will not serve you well for long. And, indeed, sometimes crummy budget performance for a given month will somehow amazingly self-correct itself the next month. But this is not usually the case. The best way to manage problems with budget performance is to get your team aligned with you in managing the budget. One way is to include financial performance measures in the supervisors' yearly performance appraisals, thus making their compensation dependent in part on these goals. Another is to share the budget performance with your staff. They may well be able to help you with ideas for cost savings or explanations for why the budget isn't performing.

The following are things I have done or heard of over the years that have had varying degrees of success at reducing operating expenses.

Recycling

The amount of disposables that we use in hospitals is shameful. There are allegedly lots of reasons we do this, and none of them strike me as very compelling. Some argue that the risk of transmission of infectious disease between patients is too great to clean reusable equipment and supplies after use. Thus, they claim, it is safer for patients to use disposables. As far as I know, no one has ever tested the assumption that there is a relationship between disposable supply usage and nosocomial infection rates. I suggest that you consider reusing certain types of disposable supplies. And don't let anyone tell you that it is somehow illegal or violates some FDA rules to reuse items marked "single patient use." There is no such injunction. However due diligence mandates that you follow all the required regulatory burdens adjacent to recycling disposables. There is a burden on you to ensure that your recycling procedures are carefully followed and that the products are tested and proven to work after reprocessing. Admittedly, for some classes of devices these burdens may be so great that it ain't worth it. There are third party companies that reprocess devices for you. One of the obvious devices to consider are disposable pulse oximeter probes, which can cost you tens if not hundreds of thousands of dollars per year and can easily be reprocessed.[5,6] You should also consider the environmental implications of how much hospitals contribute to filling up the landfills.

Reusable Products

An alternative to reprocessing allegedly disposable products is to switch whenever possible to reusable devices. If you are using disposables and there are reusable product options, you should carefully consider these. If someone tells you disposables are cheaper, don't believe it. They may be, but then again they may not be. Examine the issue carefully. Again, pulse oximetry is a good example because there are disposable and reusable sensors of almost every size from almost all manufacturers. Resuscitation bags are another item that might bear close examination. Disposables can be very expensive because a hospital can burn through a lot of resuscitation bags in a year. It has been argued that disposables are cheaper because of the labor costs associated with processing reusable devices. You must examine these claims very carefully. When I have looked at these claims they often turn out to be spurious. Besides, even if reusables versus disposables were economically a wash, I would still favor reusables for two reasons. First, if it costs the same to pay offshore disposable manufacturers versus paying local members of the community to process reusables, I would prefer to employ local members of the community. It is good press for the hospital. Second, even if costs are the same, it is still better to use reusables because of the environmental impact of heavy dependence on disposables. Reusables reduce the hospital's contributions to the local landfill or the local medical incineration company.

Hound Waste

A great deal of the consumption of supply resources in hospitals can be attributed to waste. How much? No one really knows for sure, but I estimate that it may be as high as 15–25%. Examples abound. Often, used disposable supplies in patient rooms at time of discharge are simply discarded. This should only be the practice when the patients are in isolation for infectious diseases. As an example, some hospitals put disposable resuscitators in all ICU rooms, and other hospitals put them in every patient room. Often, they are simply discarded between patients even though they are not used. These could safely be used on other cases. I know of pulmonary function labs that use MDIs for one study of bronchodilator response and then toss them because of alleged concerns about using them on multiple patients. If they were used with valved holding chambers, there could be no contamination from the patient to the MDI and thus could safely be reused. Again, if someone tells you there are regulations forbidding this, don't just believe it because someone said it was so. Check out the regulations carefully yourself.

Reduce Agency or Traveling Staff

This seems obvious, but of course dependence on temporary staffing is not an easy thing to escape from. But it can be done. It takes a long view and willpower. If you cannot recruit permanent experienced staff, figure out why. Improve your work environment. Petition administration for a better pay structure. Point out how it will save money in the long-term. If the labor market of experienced RTs in your area is just too tight, give up the search for experienced people and start hiring new graduates. Admittedly, this will take a long time to bear fruit, but at least you will be doing something that will eventually reduce your cost structure.

Improve Utilization

The truth is that unless you have worked hard on improving utilization already, about 25–50% of the routine respiratory therapy administered in your hospital is probably of little value to patients.[7] I realize this borders on heresy, but hey, heresy is my middle name. And I am not the only heretic around. Finely honed, efficient respiratory therapy treatment systems don't just happen. Unless you have developed protocols and are constantly measuring their effectiveness and adjusting them, your respiratory therapy utilization will be out of balance. You have to lean on the system all the time. You must apply steady, gentle pressure to get consistent, sustained improvements. Even if you only make a 10–15% reduction in utilization, this can have significant impacts on your cost structure. A certain percentage of the RT procedures delivered in your hospital are delivered by expensive people, such as those on overtime, from agencies, or traveling staff. If you can make even modest reductions in this top 10% of utilization, you might get some serious reductions in costs.

Decrease Frequency of Routine Checks

We do a lot of what we do because that is what we do and because it is what we have always done, etc. Sound silly? It is silly. But it is also true. The rational basis for what we do to and for patients is a bit lacking in some areas. Consider reducing the frequency of routine checks of equipment, such as oxygen rounds or equipment rounds. The frequency of ventilator checks is also a good place to examine your practice.[8] For the longest time we (the collective RT community) checked all ventilated patients every two hours. Finally this practice came under scrutiny because of how consumptive it is of resources. In many hospitals, patient-ventilator system checks every two hours have largely been to Q4 or even Q6. This is an excellent example of how deeply held spurious assumptions can be challenged and result in gained efficiencies.

Decrease the Frequency of Routine Apparatus Changes

Changing circuits, catheters, masks, resuscitation bags, and other devices is often done on an arbitrary schedule that may or may not be based on some solid science or reasoning. Examples of practices to carefully examine include the frequency of changing ventilator circuits, nebulizers, and resuscitation bags. In the case of both ventilator circuits and closed suction catheters, investigators have challenged extant practices or manufacturers' recommendations with regard to the frequency of changing these devices. They report being able to successfully reduce the costs associated with changing these disposable supplies.[9–13]

The Use of Heat and Moisture Exchangers

Heat and moisture exchangers (HME) and hygroscopic condenser humidifiers (HCH) can substantially reduce your expenses associated with conditioning inhaled gases during mechanical ventilation.[14–16] The traditional method of using vapor phase, pass-over heated humidifiers is relatively expensive when compared to the use of HME or HCH in most patients. You should examine whether this would save money in your facility.

REFERENCES

1. Bodenhimer T. High and rising health care costs. Part 2: technologic innovation. *Ann Intern Med.* June 7, 2005;142(11):932–937.
2. Chatburn RL, Primiano FP Jr. Decision analysis for large capital purchases: how to buy a ventilator. *Respir Care.* October 2001;46(10):1038–1053.

3. Clark JJ. Improving hospital budgeting and accountability: a best practice approach. *Healthc Financ Manage.* 2005;59(7):78–83.

4. Cerf C, Navasky V. *The Experts Speak: The Definitive Compendium of Authoritative Misinformation.* New York, NY: Villard Books; 1998.

5. Salyer JW, Lynch JM, Burton KK, Ballard J, Keenan JM. Adventures in recycling: the reuse of disposable pulse oximeter probes. Editorial. *Respir Care.* 1993;38:1072–1076.

6. Salyer JW. Clean em or toss em—does it matter? Editorial. *Respir Care.* 1993;38:1141–1142.

7. Stoller JK. The effectiveness of respiratory care protocols. *Respir Care.* 2004;49(7):761–765.

8. Salyer JW. Challenging assumptions: frequency of routine patient-ventilator system checks. *Advance for Respiratory Care Managers.* 2000;9:16–18.

9. Stoller JK, Orens DK, Fatica C, et al. Weekly versus daily changes of in-line suction catheters: impact on rates of ventilator-associated pneumonia and associated costs. *Respir Care.* May 2003;48(5):494–499.

10. Kollef MH, Shapiro SD, Fraser VJ, et al. Mechanical ventilation with or without 7-day circuit changes. A randomized controlled trial. *Ann Intern Med.* August 1, 1995;123(3):168–174.

11. Kollef MH, Prentice D, Shapiro SD, et al. Mechanical ventilation with or without daily changes of in-line suction catheters. *Am J Respir Crit Care Med.* 1997;156:466–472.

12. Dreyfuss D, Djedaini K, Weber P, et al. Prospective study of nosocomial pneumonia and of patient and circuit colonization during mechanical ventilation with circuit changes every 48 hours versus no change. *Am Rev Respir Dis.* 1991;143(4 Pt 1):738–743.

13. Hess D, Burns E, Romagnoli D, Kacmarek RM. Weekly ventilator changes: a strategy to reduce costs without affecting pneumonia rates. *Anesthesiology.* 1995;82(4):903–911.

14. Davis K Jr, Evans SL, Campbell RS, et al. Prolonged use of heat and moisture exchangers does not affect device efficiency or frequency rate of nosocomial pneumonia. *Crit Care Med.* May 2000;28(5):1412–1418.

15. Thomachot L, Leone M, Razzouk K, Antonini F, Vialet R, Martin C. Randomized clinical trial of extended use of a hydrophobic condenser humidifier: 1 vs. 7 days. *Crit Care Med.* January 2002;30(1):232–237.

16. Kirton OC, DeHaven B, Morgan J, Morejon O, Civetta J. A prospective, randomized comparison of an in-line heat moisture exchange filter and heated wire humidifiers: rates of ventilator-associated early-onset (community-acquired) or late-onset (hospital-acquired) pneumonia and incidence of endotracheal tube occlusion. *Chest.* October 1997;112(4):1055–1059.

CHAPTER 8

Evaluating Technology

Once technology is master, we shall reach disaster, faster.

—Piet Hein[i]

It is widely accepted that the single biggest contributor to the runaway train of rising health care costs in the United States is the alleged advancement of technology.[1,2] Yet it is not entirely clear that we are getting a reasonable return on our investment in all this gadgetry. It is inarguable that there are lots of technological advances that have substantially improved health outcomes since I started pushing IPPB machines and MA-Is around hospitals. Examples include advancements in cardiac medicine, less invasive surgical procedures, advances in cancer therapy, a phantasmagorical array of drugs, and, especially close to my heart, surfactant administration for neonates, which has played a large role in the profound improvements seen in the outcomes of neonatal care (see Figure 8-1).[3]

Consider also some of the other technologic changes that have occurred in the respiratory therapy universe. Notable among these are the growth in complexity and cost of mechanical ventilators and physiologic monitors in the last 15–20 years. Ventilators now have dual control modes, special adaptive software, visual displays of the measurement of flow, pressure and volume, sophisticated alarm packages, and the ability to export settings and measurements to computerized medical records systems. Some ventilators even measure tidal volumes in the tiniest of neonatal patients. Oops, that last part turned out, after all, not to be entirely true. Some of the ventilators widely marketed to neonates could not accurately measure tidal volume in the neonatal ranges.[4–7] Sadly, this was not widely understood by the respiratory therapy and medical communities for some time.

---

[i]Piet Hein (1905–1996) was a Dutch scientist, mathematician, and sage best known for his witty aphorisms. My favorite Heinism is, "Men, said the Devil, are good to their brothers: They don't want to mend their own ways, but each other's."

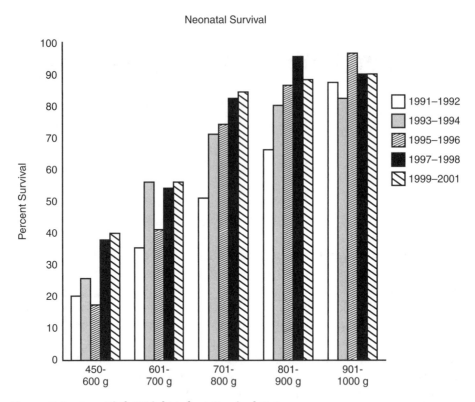

Figure 8-1. Low Birth Weight Infant Survival Rates
Survival of low birth weight infants reported from a Midwestern university department of pediatrics
from 1991 through 2001. This is prima fascia evidence that some technologies have probably been worth
the investment.
   Source: Adapted from Meadow W, Lee G, Lin K, Lantos J. Changes in mortality for extremely low
birth weight infants in the 1990s: implications for treatment decisions and resource use. *Pediatrics* 2002
May;113(5):1223–9.

   In the spirit of closing the gate after the cows have gotten out, we learned
that very little evidence was forthcoming demonstrating any benefit from
any of the dizzying array of modes and features that festooned the newer
models of ventilators, in neonates, pediatrics, or adults.[8] Thus lots of technology gets spread around the health care business without careful testing of
its impact on the processes of care. Of course devices are tested before they
are sold, under the watchful eye of Food and Drug Administration rules and
regulations. But this testing is typically focused on safety and efficacy. Lots of
questions are asked about technology before it is marketed, but
regrettably, they are often not the right questions.

You can add to the list of questionable technologic advances the nearly ubiquitous spread of advanced and costly continuous monitoring of various physiologic variables, such as heart rate, respiratory rate, temperature, every kind of blood pressure imaginable, arterial and venous oxygen saturation, partial pressure of dissolved gases in blood, pH, concentration of exhaled gases, and many others I can't recall. Oh, I forgot to mention that many of these can be measured both invasively and noninvasively. I say "questionable" because it is not entirely clear that the use of all this monitoring capability in its various manifestations has substantially changed the outcomes of disease. We simply haven't really tested the impact of much of this technology. To do so would require that we standardize the way it is used. Yeah right, like that's going to happen.

A great example of widely distributed but untested technologies is the use of continuous pulse oximetry. Now that I think about it, pulse oximetry *has* been subjected to some rigorous (and not so rigorous) testing. While pulse oximetry has an important place in the health care universe, I doubt if that is in the room of *every single patient*. When continuous pulse oximetry has been tested, it has almost always been found to have no effect on patient outcomes[9,10] unless it is used in a very carefully constructed clinical protocol.[11,12] Not only is there a conspicuous lack of evidence suggesting that pulse oximetry has any salutary effect on patient outcomes, it turns out that they create problems too, notably difficulty with lots of false alarms.[13,14] I am also convinced that the poor performance and overutilization of continuous pulse oximetry causes patient and family dissatisfaction and may contribute to unnecessary or prolonged hospitalization.

Why, you may ask, am I ranting about modes of ventilation of pulse oximetry? Because they are excellent examples of how we, as a respiratory therapy community, could have done a better job. We could have been more careful and thoughtful before we joined in promoting the spread of these unproven technologies, which I believe have added to the cost structure of inpatient care without clearly offering our patients a benefit.

We have a fiduciary responsibility to the communities we serve to be good stewards of the resources they give us. One important way to prosecute this responsibility is to be careful not to promote unproven technology and to carefully evaluate the performance claims of technology we are considering buying. Reconsider the example above of the allegedly improved neonatal ventilators that could measure exhaled tidal volume and had dual control modes of ventilation. I know of hospitals that replaced their older fleets of perfectly good, time-cycled, pressure limited neonatal ventilators for newer, allegedly sophisticated and certainly more complex ventilators based largely on the promise of a benefit to patients of volume measurement and dual control modes of ventilation. They substantially increased their cost of mechanical ventilation. If they were paying attention, they later learned that there was no real subsequent benefit to their patients. For the most part, when they got these ventilators in place, guess how they were and still are using them. Yep, in time-cycled, pressure limited modes. Had they bothered to do the most rudimentary bench testing they would have learned that the neonatal volume measurement claims of some of these devices were bogus. And without accurate measurements of tidal volume, dual control modes of ventilation aren't going to do you a whole lot of good. Thus they replaced their neonatal mechanical ventilators and are now using the new ones just like they were using the old ones.

Finally, lest I be accused of picking excessively in respiratory care technology creep alone, other disciplines are equally guilty of allowing the spread of technology for which proven benefits to patients have not been carefully established. Imaging services certainly fall into this category. Or perhaps radiology's problems might better be described as "overuse" of technology. Certainly computerized axial tomography (CAT), magnetic resonance imaging (MRI), and ultrasound imaging are nearly magical technologies that any modern hospital should have. But someone has clearly begun a long-sustained campaign that can only end, as far as I can see, in everyone who enters the hospital having a CT, MRI, and ultrasound as a screening panel at admission—kind of like vital signs. The use of these technologies is growing faster than almost any other segment of the publicly financed healthcare sector.[15] This will turn out to be fairly costly, since we are currently paying in excess of $350 per person per year for imaging services in the U.S.[16] Don't get me wrong. When I need my cardiac ultrasound, I am certainly going to want it right away. But there seems to be no meaningful movement inside the imaging community to establish some evidence-based practice regarding who might really benefit from the use of these technologies. Maybe this is because (unlike the respiratory therapy community), physicians' incomes are directly related to the volumes of these procedures done.

THE MARKETING OF HEALTHCARE TECHNOLOGY

I have lots of good friends in the manufacturing side of this business. They are good people trying to make a decent living. Many of them are former clinicians and understand the human (clinical) side of health care. But it is in their vested self-interest to represent their products in the best light possible. And shocking as this might be, some even misrepresent their products. This is not always intentional. It could well be they were given bogus or incomplete information about the products they represent by their respective engineering or marketing departments. Whatever the reason, it is safe, in fact it is really ethically required, that you assume that all manufacturers' claims are false or at least exaggerated. This is so much simpler than trying to deduce a priori, using nothing but the good offices of your astounding judgment, whether or not what you are being told is true. When you have experienced the liberating effect of deep skepticism, you can move on to the task given you: determining, as much as possible using tests and measurements, the truth about the utility and performance of the medical devices being marketed to you.

Immutable Truth #23: The burden of proof is on the advocate. The skeptic is not required to prove that something doesn't work. The burden of proof lies on the person advocating the intervention, or in this case advocating the use of a given technology. You do not have to prove that inhaled albuterol for the treatment of fever doesn't work. No, no, Dr. Kildare, the ordering physician is toting around *that* burden of proof. She must prove that albuterol *does* reduce fever.

If you think I am too dark and cynical about all this, just consider some interesting historical observations about the technology that we have embraced since I have been in the field. All of the technology and interventions I list following this paragraph have been discredited, fallen from grace, or never actually lived up to the early hype. Some of these technologies have been extensively studied for 20 years now, and you continue to find published results all over the map—there is a benefit, there is no benefit, there is a slight benefit—it all gives me a headache. In the interest of my spare time, I am not going to reference the medical literature in support of the following. But trust me on this one, anyone interested in examining the literature related to these things will find plenty to support what I am suggesting. Or you will find almost no published scientific literature at all on some of these topics, which kind of makes my point also.

- Intermittent positive pressure breathing (IPPB)—When I started in this field most departments had vast fleets of finely tuned IPPB machines, which battalions of RTs dutifully schlepped around the hospital in the belief that we were helping to minimize the effects of existing lung disease. This included such notably useless procedures as preoperative

IPPB, IPPB with normal saline, IPPB with bronchodilators for patients with no other symptoms but postoperative fever, IPPB with mucolytics, IPPB with alcohol (for fulminating pulmonary edema), IPPB, IPPB, IPPB, and more IPPB. This has (mostly) been mercifully abandoned. But not before creating a culture in the respiratory therapy community that I call *interventionism*, which is the noble, if somewhat incorrect, belief that doing something was better than doing nothing, even if the something was largely useless, consumed resources, and (we later learned) possibly was not so good for patients.

- Blow bottles—These devices were supposed to help prevent atelectasis and other postoperative pulmonary complications. Bubble bubble bubble went the blow bottles. If you are new enough in the field that you have never seen blow bottles, then count yourself fortunate.

- Ribaviran—At one time an RT department might have dozens of small particle aerosol generators humming along at the same time during bronchiolitis season to give life saving Ribaviran to infants with bronchiolitis. We even hooked these generators up to ventilators. This intervention failed to substantially change the course of bronchiolitis, and putting the devices into ventilator circuits was discovered to have a deleterious effect on the performance of the ventilators. We did not figure this out until we had spent hundreds of millions of dollars on this drug that cost about $3000 per dose.

- Endotracheal suctioning—Now I am wandering onto the thin ice of heresy. For decades we religiously inserted suction catheters into endotracheal tubes every two hours, rain or shine, morning noon and night. Oh yeah, we also poured normal saline down their tubes to loosen up those schmeehochers so we could suction them out. We were certain that this practice was essential, along with hyperinflation and preoxygenation. Unfortunately, along the route of the suctioning superhighway we forgot to do any real science about whether our assumptions were true. Now it is well understood that routine, scheduled suctioning is probably not good for patients, that every time we disconnect the ventilator for suctioning we lose functional residual capacity (FRC), that every time we use open suctioning we replace the oxygen enriched gas in the FRC with room air, and that the use of saline does most patients no good and may in fact be mostly deleterious. It is now also obvious that even suctioning with a closed catheter system significantly, if temporarily, lowers PEEP, which may contribute to atelectrauma. Unfortunately, this news is still being distributed.

- Cool and/or bland aerosols—I know of hospitals that had specially constructed mist rooms where a dense fog of cooled, bland aerosol was constantly generated and into which sick children with certain pulmonary diseases were lucky enough to get to sleep and play. This is a second cousin of the disreputable practice of hooking up a large volume nebulizer at the bedside and blowing a water aerosol somewhere almost but not entirely, close to the patient's head. Bland or cool aerosols are still used around the country, although they finally appear to be on the decline.
- Chest physical therapy (CPT)—Dateline 1990: Ninety percent of inpatient infants with bronchiolitis received CPT. In some hospitals this has now (dateline 2007) dropped to below 5%. But wait. If some hospitals use lots of lots of CPT and some don't use much at all, are their outcomes different? Does the use of CPT affect outcomes? Sorry Virginia, there is no Santa Claus, and CPT does not affect outcomes. By way of an example, Doug Wilson and Susan Horn studied 600 bronchiolitis patients receiving CPT in 10 pediatric hospitals and found that CPT utilization ranged from 4% to 71%.[17] I want to make sure you understand what this means. In one pediatric hospital, 4% of bronchiolitis patients received CPT and in another hospital 71%. Differences in severity of illness at those hospitals might explain this wide range, but the investigators found a negative correlation between resource utilization and severity of illness. In other words, it appeared that hospitals with lower severity scores were using *more* interventions.[18] This flies in the face of the argument that sicker patients have higher hospital bills because they require more interventions. This is unwarranted variation on a grand, breathless scale. The widespread overuse and misuse of CPT is no respecter of age and disease either. It is misused in adult populations as well as chronic and acute populations. There is an impressive armamentarium of percussors, vibrators, pounders, clappers, shakers, bakers, and candlestick makers marketed for administering this essential therapy. The burnished luster has worn off of CPT, which has now been shown to have no effect on outcomes of care in almost all populations, and it is detrimental in some.
- SIMV, APRV, PRVC, PSV, PAV, ASV, HFJV, HFOV, HFPPV, HFFI, PCIRV, MMV, blah de blah blah—: Yup, more heresy. There is little, if any, good controlled scientific evidence that any of these innovations turned out to make any substantial difference in the mortality and other outcomes of mechanical ventilation. To add to the ambiguity of all this, there are plenty of published papers about ventilator modes that contradict one

another. Well, of course it is nice for the clinicians to have all these tools to experiment with on patients, but I thought uncontrolled human experimentation was a bad thing. As much as you are convinced from your own experience that patients are alive who would have died without these interventions, your experience is still, regrettably, just anecdote. Remember immutable truth #4, the plural of anecdote is not data.

- Miscellaneous—This list could go on and on. I will finish by mentioning expiratory retard and its evil twin brother negative end expiratory pressure, inhaled nitric oxide, continuous pulse oximetry, indwelling blood gas instrumentation, and point of care blood gas testing. I know, I know, how can I list some of these things in this hall of shame of useless, vastly over-rated or untested technology? Because indeed they are either useless, vastly over-rated or untested. It would be a lot of fun to journey further back, say to about 1900 to 1950, and dredge up a few examples of the spread of useless or dangerous medical technology, but alas although I have the inclination and the wherewithal, I haven't got the time. One wonders what we are doing now that will be laughed at in 100 years.

My point in bringing all this up is to point out that we in the RT community could have been a little more skeptical and a little less willing to swallow the whole enchilada about the supposed utility of these interventions and technologies. Admittedly, there are a lot of people with dogs in this race, including doctors who ordered these interventions and hospital financial managers who saw a steady revenue stream. But we could at least satisfy our own ethical mandates by asking the right questions about, and doing some testing of, these "innovations" before we participated so wholeheartedly in their proliferation.

Efficacy, Efficiency, and Effectiveness

Sooner or later you will be told, either directly or indirectly, that some new technology will benefit your patients, or save you money, or make the therapists' jobs easier. As you ponder what you have been told, you might want to analyze this submission within the context of the three E's: Efficacy, Effectiveness, and Efficiency.[19] This is terminology used by researchers who conduct health technology assessments, which has become a specialized field of research. These terms have some classical definitions in terms of evaluating technology:

- Efficacy can be defined as the likelihood that a medical technology or intervention will achieve its desired effect under ideal conditions, such as a bench test or in vitro studies.

- Effectiveness is the performance of a medical device or intervention under ordinary, rather than ideal, conditions. Differences in the skill of clinicians, clinical conditions, or local disease profiles may mean that the technology does not perform as well in the real world of clinical practice as it did under ideal circumstances.
- Efficiency describes the combination of effectiveness and cost. Some things can be very efficacious but have such preposterous costs that they are not very efficient.

Case Study 14: Biphasic Quasi-Oscillatory Fusion Driven Reconditioning of Dephlogisticated Exhaled Gas Prior to Reinhalation

Woodland Hawk, the famous ventilation technology innovator, had done it again. His latest invention was causing quite a stir. The new Hyperpulmonastic Contiguous Logormorphic Ventilator with Flux Capacitor was being displayed at the Annual Corporate Conference of Expensive and Preposterous Technology (ACCEPT). It turns out this amazing new device was marketed as being able to improve oxygenation using mysterious biphasic quasi-oscillatory fusion driven reconditioning of dephlogisticated exhaled gas prior to reinhalation. According to literature provided by Mr. Hawk, this was proven in a vast series of laboratory studies using paid college students who desperately needed beer money. And indeed the device was shown to be highly efficacious because the average PaO_2 of said college students increased from 91 mmHg to 2.345×10^5 mmHg within 15 seconds of being placed on this remarkable instrument. Few, if any, people at the conference commented that otherwise healthy (although slightly pickled) college students might not necessarily represent the response of sick people to the subtleties of biphasic quasi-oscillatory fusion driven reconditioning of dephlogisticated exhaled gas prior to reinhalation.

Enter Bob Byealott, RRT, the director of respiratory therapy at the Acme Regional Medical Center in Cucamonga, California. Bob was thinking about replacing his fleet of aging ventilators and was intrigued with this new technology. His staff often had trouble oxygenating their patients, so he thought this ventilator would offer his patients a benefit. Bob got all excited about buying these ventilators. He was about to submit a capital budget request for $5 million for 10 of the new ventilators when his guardian angel tapped him on the skull one night and said, "Yo Bob, you should consider the real goal of mechanical ventilation, which is not increasing oxygenation per se but instead is supporting adequate respiration while minimizing lung injury. So

continues

Bob starting digging deeper and thinking a little more clearly about this. With this in mind it turns out the device was not quite as effective as hoped. He found a paper in the *Annals of Improbable Research (AIR)*[ii] that described a study of the use of the Hyperpulmonastic Contiguous Logormorphic Ventilator with Flux Capacitor. When placed on patients, it *did* create a considerable increase in oxygenation, but sadly had *no* beneficial effect whatsoever on length of ventilation, mortality, or morbidities associated with mechanical ventilation. Improved oxygenation alone might have been enough of a benefit to warrant acquisition of this new innovation, but alas the technology did not turn out to be very efficient, requiring as it did, a respiratory therapist to operate and a physicist to monitor the performance of the flux capacitor, not to mention a regular supply of tritium and a forklift to bring the ventilator to the patient's room.

Okay, this is a *slightly* silly example, but I had a lot of fun writing it. Let's try another one; how about inhaled nitric oxide? It certainly is efficacious, creating sustained increases in oxygenation in virtually every controlled scientific trial to which it has been subjected. But in my view, it did not turn out to be effective enough, if you broaden the definition of effectiveness to include substantially altering the course of disease, mortality, and morbidity. In the overwhelming preponderance of studies published on the gas, it appeared to have no (or very little) effect on mortality, length of ventilation, or other important morbidities. And it is certainly not a very efficient intervention, costing about $3000 per day for the gas alone, not including labor costs. More research is being done on inhaled nitric oxide and it may turn out to have other benefits not yet proven, but my goodness have we used a lot of it and spent hundreds of millions (if not billions) of dollars administering it so far.

I will describe three tools you can use in the prosecution of your due diligence in evaluating technology: (1) evaluating published evidence, (2) bench testing, and (3) clinical trials.

[ii]Don't laugh. There really is a journal called the *Annals of Improbable Research* (http://improbable.com/magazine/), which lampoons the publication of scientific papers. One of their most famous stories relates to the publication of a farcical parody of how to build a nuclear weapon. A copy of the article was reported to have been found among the papers in an abandoned Al Qaeda terrorist lair in the Middle East. For more fun with research read: Smith GCS, Pell JP. Parachute use to prevent death and major trauma related to gravitational challenge: systematic review of randomized controlled trials. *BMJ.* 2003;327:20–27.

"Measurement theory is the art of feeling confident about being in error."[20]

A great deal of the technology you will be required to evaluate as an RT manager involves devices whose design includes some aspect of measurement of the patient. Pulse oximeters measure infrared absorption of tissue beds. Mechanical ventilators measure the flow and pressure of gas. Humidifiers measure the temperature of gas. Capnometers measure the concentration of carbon dioxide in exhaled gas. Thus you very much need to be able to understand the strengths, limitations, accuracy, and precision of the measurements that are offered by the instruments and devices you are considering purchasing. *Immutable Truth #24: All measurements are erroneous.* This bloviation warrants some careful examination. In this context, "erroneous" means "containing error." When you step on your bathroom scale and it says you weigh 175 pounds, that is not your *exact* weight. You know this because you bought the cheapest bathroom scale you could down at Wal-Mart. It might misstate your exact weight by as much as two to three pounds. So what if you decide to go and get the best scale possible? You could get one of those nice medical scales ($2000) and determine your weight within about 0.2 pounds, but you still would not know your *exact* weight. In fact, if you got a scale that was accurate to within 0.0001 pounds, you still would not know your *exact* weight. But you would be mighty close. So how close is close enough?

We should stop here and define accuracy and precision. Accuracy can be described as the degree of agreement of a measured quantity to its actual or true value. Precision, which is also called reproducibility, is the degree to which further measurements will display the same or similar results. A measure may be accurate yet not precise, precise yet not accurate, neither, or both. A measurement is typically called valid if it is both accurate and precise. Figure 8-2 shows some visual examples of accuracy and precision.[iii]

What the user must figure out is if the inaccuracy and imprecision of the measurements are acceptable. In other words, how confident can you be that these errors are within a range of tolerance that still allows you to act upon these measurements? In terms of evaluating technology, you need to ask how large are the errors of the measurements of the devices that are being marketed to you? Are these errors acceptably small to allow clinical use of the

---

[iii]Further mind-boggling clarity on measurement science, accuracy, and precision can and should be added to your skills by reading Chatburn's excellent treatise on the subject: Chatburn RL. Evaluation of instrument error and method agreement. *AANA J.* June 1996 Jun;64(3):261–268.

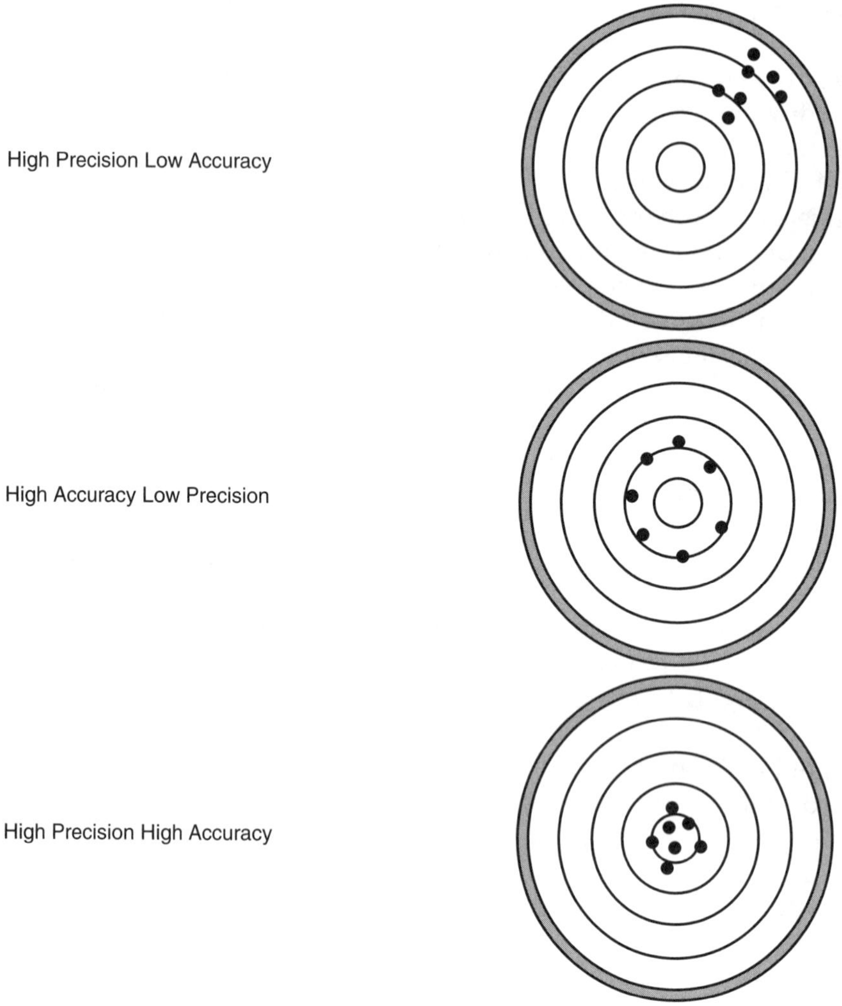

High Precision Low Accuracy

High Accuracy Low Precision

High Precision High Accuracy

Figure 8-2. Accuracy and Precision
Visual examples of accuracy and precision. High precision and accuracy can also be thought of as bias.

devices? Another aspect of this issue is figuring out whether the findings really matter. We might be able to produce a blood pressure cuff that can measure blood pressure to within an accuracy of 0.005 mmHg, but who cares? Nobody is going to make treatment decisions on differences in blood pressure of this magnitude. And you would not make dietary decisions based on changes in your weight on the order of a few tenths of a pound.

Another way I think about this is the concept I call the clinical effect size, which is the smallest clinical effect that would matter. If you are considering buying two devices that measure airway pressure and one is accurate and precise to within 1.0 cm H_2O and the other is accurate and precise to within 0.10 cm H_2O, should you go ahead and pay for the additional accuracy and precision? Because you definitely will have to pay for this added accuracy and precision? I would say no. No one will make meaningful clinical decisions based on differences in airway pressure readings of 0.1 cm H_2O.

You must also remember that all accuracy and precision statistics listed by manufacturers are determined under ideal and controlled conditions *by the manufacturers*. As soon as you start putting devices like mechanical ventilators on patients you will find that these "ideal" figures for accuracy and precision go in the tank.

Evaluating the published literature can include operating manuals, technical manuals, brochures, articles published in trade journals, masters and doctoral theses, scientific papers published in peer-reviewed journals, and the new kid on the block, Web-based information.

A thorough description of the science and art of evaluating published evidence and scientific papers are beyond the scope of this chapter. But we can take a brief journey through this forest. *Immutable Truth #25: All evidence is not created equal.* Oh my, how true this is. In fact, as true things go, this may be the truest of all the true things I have spouted. If I were speaking in Elizabethan English I would tell you, "Verily, 'tis so. Differences abound." Journals have different degrees of rigor in their reviewing process, and editors have different biases. And amazing as it may sound, researchers and scientists and journal reviewers have their biases too. I am convinced that there is no such thing as total scientific objectivity. We are all biased by our experiences and limitations. Good science acknowledges these biases and tries to design experiments and studies whose results cannot be affected by these biases. The system is far from perfect, but over time good science will determine the truth, if it is knowable.[iv] One of the most dangerous trends to emerge in recent years is the idea that science is about consensus. If this is accepted, science can devolve into an ugly political tool. While this has been happening for some time, it has grown exponentially lately and gotten very

---

[iv]Of course there is plenty of bad science out there, which some call junk science. This is mostly a result of political special interests that use pseudoscience to achieve their political ends, which usually involve lowering standards of living by assaulting your purse. Steven Milloy publishes an excellent Web site and printed materials that regularly debunk junk science. See www.junkscience.com.

scary. Consensus is about politics, not science. It only takes one scientist to be right, to change scientific truth, which is then verified by repeated experiments. Science has nothing to do with consensus. Science is about the creation of testable hypotheses that can then be verified through rigorous experiment and observation.

Some of my favorite examples of the dangers of consensus can be understood by considering the following:

- Edward Jenner (1749–1823) and smallpox vaccine—Edward Jenner was a country doctor in England who first discovered a method of vaccinating people against smallpox. His original report of his findings was rejected by the establishment (consensus), which, along with certain social and religious institutions, went on to ridicule him and humiliate him publicly for a number of years. Eventually his findings won over his opponents, mostly because his inoculated patients did not get smallpox, which was a viscious killer.[v] Of course, some say "science only progresses through the death of scientists" and many never accepted Jenner's findings.
- Ignaz Semmelweiss (1818–1865) and hand washing—Semmelweiss was a Hungarian physician who reduced maternal mortality due to infections from 17% to 1% in a Vienna hospital 20 years before Pasteur proved the germ theory to be correct. He achieved this by the then remarkable and outrageous requirement that physicians periodically wash their hands. The establishment (consensus) of the time ridiculed him and ran him out of Dodge. He died in an insane asylum.
- Repressed memory—An entire industry sprang up in the last half of the 20th century around the theory of repressed memories. The theory held that some memories, especially traumatic ones, could be stored separately from the conscious mind. While this might or might not be true, a consensus developed that these repressed memories could be recovered, and through such notable interventions as primal scream therapy,[vi] hypnosis, and group therapy, a psychological healing could take place. It was a widely believed consensus that these memories were valid, and treatments could be devised based on these repressed memories. Indeed, these rediscovered repressed memories were often used in

[v]The more cynical among us will remember the quote from the famous German physicist, Max Planck: "A new scientific truth does not triumph by convincing its opponents and making them see the light, but rather because its opponents eventually die, and a new generation grows up that is familiar with it."
[vi]OK, I admit it. I spent quite a bit of time and money in primal scream therapy, long ago when the earth was young. Details shall remain unstated, as I trust not my tongue to tell this story.

criminal and civil proceedings by plaintiffs who claimed victimhood as a result of the rediscovery of these hitherto repressed memories 15, 20, even 40 years later. This hokum has finally come under the scrutiny and skepticism that it so richly deserves. Sadly not before much damage has been done. A secondary industry sprang up that specialized, although unwittingly, in implanting (not discovering) false memories. The whole enchilada was mostly dismantled by a series of well deserved lawsuits.

• Eugenics—In 1863, Francis Galton, an English scientist, coined the term "Eugenics," which stems from the Greek word "eu" meaning good, and the suffix "genes" meaning born. This social philosophy, although probably noble in its inception, eventually came to represent the view that humanity could be improved, to the betterment of all, through selective breeding, forced sterilization, institutionalization or killing of individuals with genetic defects, and finally (in the horror of the Third Reich) genocide of "undesirable" races. For a considerable time, eugenics could be regarded as the consensus. None other than Alexander Graham Bell, George Bernard Shaw, and Winston Churchill were adherents. Bastions of enlightened thinking, such as the Ford Foundation and the Rockefeller Foundation, supported eugenics research and advocacy financially. Many colleges and universities had eugenics as an academic discipline, and the editorial boards of many "scientific" journals were adherents to this now discredited science. This is a great example of the difference between, and the dangers of, confusing science and consensus.

Anyone interested in studying the debate about consensus versus science is directed to the writings and speeches of Michael Crichton for some excellent and balanced discourse on this topic.[21]

I have to stop here for a moment and point out that I believe the most serious and potentially risky example of the consequences of confusing consensus and science is the current debate raging about the influence of humans on climate change. Way too much of what we are hearing about this debate is based on computer models and assumptions. Of course, science is always an iterative process and, although there are ups and downs, our knowledge generally increases over time. This will be true about the magnitude, consequences, and causes of climate change. But when I was a kid in Ohio and looked out the window, I could see the results of climate change. The Great Plains from Pennsylvania to Nebraska were scraped flatter than a pancake by the receding glaciers of the last ice age. The melting of these glaciers created the Great Lakes. Now *that* was climate change. It appears that the planet has been warming for some time. And, apparently, humans had nothing to do with that change. We should certainly do everything within reasonable limits to look for alternative and sustainable sources of energy. But the "consensus" of man-made global warming is and will be used as an excuse for promoting a political agenda, including a vast transfer of wealth and an increase in the power of governments, neither of which is likely to do us any good in the long run.

I got off on this tangent for a reason. Medicine is particularly prone to the dangers of confusing consensus with science, and nowhere is this truer than the practice of respiratory therapy. For example, consider the work of Branson and Johannigman.[8] In this excellent review they point out that there is really no compelling evidence to suggest that any of the newer modes of ventilation are any better than any other mode with regard to changing the outcomes of mechanical ventilation. Yet there is a strong consensus in the respiratory community about many of these modes and a widely held view that you have to have ventilators with these advanced features to offer your patients the fullest possible benefit. Beyond improving the financial performance of ventilator manufacturers and increasing the cost structure of operating hospitals, I am not sure what we have accomplished by the introduction of all this new ventilation technology. The more cynical among you might ascribe my cynicism to the encroaching effects of age combined with my own well known proclivity for the office of the curmudgeon. Maybe you are right. But I doubt it. I prefer to think of my cynicism as a "healthy" skepticism. I have bought newer generation ventilators twice in my career, not because of the availability of various modes, but because I thought they improved our ability to measure what was going on at the patient's airway, which I believe is the pathway to enlightened ventilation.

There is another caveat when evaluating and/or obtaining new technology. It involves the introduction of new risks to patients. When new technology is applied to patients it can often mean increased risk for the patients (transiently or permanently). Usually new technology adds a layer of complexity to the clinical environment. Anytime you add complexity you increase the chance for misapplication (screwing up). Something as complex as the latest generation of mechanical ventilators adds a lot more weapons to the clinical armamentarium. But this complexity comes with a cost. It will take a while for the clinical staff to really master the new devices. In the interim, patients are at increased risk of operator errors. And if the design of the device is complex enough, this risk may not go away when the staff has completed their training. There was a wildly popular ventilator from Europe that is still very widely used in the United States. It (and its ancestors) had a design feature such that control knobs were labeled in a confusing fashion. For inexplicable reasons it was decided to design a human interface where you had a knob that was labeled one thing, and when you turned it, something else happened. That is a recipe for operator errors. I suspect that it contributed to plenty of application errors, but no one knows for sure because we have no systematic way of measuring errors in the health care system. Let us hope (1) I am wrong about this ventilator and human errors and (2) that someday this paucity of error measurement changes.

This increased risk to patients might be worth it. Extracorporeal membrane oxygenation is incredibly risky, but it also offers patients an incalculable benefit—life over death. So clinicians and families are willing to risk it. In the great calculus of risk-benefit analysis, this is the equation that must be solved. You must assess the potential benefit you are offering the patients and weigh it in the cosmic balance of logic against the potential risk you are also introducing. Let me give you another example. Consider high frequency oscillatory ventilation. While opinions are divergent about the benefits of this technology, let's assume for a moment that it clearly offers a considerable benefit to patients. But it also comes with risk. The devices have a completely different set of operating parameters than conventional ventilators. They are more complex to operate. The interface between the instrument and the physiology of the patient requires a different way of thinking about the movement of gas in and out of the human lung. The average duet of physician–respiratory therapist cannot hope to operate the device with any skill whatsoever without extensive training and experience. Sadly this is not how it is usually introduced into intensive care environments where it has not been used before. I have seen some seriously bad management of oscillators by people who were dedicated and experienced clinicians; they just weren't skilled and experienced with the oscillator. This is a terrible catch-22.[vii] You cannot get skilled and experienced on the oscillator unless you use it a lot. Then it might offer a benefit to your patients. But the patients that you learn on are not offered much of a benefit. Complex technology like an oscillator or ECMO or cardiac surgery needs to be done with a frequency sufficient to keep the clinical staff competent and skilled. It has been shown repeatedly that centers that

---

[vii]Some of my readers may not have experienced the cleansing effect of reading about Captain Yossarian. *Catch-22* is the title of a novel about this World War II bombardier. I won't spoil it for you except to say that catch-22 has become a slang term referring to an unsolvable conundrum, an irreducible paradox, indeed the horns of an eternal dilemma. Warning: This book is dark, absurd, funny, and tragic.

do a low volume of complex, risky procedures have worse outcomes than centers that do a high volume of complex, risky procedures.[22]

Branson and Johannigman[8] list a useful way of thinking about grading the quality of evidence in the form of published reports. Let's examine the types of evidence they describe.

Randomized Controlled Trials

These are the gold standard of published evidence. These trials are difficult to design (properly), expensive to carry out, and consequently, with regard to studying respiratory therapy technology like mechanical ventilation, they are pretty rare. Consider this: In 2002, in the same issue of the *New England Journal of Medicine* there were two randomized controlled trials published that studied high frequency oscillation in neonates.[23,24] You might have thought this would be a happy occurrence because you can never be too rich, too thin, or have too many published trials. Regrettably it was not a happy moment because these two studies of the same intervention in mostly the same populations had divergent findings. One found a benefit to HFOV in neonates and one did not. Sigh.[viii] Still randomized controlled trials (RCTs), though sometimes flawed, remain the best form of evidence we have. Note, however, that pesky old statistical significance requirement for our results. This requirement is based on some very solid (immutable) statistical truths that underlie the theory of the design of an RCT:

- Assumption 1—You must have two (or more) randomly chosen samples of patients from the same overall population. This is a very big deal. Patients are randomly assigned to the control group or the experimental group. Great pains are taken to ensure that the allocation of patients to experimental versus control groups cannot be affected by the bias of the clinicians and researchers, who might be true believers or infidels with regard to the interventions being tested. Imagine that you are really, really sure that the intervention being tested is way better for patients, and you have a very sick patient whose best chance for

[viii]Minds immeasurably superior to mine have constructed explanations for why this occurred. It is argued that this divergence in findings was because the benefit of HFOV was limited to very low birth weight infants who had a certain severity of illness. Well, God bless them, but these ventilators are applied much, much more indiscriminately than that. I suggest that the differences in outcomes in these studies might have been related to the skill in application of HFOV, which is a great example of the difference between efficacy and effectiveness. Or, there might be no real benefit to the devices when compared to properly executed conventional ventilation.

survival was to be assigned to the experimental group. If you could game the allocation system to ensure that your patient got assigned to the experimental group, you might be very tempted to do so, albeit for very altruistic reasons. To be a truly random sample, everyone in the population studied had to have the same chance of being included in your study and the same probability of being assigned to one group or another. The entire statistical premise of the RCT is dependent on the purity of the randomization process.

- Assumption 2—These two populations of patients are equally ill and are treated the same way in every aspect of care except the intervention being tested. They *should* be equally ill if they are randomly selected from the same population of patients. A lot of the data you see presented in RCT papers is an attempt to verify this assumption. Ensuring they are treated the same way in both groups is much more challenging. In ventilation trials in particular, a lot of work is required to develop and enforce ventilation protocols for the patients in the control groups. Remember that the assumption is that these two groups of patients are treated the same way in every aspect except the intervention being tested. Any experienced respiratory therapist knows that if you ask four different physicians how to do ventilator management on a very sick patient, you might very well get three different answers. Thus, unless detailed ventilator management protocols are described for the control group, your control group might not be very controlled after all.

- Assumption 3—Whenever possible, the researchers have eliminated or seriously reduced the likelihood that clinicians can consciously or unconsciously introduce bias into the treatment of one group or another. In tests of most respiratory therapy technology, this can be challenging. The concept is referred to as blinding. In drug studies, patients are blinded to whether they are receiving the drug or a placebo. This is called "single blinded." Also the clinicians are often blinded to whether or not a patient is receiving the experimental drug. This is called "double blinded" and helps remove the opportunity for clinicians to introduce bias by treating patients differently based on whether or not they think the patient is receiving the experimental drug. In studies of a lot of respiratory therapy technology, it is very hard to achieve either single or double blinding because it is pretty hard to hide what kind of device or mode of ventilation a patient is on.

If these assumptions are met and yet you find differences in the medical outcomes of the experimental group and the control group, it is reasonable for you to conclude that these differences in outcomes were the result of the intervention you studied. But there is a fly in the ointment. There are *always* differences. Measurements are never totally precise. Human beings vary (vive la difference!). There is a certain amount of background variability in all systems. By way of example, if you randomly select two groups of mechanically ventilated ARDS patients who were treated in the same hospital over the same period of time, and you determine their mean length of ventilation, the two means will be different. This is a result of normal random variation— variation in measurement precision and accuracy, variation in sickness of the patients, variation in the quality of the gray matter of the doctors and respiratory therapists making the ventilator management decisions, and lots of other indescribable sources of variation including mysterious and inexplicable cosmic forces. Now imagine randomly selecting another two groups of ARDS patients from the same population, for example the same hospital or the same time period. When you determine the mean length of ventilation of these two randomly selected groups you will discover, lo and behold, that the means are different. And this difference between means will be different than the difference between means of the first two random groups you pulled. See what I mean (yuk yuk)? If you repeated this experiment 100 times, you would discover that the differences between the means of each of the two randomly selected groups were actually normally distributed. In other words, if you plotted the difference between the means of each pair of samples taken on a histogram it would look like Figure 8-3. This statistical truth allows statisticians and researchers to give you a certain degree of confidence about the cause of differences in your means.

Imagine a study of two modes of ventilation: one well established mode and one new mode. The established mode has been deemed by the researchers to be the control group and the new mode the experimental group. You are happily reading through the study when you encounter a statement like this. "The mean length of ventilation in the experimental group was 5.6 ± 3.1 days versus 6.3 ± 4.2 days in the control group ($P < 0.05$)." From this finding the authors concluded that the new mode of ventilation was better. But what in the world do all these numbers actually represent? The mean values are obvious. The plus or minus values may be one of two variables. The standard deviation describes the variability of the sample data around the mean and is often reported as a plus or minus value. The other plus or minus value used is the

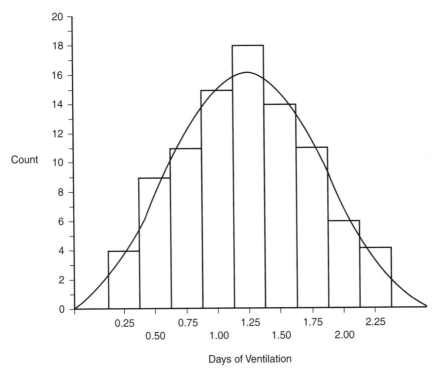

Days of Ventilation

Figure 8-3. Difference between Means of Sample Pairs
Theoretical distribution of the difference in length of ventilation between two randomly selected samples of ARDS patients, repeated 100 times. This graph demonstrates a principal feature of the central limit theorem: that such differences would be randomly distributed.

standard error of the mean, which is a measure of the uncertainty of the mean.[ix] This is an important distinction. The standard deviation is always much larger than the standard error of the mean. You will have to read carefully to figure out which is which. Some papers will not actually tell you what the plus or minus values are. This is bad form. Large standard deviations can be indicative of a highly variable measure. In the world of mechanical ventilation, the length of ventilation is often highly variable even within homogenous populations. This makes finding differences that reach statistical significance harder, and often very large numbers of patients need to be studied to ensure that your study does not have a large potential for an erroneous conclusion.

[ix]Standard error of the mean is calculated by dividing the standard deviation of the sample by the square root of number of measures in the sample.

Statistical significance *is* the take home number and is represented by the probability or P value. P values describe the likelihood (probability) that the difference between any two (or more) mean values were the result of normal random variation in your chosen measurement. If there is a low probability that the differences were the result of normal random variation, then it is safe to assume that the differences were actually the result of your experimental mode of ventilation. So how low a probability is required to reach this cherished level of confidence that is represented by statistical significance? In health care this value has been established for most types of research as $P < 0.05$. This then tells you that there is less than a 5% chance that you are wrong if you conclude that the differences in your measured samples is the result of your experimental intervention. Let's practice. If the P value had been 0.40, and yet you concluded that the difference in mean length of ventilation was the result of the new mode of ventilation, there would be a 40% chance that you were wrong.

One of the best tools for you to use in analyzing the published literature on a given technology or intervention is meta-analysis. This analytical tool is used by researchers who want to examine all the published literature on a given topic. A meta-analysis gathers all the published studies of a given topic, grades and analyzes the design and quality of the studies according to a set of a priori rules, and then attempts to pool the data and draw authoritative conclusions about the intervention being studied. You can find meta-analyses on such topics as the use of low tidal volume in ARDS, bronchodilators in bronchiolitis, high frequency ventilation, extubation readiness testing, use of steroids in various diseases, and on and on. The Cochrane Collaboration is one of the best sources of meta-analyses out there.

If you start reading a lot of meta-analyses you soon find that many of them do not draw authoritative conclusions about the topic they studied. The reason for this is there are simply not enough decent studies extant to warrant a conclusion. Another common finding is that the intervention being studied turns out to be of no discernable benefit to patients. These analyses are great tools for the health care manager trying to understand the real impact of given technologies on outcomes.

Observational Study

What if you cannot randomize your patients to one treatment group or another? Consider Dr. Casey and Dr. Zorba; each always uses his own preferred mode of ventilation when treating patients with the same disease. You decide to study the mortality, length of ventilation, and other morbidities of ventilation between these two groups of patients with hopes of finding out which mode of ventilation was better. This would be an observational study. Patients in the two groups may not be the same. Patients in one group may be sicker than the other. How patients came to be referred to or came under the respective care of each of these famous doctors may not be standardized at all and may be biased by factors that you, the experimenter, can have no control over or even knowledge of. As you might imagine, this type of research is full of potential biases, and the findings from such research do not carry the weight of credibility demonstrated by the randomized controlled trial. Besides the biases that might affect how patients got assigned to one doctor or another, you cannot have much confidence that the two doctors treat all the patients the same except with respect to the mode of ventilation chosen. A lot of observational studies get published because it is not always possible to execute randomized controlled trials. If differences are found in the outcomes of the two groups of patients studied, it could be because of a wide range of factors not measured or controlled by the experiment, and thus you need to keep this reduced level of confidence in mind when weighing the use of these kinds of findings in technology evaluation.

Studies with Historical Controls

This design is similar to an observational study except that it uses an historical control period instead of a concurrent comparison group. Suppose Dr. Romano had changed his practice with regards to managing ventilators about two years ago. Imagine that before that he used to always use tidal volumes $\cong 15$ mL/kg, but after reading a journal article or two, he got religion about using low tidal volumes and now never uses anything greater than 5 mL/kg. Further imagine that despite the fact that Dr. Romano is a despicable human being, you agree to help him study whether or not outcomes from his ventilated patients has changed since he started using a lower tidal volume. He suggests you study rates of pneumothorax, mortality, and length of ventilation for the period two years before he changed practice and compare these to the same measures for the two year period since he changed practice.

But consider all the variables to ponder. Remember the premise of studying an intervention like low versus high tidal volumes is that everything else that might affect outcomes of mechanical ventilation between then and now must be the same. The population of patients being ventilated must be about the same severity, as well as the methods of fluid management, airway management, cardiac inotrope use, antibiotic therapy, nursing care, extubation criteria, and lots of other stuff need to be the same between the two periods of time for you to be certain that any differences in outcomes of mechanical ventilation can be attributed to the change in tidal volume alone. This is particularly difficult in historical control models because of the tendency to have standards of care change over time as our knowledge and understanding grow.

Expert Opinion

Thomas Jefferson once said, "Error of opinion may be tolerated where reason is left free to combat it." When you depend only on expert opinion, you greatly increase the chances of being wrong. Everyone likes to trash "expert opinion" as a method for establishing standards of care or as a source of information when evaluating technology. But often expert opinion is all you have. The majority of health care interventions have never really been rigorously tested with regard to their effect on outcomes. Thus when you are trying to compile the best information about how to treat a given affliction, you are forced to rely on expert opinion. This kind of care modeling is susceptible to the monocular biases of whoever the experts are. The heavy reliance of the health care industry on expert opinion is what has historically contributed to so much unwarranted variation in care processes. The joke goes something like this, "If you ask four neonatologists to describe the best way to ventilate a diaphragmatic hernia patient, you will get five answers."

A recent and important example is the use of angioplasty for the treatment of angina. It has been widely believed and practiced for some time that mechanical dilation of coronary arteries using catheters (angioplasty) was the best way to relieve cardiac chest pain and reduce the subsequent risk of heart attack. Recently, a large, well constructed trial has pretty much settled the case that this invasive and expensive procedure is no better than medical management of angina, for example treatment with drugs, diet, and exercise. In the study, the patients treated with angioplasty had the same risk for further heart attacks than the patients treated medically, and the reduction in chest pain in the two groups pretty much stayed the same. But these findings fly in the face of the prevailing expert opinion. Of course, the slice of the industry whose economy is dependent on the furtherance of angioplasty is debating these findings.

One way to improve the quality of expert opinion is the use of expert panels, which are groups of recognized experts in a given area that gather to issue guidelines and statements. Many organizations sponsor such activities. The AARC has been a leader in this area by developing a wide range of clinical practice guidelines. Generally the AARC guidelines are appropriately conservative in that they do not make authoritative statements on the best way to administer given aspects of care if there are not compelling published data of a high quality to support such a position. Of course, this can be frustrating for the reader who goes to the guidelines in hopes of finding answers to perplexing questions only to find that the experts did not opine about this aspect of the question. The reason is because the answer simply is not known, and many of the best clinical scientists are reluctant to take pontifical positions without a solid base of evidence to support their positions. Other professional health associations publish guidelines of care. You can find a list of some of these organizations along with their Web sites in Appendix H.

Care must be taken when considering using any clinical practice guidelines. You need to examine their recommendations closely, including examining the references they cite to determine if these guidelines are based on expert only alone (not good) or whether they are based on a body of published science.

Another excellent resource for the director–manager who is trying to evaluate medical equipment is ECRI Institute (www.ecri.org). This organization has grown and changed over the years and has been called by *The New York Times* "the country's most-respected laboratory for testing medical products." They can be an invaluable resource for keeping abreast of the latest developments. Subscribing to their publications is rather pricey but well worth the money.

Still another resource is The Health Services/Technology Assessment Text (HSTAT), which describes itself as "a free, Web-based resource of full-text documents that provide health information and support health care decision making. HSTAT's audience includes health care providers, health service researchers, policy makers, payers, consumers and the information professionals who serve these groups." (http://www.ncbi.nlm.nih.gov/books/bv.fcgi?rid=hst)

Bench Study, Animal Study, Case Report

Bench studies use mechanical or computer models to simulate some aspect of the clinical world. In the respiratory therapy world we often use lung models to simulate ventilating a real patient. We also use models and simulators to test things like aerosol delivery, aerosol deposition, F_IO_2 delivery, intubation technology, and much more. Some commonly used models and simulators that relate to the practice of respiratory care include heart rate simulators, pulse oximetry simulators, spontaneously breathing lung simulators, intubation and CPR models, and many more. Models allow you to conduct tests on the performance of equipment or procedures that would be difficult or unethical in humans. And models are usually much cheaper than using animals. Bench testing can be a great tool for the manager–director of a department. Almost any respiratory department is equipped with enough measurement technology to do rudimentary bench testing. If you don't do some bench testing of the technology you are considering buying, you may regret it. My experience has been that it almost always yields information that you could not have gotten any other way.

Animal studies are an important part of the information base for understanding how respiratory care technology is used. I personally have no problem ethically, morally, or otherwise with well-conducted animal research. I have been in many animal labs and have never encountered any cavalier treatment or mistreatment of animals. I have never seen animals suffer any meaningful pain during the kinds of research I have seen or been involved in. Indeed to the contrary, the researchers and laboratory staff I have seen take painstaking care to ensure the best possible treatment of animals. I much prefer to refine and improve our medical technology using well crafted animal research than to put insufficiently tested technology on Aunt Mabel or Little Billy-Bob. The currently popular myth that we can reduce or even replace animal testing with computer models is so preposterous that it reminds me of Stalin's proclamation that the bigger the lie, the easier it is for people to swallow. The more we learn about the frightful complexity of biological systems, the more I doubt our ability to create meaningful computer models for testing technology. No one enjoys or relishes the prospect of doing animal research. My family has had a wide variety of pets including a lovable basset hound, numerable fish, cats, parakeets, hamsters, guinea pigs, an iguana and a cockatiel named "Gimli". I always felt a certain unease in the lab, but I knew that on the great cosmic scales, what we were doing would be deemed a good thing. There, now I feel better.

But animal research is a form of modeling too. Animals are approximations of humans with regard to the effect of interventions. I was involved in a project once where dogs were used to attempt to model asthma in humans. It was not possible to do widespread screening of dog populations for the presence of canine airway obstruction because doggy peak flow meters and normal values for peak flow were not widely available. So dogs slated for destruction at the dog pound were obtained and (after anesthesia) given large doses of metacholine to induce bronchoconstriction. Many of the dogs had no change in airway resistance. Thus this was not the best animal model around. On the other hand, much of the basic science behind the development of surfactant replacement therapy was done in animal models. This drug has been one of the great success stories of health care research.

In the end of deliberations about the published literature about a given technological intervention, you could sift it down to two questions. Does the technology perform the way the manufacturer says it does? And if so, does that matter? In other words, will this technology really improve processes and outcomes for our patients?

DESIGNING YOUR OWN TECHNOLOGY EVALUATION

When considering the purchase of a complex technology, a lot of good planning and analysis ought to precede actually having the devices in the hospital for clinical trials. For the sake of simplicity, I am going to focus on a ventilator as an example of how to design an evaluation. Everything I discuss here are ideas and principles that I have developed over the span of my so-called career. Upon reflection, I realize that I have led teams that did careful (and not so careful) evaluations of 10 different models of mechanical ventilators, conducted a number of clinical trials, and then finally made purchasing decisions of over 70 mechanical ventilators of various types. Over this period I have developed a basic process for technology evaluation. In the previous chapter we reviewed the tools for analyzing the financial implications of a large capital purchase, and I would again remind anyone working in the area of technology assessment to carefully review the work of Rob Chatburn.[20] The remainder of this chapter will primarily focus on the tools you can use. Here is an outline of the basic process, which I will then expand on:

1. Why purchase new technology?
2. Creating an evaluation team and format
3. Survey of the ventilator market
4. Bench testing
5. Clinical trial
6. The decision
7. Implementation planning

Why Purchase New Technology?

Believe it or not, the quality of the evaluation and selection of new respiratory care technology often falls apart right here. Think real hard about why you are considering new technology. In the case of ventilators, do not allow yourself to be the victim of slick marketing and ventilator envy. Respiratory technology is marketed. Just like automobiles, lawnmowers, and sneakers. All these products have something in common. They have a basic function, which for the most part, all of them perform with adequate utility. Any car will get you down to the 7-Eleven to buy a six pack. Any lawnmower will trim your estate, and pretty much any sneakers will allow you to drive the lane and toss up a prayer. So to get you to buy a particular car, lawnmower, or pair of sneakers, they either create an image of their products that makes you feel special when you use them, or they festoon their products with features.

It is said that image is everything, and there is some truth to this. I remember a manufacturer who ran a magazine ad for their over-priced and over-engineered ventilator in the 1980s that was all about image and a teensy tiny bit short on substance. The ad showed a picture of the ventilator with a superimposed artist rendering two terminal respiratory units. One unit looked healthy and normal, and one unit was exploding outward as if ruptured by over expansion. It was a beautiful drawing, and overall the ad was gorgeous. The text of the ad has been lost in the dark corridors of my increasingly faulty memory, but I clearly remember that the ad was intended to make you think that if you purchased this ventilator you would most certainly avoid over expanding the alveoli of your patients and would have less ventilator induced lung injury. This was predicated on their new feature, pressure regulated volume control, which could allegedly deliver the same tidal volume with less airway pressure and thereby reduce the potential for lung injury. Sadly it had absolutely no foundation in truth, mom, apple pie, or the American way. Some of us knew then and lots of people know now that lung injury is caused by volumetric over distention. Thus if a mode of ventilation gave the same volume using lower proximal airway pressure, there was no real reduction in the risk of lung injury. But their marketing sure was convincing.

There was then, and is now no published scientific evidence that I am aware of that any one brand of ventilator has any better effect on outcomes than any other. As I have said before, this is also true of all the different modes available on ventilators then and now. Any fool can explode an alveoli or two with any ventilator. Just like a particular brand of sneaker cannot make you a better shooting guard (I know, I have tried), the vast majority of features on a mechanical ventilator generally cannot make you a better clinician.

However, there are differences in ventilator *performance* between manufacturers and models. The one I want to focus on here for a moment is measurement. Ventilators measure gas flow and pressure, and through the mathematic treatment of these measurements, volumes of gas are determined. We now know that keeping tidal volume within a certain range (low relative to historical practice) improves outcomes from certain diseases. Thus how accurately ventilators measure tidal volume is an important performance difference, and I would recommend that when you are considering buying a ventilator or any other piece of health care technology.

I would also again point out that the manufacturers' published accuracy and precision statistics are obtained under very controlled and ideal conditions, and ventilator measurement systems almost never perform this well in the real clinical environment.

So the very first thing to do in any technology assessment with an eye toward purchase is to utterly question the assumptions about why you need to buy the new technology in the first place. *Immutable Truth #26: All assumptions are suspect until proven otherwise.* You must challenge all assumptions. After all, they are just assumptions. This is true in all aspects of your management career, but nowhere is it more important than in the process of acquiring new technology. The Toyota production system, perhaps the most effective and efficient method of analyzing business processes on the planet, teaches managers who are analyzing a complex issue to ask *why* at least five times.[x] Let's try it:

1. I need new ventilators.
   - *Why?*
2. Because my ventilators are old.
   - *Why* does this matter?
3. Because I don't have the latest technology.
   - *Why* does this matter?
4. Because new technology is better.
   - *Why* is it better?
5. Because newer technology gives better care.
   - *Why* do you believe this is true?

---

[x]From: *The Toyota Way Fieldbook* by Liker and Meier, published by McGraw-Hill in 2006. If you want to get ahead of the curve, start reading about lean manufacturing processing, or the Toyota Way. It has already arrived in many hospitals and is on its way to many more. It is essentially a set of principles and analytical tools for improving the processes that constitute any logistics and production system, which, whether you like to admit it or not, is what a hospital is.

Do you see how this works? Many arguments start to fall apart when drilled down to this level. Before you set out to evaluate technology, make sure your assumptions about why you want new technology are valid. As I have already repeatedly ranted about, we have a somewhat dismal track record of trying to fix problems within the health care universe with unproven and untested technology. I am beginning to realize that most of our problems relate to badly designed processes over which we superimpose technology in the hope that it will help improve things. Instead what you usually end up with is a highly advanced, computerized, electronic, sophisticated process that remains screwed up.

Most of our technology will last much longer than the customary depreciation period (5–7 years). This is clearly true because most of our old equipment is like our old military hardware. It is resold overseas and remains in use for many more years after we have discarded it. So the "old" argument for replacing technology is usually a little flaccid. And since most of the advancement in features in the last 20 years hasn't borne much fruit, the "features" argument turns out to be pretty flaccid too. The last two wholesale ventilator replacements that I have promoted and executed were in search of improved measurement performance, not for features.

Creating an Evaluation Team and Format

One of the worst things you can do when setting out to evaluate and possibly acquire new technology in respiratory care is to have the hubris to go it alone. Respiratory therapy departments tend to take ownership of ventilators and monitors and the other technology of respiratory therapy. This is as it should be. I like ownership. It creates clear lines of accountability. But do not take this ownership too seriously. Lots of other disciplines interface with respiratory therapy technology. Some of the most famous career ending moves of directors–managers that I know of were related to acquiring ventilator technology without getting buy in of all the stakeholders.

Keeping with the ventilator example, the first thing you should do when considering the evaluation and selection of new ventilators is the creation of a team to help you with this complicated project. You should carefully consider the stakeholders. They typically include representatives from medicine, nursing, clinical engineering, and respiratory therapy. For hospitals with multiple intensive care units, be sure to include physician representatives from each of the intensive care units and your own medical director. And in some hospitals you may want to include anesthesia, pulmonology, and surgery representatives. They may not want to participate, but it is much better to have asked them and had them decline than to have to explain later why they were never asked to participate in the project. One way to think of this group is as a guidance team that will help oversee the evaluation project.

Take some time to think about who the right players are for this team. I know of a respiratory director who did not include the neonatologists in the process of selecting new ventilators. This probably helped contribute to the selection of a ventilator that really wasn't very good for neonates. The director was understandably trying to standardize technology across the ventilation continuum from neonates to adults. But he did not do a sufficiently rigorous evaluation. When the new ventilator showed up in the NICU, it quickly became obvious that it wasn't suitable for neonates. The neonatologists soon banned the ventilator from the NICU, and before long the director was dusting off his resume.

I know of another example of a director–manager who bought some new ventilators as additions to the current fleet. Unfortunately there did not appear to be much of a detailed evaluation done, and there was very little staff participation in the process. I suspect they were purchased mostly because of: (1) the reputation of the company, (2) the skill of the local ventilator manufacturing representative, and (3) the irresistible lure of new features. Predictably, the ventilators sat around and did not get used by the staff. The director–manager eventually moved on to another job in the hospital and rumor on the street was this ventilator issue helped contribute to this.

You should do some prep work before the first meeting of this team. Outline a rough plan for your evaluation. It is always better to come to a meeting with something for people to react to. It is very difficult to create plans from scratch in a meeting environment. Remember that one of the biggest problems with carefully executed, collaborative planning in hospitals today is getting everyone in the room at the same time. Scheduling meetings has become very difficult. Pay close attention to not wasting anyone's time, and do as much work as can be done outside the framework of the meetings.

Appendix F contains a series of documents that were developed to support an evaluation and selection process for new mechanical ventilators. The original plan (document F-1) was a general roadmap for our evaluation process. We got lost a few times along the way and did not follow the map precisely, but it helped to clarify our thinking. Also in Appendix F are a bench testing protocol, detailed plans for implementation, guidelines for how to use the ventilator, and training requirements and documentation.

It is really tragic how much managerial pain and suffering could be alleviated by two things with regard to planning. First, actually doing some planning can really help you avoid heartache. I know managers who carry a lot of plans around in their head. Get yours onto paper in detail. This process of writing down your plans in detail is a clarifying process. This may sound pretty pedant and obvious, but I have seen some fairly large projects attempt to be prosecuted without any real detailed written plans. Second, you must be willing and able to nimbly modify your plans slightly or significantly when necessary. *Immutable Truth #27: The "Six P Principle": Proper Planning Prevents Piss Poor Performance.* Here are some other thoughts on plans.

- Definition of Planning: To bother about the best method of accomplishing an accidental result. (Ambrose Bierce, 1842–1914)
- I have never yet seen any plan which has not been mended by the observations of those who were much inferior in understanding to the person who took the lead in the business. (Edmund Burke, 1729–1797)
- To be prepared is half the victory. (Miguel de Cervantes, 1547–1616)
- It is a mistake to look too far ahead. Only one link in the chain of destiny can be handled at a time. (Winston Churchill, 1874–1965)
- I'm just preparing my impromptu remarks. (Winston Churchill, 1874–1965)
- Before beginning, plan carefully. (Marcus Tulius Cicero, 106–43 BC)
- A man who does not think and plan long ahead will find trouble right at his door. (Confucius, 551–479 BC)
- To have his path made clear for him is the aspiration of every human being in our beclouded and tempestuous existence. (Joseph Conrad, 1857–1924)
- A good plan violently executed now is better than a perfect plan next week. (George S. Patton, 1885–1945)
- In preparing for battle I have always found that plans are useless, but planning is indispensable. (Dwight David Eisenhower, 1890–1969)

Survey of the Ventilator Market

An important part of the process of evaluating new technology is knowing the market. This can be challenging. Some segments of the market change very fast. Staying on top of the published literature is essential. But PubMed alone has over 16 million citations. Then there is the combined index for allied health (CINAHL), which is a commercially available database of over

924 journals dating back to the early 1980s. Many of these journals are not listed in PubMed. There are approximately 11 major manufacturers offering over 22 different models of mechanical ventilators in the United States.

Some peer-reviewed journals you might want to watch carefully for information about mechanical ventilators and other respiratory care technology are provided in Appendix H. This is not intended to be a comprehensive list, so your favorite journals might not be listed here. If you have access to a table of contents service (TACOS), all or some of these journals would be good ones to include in your TACOS list. I would also recommend reading the abstracts published in the front of each issue of *Respiratory Care*. The editor reviews a lot of literature and shakes and bakes it down to a list of abstracts that are thought to be of interest to respiratory clinicians. Also to get some of the latest information about new technology, I suggest scanning all the abstracts published each year in *Respiratory Care, Critical Care Medicine,* and *Chest.* By this I mean the abstracts that were presented at their respective annual scientific conferences, which each organization publishes in one issue of their journal. If you are a member of the AARC, you can get all the abstracts on a CD.

The other obvious place to learn about new technology is at conferences. The two big ones for respiratory therapists are the International Respiratory Congress put on each year by the AARC and the Focus on Respiratory Care and Sleep Medicine Conference put on by Focus Publications. Depending on exactly how you count people, there are somewhere between 2500 and 5500 respiratory therapists at these meetings. The manufacturers are out in force, and all the latest technology will be displayed. To be an effective respiratory therapy director–manager, you simply must regularly attend these meetings and your state society meetings, many of which are excellent. If you are not attending these meetings, you are coasting, and if you are coasting, you are probably going downhill (Immutable Truth #13).

When you get a feel for what products are out there, start setting up demonstrations. The classic approach to demonstrations has been to call the product rep and set up an appointment with little other preparation. A little more planning will help you save time. When setting up a demonstration, keep the following points in mind:

- Ensure the key formal and informal opinion setters are there. Remember to keep your friends close and your enemies closer.
- Require the product reps to make sure that someone with a clinical background represents the product and makes the demonstration. I have had sales reps with no clinical background conduct demonstrations

of some fairly complex clinical equipment. I know, I know, nonclinicians are people too, but I need *clinicians* to talk to about *clinical* technology.

- Require the manufacturers to come at your convenience, not theirs. Start establishing who is boss. This might save you some trouble later.
- Require manufacturers to bring exhaustive bibliographies and user lists for their products. Be sure to ask for complete user lists so they cannot cherry pick accounts that they want you to talk to.
- Talk with the manufacturers up front and warn them to minimize the shtick and just focus on the essentials of why their technology is better than what you already have.
- Grill them. Ask lots and lots of questions. Be tough but pleasant. There is no need, other than the obvious sick thrill you get, to publicly humiliate and embarrass product reps. Treat them with civility. I have seen some directors–managers that were just downright rude to reps just as a matter of principle.
- Believe nothing. Challenge all assumptions.
- Require repeated demonstrations for each product evaluated. This is separate from training in preparation of a clinical trial. Several repeat demonstrations will give more members of your staff a chance to get involved. It will also give you and your evaluation team a chance to better master an understanding of the technology, which is growing in complexity.

It is at about this point when the manufacturers will realize you are serious about evaluating and purchasing new technology. When this happens, the gravy trains will start arriving at the station. I have been offered and accepted, to varying degrees, all of the following during the evaluative phase of acquiring new technology at various times in my career:

- Lots and lots of free lunches
- Cute little gifts like calculators, alarm clocks, golf balls and tees, pens, bags, baubles, bangles, and bright shiny beads
- Free dinners, sometimes at some pretty swank joints that I wouldn't be frequenting if I was paying the bill myself
- All expense paid trips to the factory
- Honoraria to look at new product designs that are at various stages of development

Early on in my career I accepted some of these without a second thought. I figured I was tough minded enough to enjoy all of these benefits without having my judgment clouded. I am not so sure anymore. The more you hang with these reps, the closer you get to them. The chummier you get with them, the harder it is to remain totally objective. And some reps are shameless in the subtle and not so subtle tools they will use to try to manipulate you. Ego stroking is one of their favorites, and they use it on me endlessly. My ego being somewhat oversized already, it is an easy target. I had a rep tell us that we were taking food out of his children's mouths when we told him we weren't selecting his product. I also once had a rep tell me that he would lose his job if I didn't do further testing on his product. Mostly though, my experience with product reps has been pretty positive.

Many hospitals have now put some strict rules in place about how many of these benefits you can enjoy. I think this is a pretty good idea. In my last round of evaluating and purchasing mechanical ventilators, all the manufacturers offered to fly me and key members of my team to their manufacturing plants, put us up in hotels, wine and dine us, and give us a tour. I declined. I told them that if, after we had decided which products to buy, they were still interested in taking us to their plant for a tour, well, then we could talk about it.

However you can go too far with this ethical purity business. There is nothing wrong with manufacturers bringing in food to demonstrations and training sessions. It generally improves attendance, which can be problematic.

Bench Testing

When it comes to bench testing, I am admittedly on the lunatic fringe. I think any respectable respiratory therapy department ought to, whenever possible, design and carry out a series of bench tests on any devices that are being considered for purchase. Respiratory therapists ought to be the undisputed experts in the hospital on any technology they are operating. By bench testing devices you are considering purchasing, you learn a lot about how they work, perhaps identify some conditions where they don't necessarily work so well, and hopefully verify the credibility of manufacturers' claims. The basic equipment you need for bench testing are simulators and measurement instruments. Simulators help you mimic clinical conditions, and measurement instruments help you verify the performance of the devices you are testing. Typical simulators that you can get your hands on without too much expense are test lungs. They range in complexity from rigid bottles and containers to simple bellows to pistons and all the way to very sophisticated, programmable breathing simulators. Here is a list of companies (and their Web sites) that make test lungs and breathing simulators:

- IngMar Medical (www.ingmarmed.com)
- Michigan Instruments (www.michiganinstruments.com)
- South Pacific Biomedical (www.southpb.com)
- Hans Rudolf (www.rudolphkc.com)
- VacuMed (www.vacumed.com)

In addition, many ventilator manufacturers make simple static test lungs that come with their ventilators that are used for operational verification procedures before applying the ventilator to patients. The capabilities of the lung you would use will of course depend on the design of your testing.

Measurement instruments in the typical respiratory care department include oxygen analyzers and computerized pneumotachometers, of which there are several brands. Two widely available pneumotachometers, the Ventrak and the CO_2SMO (both made by Novametrix Inc.), have been repeatedly used as research instruments.[25-28] They can be bought used for a very modest price and rented for as little as $18 per day. I found one on eBay with a current bid of $179. With a computerized pneumotachometer you can measure a lot of aspects of ventilator performance. Most of the bench testing of products we have done was with one of these two instruments. Other measurement devices for equipping a bench testing lab include pressure manometers, flowmeters, thermometers, barometers, and hygrometers.

What you are about to read is all true to the best of my recollection. It is the story of two bench test series that I conducted, with the help of a lot of very skilled people, in the pursuit of information about product performance. Both led to big changes in practice.

Bench Testing Saga #1: This Just Ain't My Bag

We were trying to determine which type of resuscitation bags were the best to use for manual ventilation of infants and children. There were three distinct camps. Camp one was the true believer in flow-inflating bags (FIB). Camp two preferred the self-inflating bags (SIB), and the third camp didn't give a rip either way. My own experience told me that maintaining PEEP and PIP with a FIB was pretty challenging. I had been told all my career that FIBs were better because they offered the clinician a better feel for changes in lung compliance, allegedly because the compression chamber of an FIB is made out of much thinner material than an SIB, allowing the better feel. As a full-time card carrying, lifelong, charter member of skeptics anonymous, I had my doubts about this. As we began to learn more and more about the importance of strict control of tidal volumes, I began to worry that the FIB caused unacceptable variation in ventilation parameters when compared to SIB. I decided to do some bench testing of products. I collaborated with my equipment manager. We compared a SIB (Baxter) and a FIB (Drager-Rusch). We tested 5 RCPs and 20 nurses on each bag type. We used a Siemens test lung and monitored proximal airway pressures with a pressure manometer. Subjects were asked to manually ventilate the test lung using PIP = 30, PEEP = 4, f = 30. Data were gathered for 8–10 minutes. PIP, PEEP, and tidal volume were measured using a Ventrak. We interfaced the Ventrak with a computer and used software that was given to us by the manufacturer to acquire tidal volumes and pressures for every breath, and we dumped them into a spreadsheet format. Students from the nearby respiratory therapy school were used to help carry out the project. We found that the SIB produced considerably less variability in tidal volume, PIP, and PEEP than the FIB when used by either nurses or RTs. By the way, RTs exhibited less ventilation variability than did nurses on either bag tested. We then crafted these data into monographs, which we published in abstract form.[29,30] I had only partial success in getting medical staff to pay much attention to our findings. They apparently did not want to be bothered and possibly confused with the facts. We did change to SIB in parts of the hospital but not all of it. I had virtually no incremental increase in expense.

But the story does not end there. I subsequently changed hospitals and encountered additional pockets of resistance regarding the use of FIB versus SIB. I kept hearing the argument that lung compliance changes could be felt better with a FIB than with a SIB. I set out to test this assumption. Once again, members of the leadership team helped me devise a bench test. An IngMar test lung was modified so that compliance could be increased or decreased by placing steel weights on top of the bellows, making it more difficult to inflate. The lung was encased in a cardboard box so that the test subjects could not see whether weight was added to or removed from the lung. Test lung pressure was displayed for the test subjects on a pressure manometer mounted in the side of the box. A visual analog of movement of the bellows was created by attaching an 8-inch tongue depressor in such a fashion that one end of the piece of wood passed through a slit and could be seen outside the cardboard box and rose and fell with the movement of the bellows, thus mimicking chest wall motion. Test subjects were 13 neonatal-pediatric respiratory therapists with a mean of 13 years of experience. Subjects were asked to manually ventilate the test lung to PIP = 25 cm H_2O, PEEP = 5 cm H_2O, f = 30/min while watching the manometer and chest rise analog. The investigator(s) then added or removed weights to the lung to simulate increases and decreases in compliance. Seven different changes were simulated: (1) increase of 20%, (2) decrease of 20%, (3) increase of 40%, (4) decrease of 40%, and three false changes, for example noise was made behind the cardboard to simulate adding or removing weights, but no actual change in compliance was made. This process was repeated for two brands of SIB and one brand of FIB. Overall subjects were able to correctly identify compliance changes 65% of the time. Table 8-1 shows the correct percentage sorted by bag type.

Sacred cows make the best hamburger, and this one was mighty tasty. We discovered no difference in the rates of correctly identifying compliance changes between bag types.

Because prophets are seldom recognized in their hometowns,[xi] we also repeated the study on ventilation variability we had done at my previous

Table 8-1. Bench Test Results of Resuscitation Bag Types

Sequence	SIB Brand #1	SIB Brand #2	FIB
False change	85%	69%	85%
Increase 20%	38%	62%	69%
False change	54%	46%	54%
Decrease 20%	77%	46%	54%
Increase 40%	77%	77%	69%
False change	54%	62%	46%
Decrease 40%	77%	85%	77%
Average	66%	64%	65%

Results of bench testing of resuscitation bag types and the ability of clinicians to detect changes in compliance sorted by bag type. Percentages indicate the number of subjects tested who could correctly detect changes in compliance.

[xi]Book of Luke 2:24 (Common English Version). "But you can be sure that no prophets are liked by the people of their own hometown."

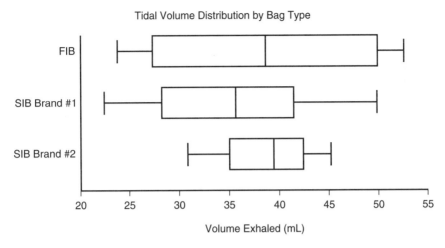

Figure 8-4. Tidal Volume Distribution by Bag Type
Results of a bench test; distribution of tidal volumes when using three different types of manual resuscitators. SIB = self inflating bags, FIB = flow inflating bags.
   Source: Adapted from Salyer J, Foubare D. Ventilation variability using flow-inflating versus self-inflating manual resuscitators in a neonatal lung model. *Respir Care* 2005;50:1498.

hospital. The findings were similar. Tidal volumes were more variable with a FIB than with a SIB (see Figure 8-4).

Thus we determined that SIB gave more consistent ventilation than FIB and that being able to feel changes in compliance better with one bag or another was a myth. We crafted the results of both of these tests into monographs that were published in abstract form.[31,32]

I used all of these combined data to convince the last pockets of resistance that we needed to change practice and switch from FIB to SIB, and indeed the hospital converted all inpatient beds and the emergency department to SIB. These bench tests also helped us select between two brands of SIB. There remain a few anesthesiologists who hold out, but I am working on them. The point here is that bench testing is very feasible and can improve the quality of your decision making and thus your clinical operations.

I later learned that the myth about feeling changes in compliance had actually already been dispelled. Spears, Yeh, Fisher, and Zwass reported a study in 1991 in which they demonstrated that only 14% of a group of 24 anesthesiologists, both faculty and residents, pediatric and adult, could correctly identify a complete occlusion of the endotracheal tube while ventilating a neonatal and pediatric test lung with flow-inflating bags in anesthesia circuits.[33] This in no way diminished the full beefy flavor of my hamburger.

Bench Testing Saga #2: Would the Real Tidal Volume Please Stand Up

One day a respiratory therapist came to me with copies of a ventilator flow sheet and a story. He was caring for a 900 gram neonate on a Servo 300, the only neonatal ventilator used in that NICU at the time. The corrected exhaled tidal volume was running 6 to 8 mL/kg. Corrected tidal volume was determined by the following formula:

$$VT_C = VT_E - [(PIP - PEEP) \times C_T]$$

Where:

VT_C = Corrected tidal volume
VT_E = Displayed exhaled tidal volume from Servo 300
C_T = Tubing compliance factor

The RT went on to say that he had his doubts about the veracity of the corrected tidal volume data. His clinical observations led him to believe that the tidal volume was much larger. So he put a computerized pneumotachometer at the proximal airway (CO_2SMO). The pneumotachometer indicated that the patient was getting a tidal volume in the 14–16 mL/kg range. This had been going on for the biggest part of 24 hours. This story, combined with a string of other anecdotal reports and published papers, convinced me that the Servo 300 was not so good at measuring neonatal tidal volumes. This was not surprising because it did not measure at the proximal airway.

We set out to test the accuracy of the tidal volumes displayed by the Servo 300 in a bench test model. It was an elegantly simple test. We used a static neonatal lung model and a typical circuit setup. The lung was ventilated with a Servo 300, and tidal volumes were collected for each breath in two ways. One way was to determine the corrected tidal volume as described above and the other was to use a computerized pneumotachometer placed at the proximal airway (CO_2SMO). Table 8–2 shows the results of our bench test.

These data, and some other design concerns we had about the user interface with the Servo 300, led us to wonder if we could do better, such as find a ventilator that could accurately measure neonatal tidal volumes.

I want to stop and point out that we were testing the Servo 300 at the extreme lower end of its operating limits. This narrative is intended to

Table 8-2. Bench Test Results of the Servo 300

Ventilator mode	V_T actual (CO_2SMO)	V_T displayed (Servo)	V_T displayed error (Servo)	V_T corrected	V_T corrected error
PRVC high	8.7	31.0	258%	−1.1	−113%
PRVC low	3.3	12.3	268%	−0.9	−127%
TCPL high	9.9	35.1	255%	1.7	−83%
TCPL low	4.0	10.2	157%	−3.2	−180%
VC high	11.2	35.0	213%	−0.9	−108%
VC low	3.8	13.8	261%	0.0	−101%

Results of a bench test of the accuracy of the displayed and corrected tidal volumes (V_T). PRVC = Pressure regulated volume control. TCPL = Time cycled, pressure limited. VC = Volume controlled. All volumes are exhaled. CO_2SMO is a computerized pneumotachometer. Error calculations were (displayed-actual)/actual. V_T corrected = VT_E − [(PIP − PEEP) × CT)], where VT_E is displayed exhaled tidal volume and C_T is the tubing compliance factor. High and low refer to the targeted tidal volume in a 1 kg infant, which were targeted to be ≅ 5 mL (low) and 10 mL (high).

point out the value of bench testing, not to besmirch the reputation of the Servo ventilators in general, which are widely respected in the RT community. This test was narrowly focused on the accuracy of displayed tidal volumes in the neonatal range, something that the Servo 300 was not principally designed to do. Ditto for much of the rest of the data you will see in this example. All of the ventilators we tested are technological marvels. They are great devices that have helped countless thousands of patients. And they probably work very well in nearly any population they would be used on. Our focus was on one very narrow aspect of their function—accuracy of tidal volume displayed at the very lowest ends of their operating limits.

We set out to bench test the displayed tidal volume accuracy of a range of ventilators that were considered to be neonatal. We kept in mind an overarching goal—to have one critical care ventilator that was suitable for use across the entire range of patient sizes ventilated in our three critical care units. These ranged from 600 grams (in the NICU) to 114,000 grams (in the PICU). The benefit of a single ventilator was the value of standardization. The staff would only have to master the operation of one critical care ventilator. This was thought to be a benefit to the patients from a safety perspective.

So we surveyed the ventilator market and selected a group of ventilators to test that included the Viasys Avea, Puritan Bennet PB 840, Hamilton Galileo, Maquet Servo-i, and the Drager Baby Log. Actual V_T was determined independently of the ventilator display with a pneumotachometer (CO_2SMO Plus) placed at the proximal airway. The ventilators were set to operate in volume-targeted, decelerating flow modes and connected to a static neonatal test lung. Ventilators were set to deliver either 5 mL (low V_T) or 10 mL (high V_T) with the exception of the Galileo, which was only tested in the high V_T setting because 10 mL is the lowest volume setting on the device. The percent of error was calculated as [(Mean Displayed V_T) − (Mean Actual V_T)] ÷ [Mean Actual V_T]. We used exhaled volumes for all measurements and computations. We found important differences in the displayed V_T accuracy of these neonatal ventilators in volume-targeted modes. This bench research was an important part of our process of ventilator selection. The laboratory work was done by one of the RT clinical supervisors who had an interest in computers and ventilator technology. He was willing to work the extra hours necessary to carry out the project, and he was very self-directed and self-taught, which are pretty important attributes when selecting someone to help you with such a project. Table 8-3 describes our results, which we also described in a monograph and published in an abstract.[34]

Table 8-3. Bench Test Results of the Accuracy of the Displayed Tidal Volumes on Several Neonatal Ventilators

Ventilator	Overall error rate (%)	Low V_T error rate (%)	High V_T error rate (%)
Avea	10.1 ± 9.6	14.1 ± 11.7	6.2 ± 4.2
Baby Log	16.8 ± 4.4	19.3 ± 4.5	14.4 ± 2.6
Galileo	−19.6 ± 0.9	NA	−19.6 ± 0.9
PB 840	74.3 ± 127.1	47.9 ± 10.2	106.9 ± 185.9
Servo-i	20.5 ± 28.4	3.5 ± 29.9	37.2 ± 12.7

Data are represented as mean error rates ± standard deviation. Error rates are calculated as (actual V_T − displayed V_T)/actual V_T.

These results were important factors in helping us decide which ventilators, if any, to evaluate in a clinical trial.

We were also interested in evaluating a second aspect of ventilator performance in the neonatal range. Each ventilator had the capacity to deliver volume targeted breaths with a decelerating flow profile. But we knew that each company had different computer algorithms that controlled the ventilator's response to rapidly changing lung mechanics in spontaneously breathing infants. So we set out to model erratic spontaneous breathing in a neonate.

We used the IngMar Active Servo Lung 5000 (IngMar Inc.) simulator to mimic neonatal breathing. The simulator allows programming of individual breaths or groups of breaths. The spontaneous breathing model was programmed for 196 second runs including epochs of apnea, eupnea, and tachypnea, with varying tidal volumes. Again the same pneumotachometer was used to independently measure V_T. Ventilators tested included Viasys Avea, Drager Baby Log, Drager Evita XL, Puritan Bennet PB 840, and the Maquet Servo-i. Each ventilator was set up with a typical circuit to give $V_T = 5$ mL in their respective modes for volume-targeted ventilation with decelerating flow.

Our assumption was that the best ventilator performance would result in the tightest distribution of tidal volumes. As the baby (lung simulator) breathed erratically, the ventilator would have to make rapid changes in the dynamics of flow to try to keep the tidal volumes in the targeted ranges. Figure 8-5 shows you the distribution of tidal volumes for each ventilator tested, which we also published.[35]

There were clearly very important differences in the distribution of tidal volumes. The reason the Avea had such a tight distribution of tidal volumes is that it has a unique feature called volume limit. This allows you to set a maximum tidal volume that the ventilator will not exceed, *no matter what,* which is an intriguing feature in light of the growing body of evidence about lung injury caused by over distention. But it is not yet clear how to use this feature.

These data were very important in our decision making about which ventilators to select for a clinical trial. The total incremental increase in costs related to our bench research was approximately:

- Breathing simulator leased for three months—$1500
- Labor cost to pay my staff for training and bench time—$2000
- Other miscellaneous costs—$1000

Thus we had a total of about $4500 spent to determine if, and how, to spend nearly $1 million for new mechanical ventilators.

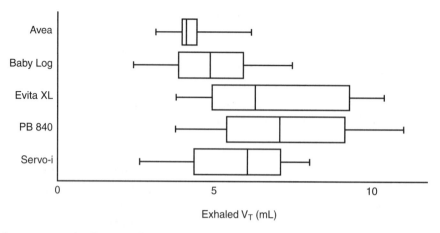

Figure 8-5. Distribution of Tidal Volumes for Tested Ventilators
Results of a bench test of tidal volume variation in a spontaneously breathing neonatal lung model.
    Source: Salyer JW, Jackson C. Accuracy of tidal volume (VT) displayed during volume targeted ventilation in neonatal ventilators. *Respir Care* 2005;50:149.

At this point it is time to talk about how we managed the manufacturers through this process. We included them at every step. We shared the testing protocols with them, offered them the chance to suggest changes to our protocol, and invited the local reps and anyone they wanted to bring along to come and be present for testing. In fact the product managers and local reps made our bench testing better. Well, mostly they made it better, with the exception of one company that did not conduct themselves very well throughout this process.

This is a good point to talk about the role of clinical engineering in this bench testing saga. Early on, I met with the manager of clinical engineering, who was an outstanding engineer and a very smart guy. He helped design some very cool test equipment for us that was an important part of our testing. He reviewed all our designs and was invited to come and observe the testing, which he sometimes did. By having him involved it gave our work more credibility. He supported the design of our studies, and when a letter came to administration from one of the ventilator manufacturers accusing me of bias, he backed our testing and described our ventilator evaluation as the most rigorous he had ever seen. The lesson is that you should work closely with your clinical engineering department.

Clinical Trial

Based on our data and judgment we decided to conduct clinical trials on two ventilators: first the Viasys Avea and then the Drager Evita XL. A lot of planning went into our preparations for this trial. There was a time in this business when ventilator evaluations would go like this: A single ventilator would be brought in and a handful of people would get some rudimentary training, usually for 20 minutes at change of shift, often at the bedside. Then the ventilator would get put on a handful of patients over a period of a couple of weeks. Then, abracadabra, a decision would come forth. I decided that this would happen over my dead lifeless corpse. As we began planning our clinical trials my number one concern was patient safety. I knew that these ventilators were complex and different and that this posed a real risk for patients because it greatly increased our chances of operator error.

So we did a lot of careful planning related to when and how we would introduce the ventilators into clinical practice. Because we were going to live (or die) with this decision for many years, I wanted to ventilate enough patients of various kinds to get a good assessment of how well the ventilators would meet our patients' clinical needs. Here are some important considerations we developed before the Avea clinical trial:

- No one would be allowed to operate the ventilator who had not been trained and demonstrated basic competency. Here is what this really meant. Staff therapists could not skip in-service training, show up for duty, and get trained by the therapist who was going off duty at the bedside at change of shift during report.
- Training was mandatory for *all* respiratory therapists working in critical care at the time. We decided to train everyone for the clinical trial because, presumably, everyone would be using the ventilators if we bought them, and we wanted lots of interaction and experience with the ventilators. Training included return demonstration competency assessment. This was a large commitment, but we were determined to minimize patient risk and conduct a thorough assessment. Thus it took weeks and weeks of training before we could even put a single ventilator on a patient.
- All training took place outside the clinical environment. By this I mean in controlled space where interruptions were minimized. Staff members were trained during hours when they were not actively taking patient assignments, for example after their shift (not good), before their shift (better), or on their days off.
- We selected a group of volunteer respiratory therapists to receive advanced training. They were designated "Aces" and we selected and scheduled them in such a fashion that at least one was on duty at all times.

- We required a nearly constant on-site clinical presence from the manufacturer's reps during the trial. After negotiation they agreed to bring in a team that pretty much managed round the clock coverage. There were occasional uncovered periods in the wee hours, but the reps stayed in nearby hotels and could be back in the hospital in a few minutes. It took slightly longer if we wanted them dressed and awake.
- Our clinical coordinator was designated by me as responsible for this clinical trial. Of course in the end we would all be held accountable if we screwed it up. Ultimately the buck stopped on my desk because I dreamed up this hair-brained scheme to begin with. But he was identified as the front line platoon leader. I made this clear to him, and he rose to the occasion and really focused on the success of this trial. He worked many extra hours, took many phone calls at home on his time off, and was instrumental in the success of this trial. Remember, all successful projects are owned by someone. If they are not owned, they are never successful.
- We did some careful planning with our medical staff about the kinds of patients that would be put on the ventilator, whose permission had to be obtained to switch the patients to the ventilator being tested, and what would be said to patients and families about what we were doing. We also wanted to describe a set of criteria that would define if and when the patients should be removed from the ventilators (prior to extubation). This resulted in a set of guidelines that are in document F-3 in Appendix F. We were pretty strict in enforcing these. We wanted to limit the use of some of the ventilators' advanced features because they were new and thus we were not experienced in how to use them. We felt this reduced potential risks to patients.
- One thing that somewhat rocked the manufacturer's world was how many patients we wanted to ventilate. Our goal was 40 to 50 patients, and we thought this might take 1–2 months. I later learned that they dubbed our evaluation the "trial that would never end." This brought a crooked smile to my grizzled old face.

The Decision

Recall Eisenhower's great comment that "plans are useless, but planning is indispensable"? That was somewhat true for us. I am forced now, finally, after so many years, to admit that I always aim a little too high. I can never quite execute the plans I make to their completion. But because I aim so high,

I have often managed to achieve something or another, even if it wasn't what I originally set out to do. Such was the case with our program of clinical trials. Remember that we were going to test two ventilators and try to ventilate 40–50 patients on each ventilator. We ended up ventilating 10 patients with the Avea for a total of about 400 hours. Still we were pretty much exhausted by this effort and wanted to stop and evaluate our progress.

At first the word on the street was positive. The anecdotal evidence was that the staff, both therapists and nurses, very much liked the ventilators being tested. But the plural of anecdote is not data, so we set out to try to get a more quantifiable assessment of staff perceptions of the clinical trial. We constructed separate survey instruments to be administered to respiratory therapists and nurses respectively to measure their experience with the Avea. The survey instrument for the respiratory therapists is document F-8 in Appendix F. They had all been working with the Servo 300 for years, and we sought to use that ventilator as a standard against which we would compare the experience with the Avea. Figure 8-6 shows the respiratory therapy results of the survey.

The fact that the staff was not yet very comfortable with the new ventilator and yet rated it so highly compared to the existing ventilator was a very important finding.

We had planned to do two clinical trials. Our concerns about patient safety led us to rethink this part of our plan. There had been some episodes of care during the Avea trial that were very concerning. In two separate instances the ventilator had been misapplied, and temporary derangement of ventilation had occurred. In both cases, these respiratory therapists were experienced, had completed all the required training, and demonstrated competency on the Avea. Both mishaps were deemed to have been caused by unfamiliarity with the device. We knew that if we brought a second ventilator in for trial, we would expose our patient population to these kinds of errors again. The results of our clinical trial of the Avea convinced us that we had enough information to determine that the Avea was demonstrably better than our existing ventilator technology. While another clinical trial might have given us more information, we already knew that the Avea performed better in bench testing than the Evita XL. Based on this, we were unwilling to expose our patient population to the risk of another clinical trial.

This narrative was not intended to be a testimonial about the qualities of the Avea. As I pointed out, all the ventilators tested well and are excellent devices. Instead, I am sharing the process by which we conducted this evaluation.

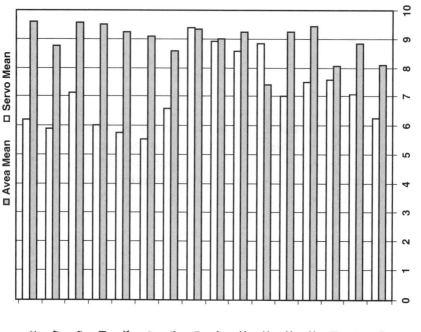

Post Clinical Trial Ventilator Evaluation n = 12

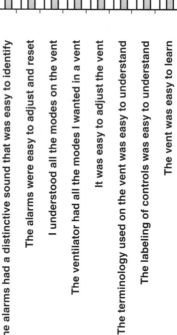

Figure 8-6.   Postclinical Trial Ventilator Evaluation

Results of a survey designed to assess staff impressions of the clinical trial of the Viasys Avea ventilator. The Avea was compared to the existing ventilator, the Servo 300. Questions were asked on a 10-point ordinal scale. There were 12 respiratory therapists who responded.

Finally, there were other factors to consider in this decision, and you can review them in the documents in Appendix F. But the respiratory therapy department was convinced that a replacement of our fleet of Servo 300s with Viasys Aveas was warranted. We took all our data and transformed it into information that we then crafted into a crisp, clean, frightfully compelling PowerPoint presentation and started sharing our conclusions. I believe the thorough and methodical nature of our evaluation made the outcome a foregone conclusion—whatever we recommended to the hospital would probably be endorsed. Twenty-eight Viasys Aveas were purchased.

Implementation Planning

Of course there was still a lot of work to do, including retraining of all the respiratory therapy staff and training of the nursing and medical staffs when the ventilator was introduced, which was many months after the clinical trial. We had two choices with regard to implementation of this new ventilator technology. We could slowly phase the ventilators into use over a period of several months or pick a point in time and start at one end of the intensive care units and convert all the patients to Aveas. We chose the latter. Our reasoning went like this: The overall risk to patients of operator errors would be reduced if we trained everyone within a short period of time and required them all to start using the ventilator right away while the training was still fresh in their minds. This was compared to training everyone and then slowly rolling out the ventilator over a period of months and having all the initial training go stale. Minimizing risk to patients required extensive training and competency demonstration for all nurses and respiratory therapists. Physicians had to be trained too. The checklists and documents used for training and competency can be found in Appendix F. Do not underestimate the amount of planning and work that this phase of this project will take.

REFERENCES

1. Ginsburg PB. Controlling health care costs. *N Engl J Med.* October 14, 2004;351(16):1591–1593.
2. Bodenheimer T. High and rising health care costs. Part 2: technologic innovation. *Ann Intern Med.* 2005;142:932–937.
3. Meadow W, Lee G, Lin K, Lantos J. Changes in mortality for extremely low birth weight infants in the 1990s: implications for treatment decisions and resource use. *Pediatrics.* May 2004;113(5):1223–1229.

4. Cannon ML, et al. Tidal volumes for ventilated infants should be determined with a pneumotachometer placed at the endotracheal tube. *Am J Respir Crit Care Med.* 2000;162:2109–2112.

5. Neve V, Leclerc F, Noizet O, et al. Influence of respiratory system impedance on volume and pressure delivered at the Y piece in ventilated infants. *Pediatr Crit Care Med.* 2003;4:418–425.

6. Castle RA, Dunne CJ, Mok Q, et al. Accuracy of displayed values of tidal volume in the pediatric intensive care unit. *Crit Care Med.* 2002;30:2566–2574.

7. Salyer JW, Jackson C. Accuracy of tidal volume (V_T) displayed during volume targeted ventilation in neonatal ventilators. *Respir Care.* 2005;50:149.

8. Branson RD, Johannigman JA. What is the evidence base for the newer ventilation modes? *Respir Care.* 2004;49(7):742–760.

9. Ochroch EA, Russell MW, Hanson WC, et al. The impact of continuous pulse oximetry monitoring on intensive care unit admissions from a postsurgical care floor. *Anesth Analg.* 2006;102:868–875.

10. Salyer JW. Neonatal and pediatric pulse oximetry. *Respir Care.* 2003;48(4):386–396.

11. Durbin CG Jr, Rostow SK. More reliable oximetry reduces the frequency of arterial blood gas analyses and hastens oxygen weaning after cardiac surgery: a prospective, randomized trial of the clinical impact of a new technology. *Crit Care Med.* 2002;30(8):1735–1740.

12. Chow LC, Wright KW, Sola A, CSMC Oxygen Administration Study Group. Can changes in clinical practice decrease the incidence of severe retinopathy of prematurity in very low birth weight infants? *Pediatrics.* February 2003;111(2):339–345.

13. Lawless ST. Crying wolf: false alarms in a pediatric intensive care unit. *Crit Care Med.* 1994;22:981–985.

14. Poets CF, Urschitz MS, Bohnhorst B. Pulse oximetry in the neonatal intensive care unit (NICU): detection of hyperoxemia and false alarm rates. *Anesth Analg.* 2002;94:S41–S43.

15. Iglehart J. The new era of medical imaging—progress and pitfalls. *N Engl J Med.* 2006;354:26.

16. Farnsworth C. Testimony March 17, 2005, before the House Ways and Means Subcommittee on Health. Washington, D.C.

17. Wilson DF, Horn SJ, Hendley JO, Smout R, Gassaway J. Effect of practice variation on resource utilization in infants hospitalized for viral lower respiratory illness. *Pediatrics.* 2001;108(4):851–855.

18. Salyer J. Respiratory care of bronchiolitis patients: a proving ground for process improvement. *Respir Care.* June 2004;49(6):581–583.

19. Brook RH, Lohr KN. Efficacy, effectiveness, variations, and quality. Boundary-crossing research. *Med Care.* 1985;23(5):710–722.

20. Chatburn RL. Evaluation of instrument error and method agreement. *AANA J.* June 1996;64(3):261–268.

21. Crichton M. *State of Fear.* New York, NY: Avon Books; 2004.

22. Halm EA, Lee C, Chassin MR. Is volume related to outcome in health care? A systematic review and methodologic critique of the literature. *Ann Intern Med.* 2002;137:511–520.

23. Courtney SE, Durand DJ, Asselin JM, et al. High-frequency oscillatory ventilation versus conventional mechanical ventilation for very-low-birth-weight infants. *N Engl J Med.* 2002;347:643–652.

24. Johnson AH, Peacock JL, Greenough A, et al. High-frequency oscillatory ventilation for the prevention of chronic lung disease of prematurity. *N Engl J Med.* 2002;347:633–642.

25. Szymankiewicz M, Vidyasagar D, Gadzinowski J. Predictors of successful extubation of preterm low-birth-weight infants with respiratory distress syndrome. *Pediatr Crit Care Med.* 2005;6(1):44–49.

26. Tracy M, Downe L, Holberton J. How safe is intermittent positive pressure ventilation in preterm babies ventilated from delivery to newborn intensive care unit? *Arch Dis Child Fetal Neonatal Ed.* 2004;89(1):F84–7.

27. Sasaki C, Hoshi K, Wagatsuma T, Ejima Y, Hasegawa R, Matsukawa S. Comparison between tube compensation and pressure support ventilation techniques on respiratory mechanics. *Anaesth Intensive Care.* August 2003;31(4):371–375.

28. Al-Majed SI, Thompson JE, Watson KF, Randolph AG. Effect of lung compliance and endotracheal tube leakage on measurement of tidal volume. *Crit Care.* December 2004;8(6):R398–402.

29. Keenan J, Salyer JW, Ashby T, Withers J, Bee N. Manual ventilation technique variability in a pediatric lung model. *Respir Care.* 1999;44:1252.

30. Keenan J, Salyer JW, Ashby T, Withers J, Bee N. Ventilation variability using self-inflating and nonself-inflating resuscitation bags in a neonatal lung model. *Respir Care.* 1999;44:1253.

31. Salyer J, Foubare D. Ventilation variability using flow-inflating versus self-inflating manual resuscitators in a neonatal lung model. *Respir Care.* 2005;50:1498.

32. Salyer J, Foubare D. The myth of "feeling" compliance during manual ventilation. *Respir Care.* 2005;50:1512.

33. Spears RS, Yeh A, Fisher DM, Zwass MS. The "educated hand": Can anesthesiologists assess changes in neonatal compliance manually? *Anesthesiology.* 1991;75:693–696.

34. Salyer J, Jackson C. Accuracy of tidal volume (V_T) displayed during volume targeted ventilation in neonatal ventilators. *Respir Care.* 2005;50:1498.

35. Salyer J, Jackson C. Precision of tidal volume (V_T) delivered during volume targeted ventilation in a spontaneously breathing neonatal lung model with different neonatal ventilators. *Respir Care.* 2005;50:1498.

CHAPTER 9

Staff Development

Excellence is an art won by training and habituation. We do not act rightly
because we have virtue or excellence, but we rather have those because
we have acted rightly. We are what we repeatedly do. Excellence,
then, is not an act but a habit.

—Aristotle

The beautiful thing about learning is that no one can take it away from you.

—B.B. King

The single most important duty of the director–manager of a respiratory care department is to put the right therapist at the bedside of the right patient at the right time to give the right therapy. All the systems for staffing, budgeting, designing, measuring, structuring, and such are for naught if they are not toward this end. But who is the "right" therapist? I suggest that it is someone who is properly trained, motivated, supported, and supervised. This is the stuff of *staff development.* It is the combination of training, education, orientation, mentoring, and nagging that will serve to transform your everyday, pedestrian therapists into sharp edged clinical wonders. You can nail all the other systems, but if your clinicians are not rigorously trained and highly motivated, the rest of the systems you have crafted won't do you much good. And why shouldn't your staff be "clinical wonders"? Aim high. It is my experience that people tend to live up (or down) to whatever expectations are set for them. Do not misconstrue my remarks. I am not one who would motivate you by telling you that you can achieve anything that you can set your mind to. What a crock. For example, I was destined in life never to be able to slam dunk (at a regulation height rim). I could set my mind to dunking all day for 20 years and it will never be. But you can achieve a lot more than you generally think you can. So too can your staff achieve much more than they might believe.

Immutable Truth #28: It is very hard to have too much training. It's all about training. A vital staff development program is a hard thing to create and even tougher to sustain. It requires a lot of hands on attention and steady gentle pressure to keep it from becoming stagnant, slowing down, and fading away. Our human tendency is to believe, after a while, that we know it all, and there is little left to show us. An avocation like respiratory therapy can promote this kind of intellectual lethargy. Your job as a leader is to oppose this every chance you get. Keep yourself freshly interested in your field and require it of others.

You are required by regulatory fiat to ensure the competency of your staff, so most departments have some form of training and development activity. But it is sometimes pretty minimal and is focused on procedural skill. The field has undergone tremendous change since I first began disassembling IPPB setups during the previous century, oh so many decades back. The complexity of equipment and intensity of care have increased dramatically. In many care models the respiratory therapists are now expected to function at a pretty high level with regard to patient assessment and critical thinking. This requires a lot of training and practice, most of which RTs do not possess when they emerge from two year training programs. My view is that this is just not enough time. The schools do a respectable job considering the constraints they have to operate within, and there are some schools that turn out remarkably prepared students, all things considered. But still a four year degree ought to be our minimum entry level training requirement. I think the majority of leaders in this field agree with this, but getting from here to there will take some time, and the passage will be wind swept and strewn with jagged rock.

The evolving duties of respiratory therapists and the limited amount of time the schools have available have shifted some of the training and development burden away from the schools and toward hospitals. Hospitals end up doing a fair amount of what I consider to be remedial instruction of new graduates in the basics of patient assessment, basic aerosol science, oxygen transport, and respiratory physiology. Please do not regard this as a criticism of the two year schools. It is simply the truth. If you want respiratory therapists to function at the highest possible levels, such as autonomous practice using protocols and guidelines, they are going to require a lot of training after graduation.

Of course you could skip hiring new graduates and presumably skip this aspect of the training and development burden. Good luck with that. Early on in my so-called management career I thought the hospitals I was in should not hire new graduates. I reasoned that the practice environments at the tertiary academic medical centers were too demanding and risky and that new graduates ought to go hone their skills somewhere else. So I decided to only consider experienced candidates for hire. After a few years of chronic inability to find qualified experienced candidates, I gave this up. And the truth is that I have much better outcomes in the long run hiring new graduates.

A much larger proportion of new graduates that I have hired turned out to be good clinicians and employees than did the experienced people I have hired. Besides, believing that experienced respiratory therapists will come to you with solid fundamentals is spurious. There are a lot of experienced therapists out there who could use some remedial instruction too.

The need for advanced training for respiratory therapists has been clearly demonstrated by a number of studies related to the application of therapist driven protocols (TDPs). An editorial in the journal *Chest* said, "Institutions approving TDPs should restrict participation to experienced RCPs proven to have specialized knowledge and skills."[1]

One of the very best respiratory therapy departments in the world is the program at the Cleveland Clinic. They suggest that, "Consult evaluators need to have well-developed respiratory care skills, but also should be ambassadors for the program and educators to other health care providers regarding the delivery of appropriate respiratory care."[2] They go on to point out that TDPs call on therapists to go beyond the technical expertise of administering treatments, namely the following:[3]

- Knowledge about the science of respiratory care and clinical indications for specific therapies
- Excellent skills in assessing patients and their response to therapies
- Self-confidence and communication skills that permit useful interaction with other health care providers

Failure to do a lot of rigorous training of your respiratory therapy staff and then expecting them to administer care in complex environments using assessment skills and TDPs just doesn't work very well. It has repeatedly been shown that even when respiratory therapists are given TDPs to guide their practice, the care they recommend for patients can be discordant with the best practice. This rate of discordance has been shown to range from 15% to 79% depending on the level of experience and amount of training of the respiratory therapy staff.[4–9]

COMMUNICATION

"What we have here, is failure to communicate."[i]

I have come to believe that the single largest intrinsic, ubiquitous, unfailing, constant barrier we face in organizational life is communicating effectively

---

[i]From my favorite prison film, *Cool Hand Luke.* If you have not seen Strother Martin deliver this line as the "Captain," then you have missed a great piece of Americana.

with one another across dimensions of time and space. Consider these fine examples of signs spotted recently:

- In a toilet of an office: "Toilet out of order. Please use floor below."
- In an office: "Would the person who took the step ladder yesterday please bring it back or further steps will be taken."
- In an office: "After tea break staff should empty the teapot and stand upside down on the draining board."
- Seen at a notice board: for anyone who has children and doesn't know it, there is a day care centre on the first floor.
- On a repair shop door: "We can repair anything (please knock hard on the door—the bell doesn't work)."
- Outside a shop selling secondhand items: "We exchange anything—bicycles, washing machines, etc. . . . Why not bring your wife along and get a wonderful bargain?"

Good communications can be an elusive thing. You can work at it and work at it and think you have it figured out only to realize, sometimes at the most inopportune time, that you really haven't communicated what you wanted to at all. Or conversely you can listen to what someone is saying to you, act on it, and then later realize you missed what they were really trying to communicate.

The explosion of information and communication technology ought to have helped us with this. I am not so sure. The trouble is the low signal to noise ratio. So much of the communication that comes to us in corporate life is low priority noise, and we have trouble sorting that out from the more important messages that we ought to pay attention to.

It is useful to think carefully for a moment about communication theory. Peter F. Drucker (1909–2005) was a noted management theorist and author. He said that the following are fundamentals of communication:[10]

1. Communication is perception of the recipient not the utterance of the instigator—Wow is this ever true. What you meant to say or write or present is one thing. What the listener comes away with may be something else entirely. In conversations like interviews or coaching sessions I often repeat the key things I was trying to get across. Sometimes I repeat them several times to help ensure receipt of the message. In long, complex conversations it is also very useful to summarize the discussion at the end so there is minimal confusion about what transpired. This goes both ways. You have to listen very carefully to what people

are trying to say to you. If you are not *actively* listening you may confuse what people *actually* say to you with what they *meant* to say to you. I am articulate and something of a loud mouth and have always talked a lot. You would think I would be good at communicating. Not. Early on in my career and personal life I (at first reluctantly) took a number of communication classes. I eventually was forced to admit how much these helped me.

2. Communication is expectation in that recipients will heed only what they are expecting to hear—Expectations can be barriers to overcome in communication. I used to think I had it all figured out. People were easy to read. Why, in fact, after listening to the first few words out of someone's mouth, I thought I already knew the substance of what they were going to say. So while they were still talking, I was busy planning what I was going to say back to them. This is very bad form and risky business. I missed a lot. I had expectations of what I was going to hear, indeed of even what I wanted to hear. So often communication was garbled, incomplete, or ineffective. Usually on the receiving end. Unless I really actively concentrate, this still happens to me. Good listening takes work.

3. Communication makes demands of the recipient that they become someone, do, or believe something—This is certainly true in corporate communication. Generally communication is intended to elicit action in others whether it be to change behaviors or beliefs. It might be argued that this is the essence of true communication and everything else that happens under the guise of talking and writing is just the exchange of information, which in and of itself is not really communicating.

Clinical Communication

If you really want to deeply and fundamentally improve the quality of your clinical processes you should spend a lot of time working on seamless systems of communication. This is the heart of staff development because you cannot help them develop if they are not communicating effectively with one another or with you or with other disciplines. The lack of effective communication has been identified as a major cause of errors and mishaps in the health care system. The JCAHO analyzed 3000 reports (Sentinel Events) from 1995 to 2004 and found that 65% were caused by communication problems. In 2005 it rose to nearly 70%.

One place that communication repeatedly breaks down is at the points where responsibility for patients is passed from one entity to another. When patients are transferred between units, when a report is given from one shift to another, or when management of patients passes from one medical service to another, this is often called a "hand-off." This is where lots of errors occur as a result of poor communication. The JCAHO has issued a National Patient Safety Goal related to improving the quality of communication. These guidelines warrant review even if you have already seen them.

- Goal 2—Improve the effectiveness of communication among caregivers.
    - 2A—For verbal or telephone orders or for telephonic reporting of critical test results, verify the complete order or test result by having the person receiving the information record and read back the complete order or test result.
    - 2B—Standardize a list of abbreviations, acronyms, symbols, and dose designations that are not to be used throughout the organization.
    - 2C—Measure, assess, and, if appropriate, take action to improve the timeliness of reporting, and the timeliness of receipt by the responsible licensed caregiver, of critical test results and values.
    - 2D—Implement a standardized approach to hand-off communications, including an opportunity to ask and respond to questions.

Obviously respiratory therapists are deeply involved in areas of practice related to all of these standards. Respiratory therapy is particularly guilty of using a dizzying array of homegrown abbreviations. We report lots of critical lab values, and we give and receive (hopefully) complex, detailed reports on many patients every time we work. These national patient safety recommendations all came out of the painful experience of learning from our mistakes. Of course, our pain ain't nearly as acute as that of our patients on whom we practice our imperfect arts. I know of a number of very bad outcomes related to botched or nonexistent communications across shifts and between and within clinical disciplines.

The American Association of Critical-Care Nurses (AACN) has collaborated with a commercial consulting company to publish a report entitled "Silence Kills." This is an excellent review of the contribution of poor communication to errors and breakdowns in our health care systems. I highly recommend a careful review of this excellent monograph.[11]

It has been suggested that a major contributor to dangerous breakdowns in communication is the hierarchical nature of our team structures. Typically doctors lead the team, and nurses, therapists, and technologists are on various rungs of the descending food chain. This hierarchy is intended to place the people with the most training, skill, and experience in positions of authority, and some would argue that such a hierarchical system is very valuable and ought to diminish errors and mishaps. But some theoreticians in health systems design have speculated that this hierarchical structure may actually contribute to errors because of "authority gradients."[12] These gradients cause more junior members of the team to be reluctant to speak up when they have doubts about what is happening, and these same gradients cause more senior members to be too dismissive of the suggestions and observations of junior team members. The military has learned that authority gradients in the cockpit can be deadly.[13] Cosby and Croskerry put it very well and I will quote from them.[12]

When officers of different ranks occupy a helicopter cockpit together, the rate of aircrew mishaps increases. As the transcockpit authority gradient increases, so does the number of incidents. As many as 40% of junior ranking copilots reported a failure to relay significant doubts about safety to their pilots. When junior officers do offer their concerns, their senior-ranking officers may dismiss them without careful consideration. The failures of subordinate first officers to challenge their captains despite dangerous actions and violations of safety rules, and the failures of captains to heed warnings from crew members, are cited as factors in a number of airplane crashes, including the runway collision of two airliners at Tenerife in 1977 in which 583 people died.[ii]

This has direct bearing on the practice of respiratory therapy. The respiratory therapists practice in a team environment where the therapist–nurse–physician team manages the patient. If any member of the team feels uncomfortable speaking up or does not possess the basic communication skills to clearly articulate their concerns, mistakes and bad outcomes can happen. Why talk about all of this in a chapter on staff development? Because you have to inculcate these ideas in your staff. These philosophies and skills do not just happen, they have to be developed. Leading this charge is *your* job as a director–manager.

This idea that anyone on the team should and can speak up with impunity about any patient safety concerns has several names. Some hospitals refer to the practice as "stopping the line," in which all staff are encouraged to speak

---

[ii]My younger readers may not remember this tragedy. In the Canary Islands, one fully loaded 747 was taking off in limited visibility and struck another fully loaded 747 that was taxiing on the only runway at the airport. Everyone on the plane taking off died, but incredibly some passengers on the taxiing aircraft survived.

and stop whatever process or procedure is happening if they have concerns about the appropriateness of what is happening. This term came out of manufacturing production theory in which the highest possible quality is ensured by empowering anyone on the production line to stop the line if they see a problem. Conceptually this is similar to the aviation philosophy of "crew resource management." This term refers to the practice of fully utilizing all the resources of your crew by maximizing their training and communication skills as well as empowering them to communicate with those above them in the authority gradient and ensuring that those above them listen carefully to all concerns voiced by junior crew members.[14] I once heard a grand rounds lecture given by a commercial airline pilot. He was married to an anesthesiologist and thus got connected to the academic medical community. He told a harrowing story. He was in command of a jetliner during bad weather. Before takeoff they drove the aircraft to the deicing area. After deicing they were about to take off when the copilot voiced concerns that something didn't seem right about the deicing. He couldn't quite say what it was, but something about it bothered him. The pilot thought for a moment and decided to stop the line. They aborted their takeoff and reinspected the outside of the aircraft. They then discovered that the deicing equipment had malfunctioned, and if they had taken off, the aircraft would most certainly have crashed. Had the pilot dismissed the vague and undifferentiated concerns of the copilot, a great tragedy could have occurred. Consider the pressures the pilot is under to take off on time. It is this kind of leadership and team cohesiveness we need to foster in the health care environment. And as a leader of the respiratory therapy service, you need to be on the leading edge. You must encourage your staff to speak up, and you must back them up when they do, whether they are speaking up with one another, with nurses, or physicians.

Cosby and Croskerry[12] have developed a list of proposed system changes and educational recommendations to minimize the risk of authority gradients causing dangerous communications breakdowns:

1. Trainees should be empowered to present their opinions and information they consider relevant.
2. Authority figures need to recognize that valuable information comes from many sources and to carefully consider the contributions others provide.
3. Experienced clinicians should use clinical narratives to illustrate their own vulnerability to error.
4. Teamwork factors and patient safety should take precedence over authority roles.

5. Changes in medical education should begin early and continue throughout the professional lives of physicians to help them adopt healthy communication styles.
6. Systems should be designed to facilitate effective teamwork and provide support for clinicians.

Clearly these recommendations are appropriate for any clinical discipline. I particularly like number 3. We have to model the behavior we want to induce in others, including telling our own stories of mistakes.

The AACN has also published a very interesting report on recommendations for creating a healthy work environment, which speaks directly to the issue of creating good communications systems.[15] The report is focused on nurses, but the ideas expressed therein are universal and merit consideration. Table 9-1 lists their standards for establishing and sustaining healthy work environments. I suggest that you obtain both of these AACN reports and review them very carefully.

Table 9-1. AACN Recommendations for Sustaining a Healthy Workplace[15]

Skilled communication	Respiratory therapists must be as proficient in communication skills as they are in clinical skills.
True collaboration	Respiratory therapists must be relentless in pursuing and fostering true collaboration.
Effective decision making	Respiratory therapists must be valued and committed partners in making policy, directing and evaluating clinical care, and leading organizational operations.
Appropriate staffing	Staffing must ensure the effective match between patient needs and therapists' competencies.
Meaningful recognition	Respiratory therapists must be recognized and must recognize others for the value each brings to the work of the organization.
Authentic leadership	Respiratory therapy leaders must fully embrace the imperative of a healthy work environment, authentically live it, and engage others in its achievement.

These recommendations were first published for nurses. I have adapted them by cleverly substituting the term "respiratory therapists" wherever it said "nurses."

Communication within Your Department

One of the very best pieces of advice I can give you on improving the quality of your communication is to keep it lean and clear. I cannot tell you how many times I have fallen into a deep and restful sleep sitting at my desk trying to read through some dense, turgid memo or e-mail that was carefully and thoughtfully constructed. E-mail writers often operate under the assumption that the best way to get my attention and spur me to action or get my support is to include a mind boggling amount of detail. Because some information appears to be good, well then, more information must be better. This premise is sometimes carried to a nearly absurd length. Do not give in to this temptation when communicating with your staff either orally or in written form. Keep your messages few and simple. Otherwise it just gets lost in the clutter.

But what about the mechanics of communication? How best to get the message out? Here is a description and assessment of the currently available methods:

- Bulletin boards—These are effective only if maintained by debriding them regularly of accumulated detritus. If you do not clear these boards off regularly, their utility drops to near nil. Don't be afraid to remove the latest hospital flyers on yoga classes and diversity training. This is your bulletin board, so own it. However, even under the best of conditions, the bulletin board is only marginally effective. If you do use one, be sure to use visual clues like color or large fonts to grab the reader's attention.
- Paper memos—The hit rate here is rather low, especially if you use the traditional mailbox method for each staff member. Many therapists only check their snail mail occasionally in this enlightened digital age. Paper memos are slightly more effective if manually passed out by the leadership team. I know of departments that have a list of all staff members, and they have the staff members initial this list when they are given a memo. This is supposed to minimize the frequency of episodes when someone says, "No one ever told me," which drives most supervisors and managers to distraction.
- Marker board messages—If your staff room has a marker board this is a pretty effective way of communicating, although it is technically informal in that it cannot really be used later as a proof of communication.

You will see later in this chapter the role that proof of communication plays in staff development.

- E-mail—As I have said before, I have a love/hate relationship with e-mail. Remember, sending e-mails is only marginally effective. Yes, yes, you can rant and rave if you want to about how staff members don't read their e-mails, and what in the world is wrong with them, and it is a crying shame, etc. While this offers you temporary emotional satisfaction, in the end you still have to admit that e-mail has not lived up to its potential. As I have said, it is all about information glut.

- Talking—It is surpassingly easy to slip into the path of least resistance and not spend much time talking to your staff. I go through these cycles where I seem to be caught up in the daily grind of meetings and documents and spreadsheets and voice mail and e-mail and incident reports and projects and this and that and that and this. When this happens, I don't spend enough time just talking with my staff. This usually results in confusion, misunderstandings, and discontentment. When this happens I try to reassert myself. This is a battle you will never win, but is also one you can never give up on. "Cut and run" doesn't work here either.

If I had to pick the most effective technique for communication within your department, my answer would be: all of them. If it is a really important issue that needs to be communicated, I would send an e-mail, post a notice on the bulletin board, put a memo in everyone's snail mail box, write a message on the staff room white boards, and talk to everyone I could to deliver the message in person. This will give you maximum coverage. Of course you do not want to do this too often because the Chicken Little/boy who cried wolf coefficient will eventually reduce your communication to just more noise.

CREDENTIALS: THE END OF THE ENDLESS DEBATE

I could be more tired of the debate about credentials, but I would have to work at it. It is inconceivable to me that otherwise rational people in my field still take the untenable position that advanced practice credentials don't really make any difference. For those of you young enough not to have suffered through 20 years of this debate, allow me to summarize for you.

- There are still a lot of CRTTs (now CRTs) out there who either couldn't or didn't ever sit for the RRT exam. A lot of them have a sort of dualistic syndrome, which I am calling "professional identity crisis/inferiority complex."[iii]
- Every so often, this topic percolates up in letters to the editor and on e-mail Listservs like RC_World. The debate principally devolves into two camps. Those with advanced practice credentials and those without. The certified crowd gets mortally offended when anyone suggests that registered respiratory therapists (RRTs) make better therapists or give better care or function at a higher clinical level than do CRTTs.

The debate is preposterous. Why, don't you know that every single CRTT can tell you stories about RRTs who were crummy therapists and conversely can tell you about CRTTs who practiced better than Dean Hess, Mike Czervinski, Bob Kacmarek, Rob Chatburn, and Rich Branson all rolled into one? FYI gang, these arguments usually come from those without advanced practice credentials. It's probably just a coincidence. The problem with this argument goes back to *Immutable Truth #4: The plural of anecdote is not data.* Yeah, so there are lots of these stories around. But so what? There is no doubt in my mind that if I could find a way to administer an assessment of the clinical performance of 1000 randomly selected CRTTs versus 1000 randomly selected RRTs that the registered crowd would score better. This is not because they *have* an RRT credential. It's because they *got* an RRT credential. It is the journey that matters here much more than the destination. The studying that staff members will do to prepare themselves to pass an advanced practice examination gives them a better foundation upon which to build excellent clinical practice. I am not suggesting these exams are perfect nor that there are not many gifted clinicians who have only a CRTT (CRT). But here is the truth of this for me. If you come to apply for a job in my department, and you never bothered to get your RRT credential, then I am immediately a little suspicious. The RRT credential tells me, among other things, that you are motivated. And blaming others or the system for your lack of credentials is pretty self-serving.

[iii]Come to think of it, the respiratory therapy profession as a whole has more than its share of folks who seem to be hung up a bit about not getting respect from hospitals, doctors, nurses, pharmacists, phlebotomists, whomever. I am pretty much sick to death of hearing about how badly treated respiratory therapists are. If you are not getting the respect of your colleagues on the health care team, it might be time to look in the mirror. If you want respect, you might try getting it the old fashioned way—by earning it. You do this by continually working on your professional development. Reading, studying, developing a spirit of inquiry and a search for excellence—that is how you get respect.

To argue against this is delusional. Think of it this way. When you finally plug off your left anterior descending coronary artery, will it matter to you whether the doctor who is about to crack your chest is fully credentialed? You bet your sweet bippy it will.[iv] To my many friends and colleagues who never bothered to go ahead and get the advanced practice credentials, I say "absit invidia."[v]

Because your first duty is to your patients, you should build a practice model that offers your patients the best opportunity to get the highest level of care possible. This is partly achieved by offering them the highest credentialed and trained staff you possibly can. You may be constrained by the culture and workplace realities of your hospital, but you should do all in your power to get all your staff to hold advanced practice credentials. I am personally not a big fan of setting up different pay scales for certified and registered therapists. My opposition stems from the observation that the therapists in these different pay scales are often used interchangeably in the day-to-day bump and grind of staffing assignments. Thus staff members are side by side giving ostensibly the same kind of care to the same kinds of patients, and yet they are getting different rates of pay. This constitutes unfair labor practice in my book. But lots of different departments get away with this. God bless them. It is probably better than not having any system that has financial incentives that promote advanced practice credentials.

I think a better system of pay for credentials is to design different jobs within the department that have different minimal levels of required credentials. This is sometimes called a clinical ladder. The jobs are designed differently, and work is assigned differently based on the job descriptions, and thus, pay is different.

As an example, I know of a pediatric respiratory department that has two job descriptions:

- RT-I—Minimal requirements include being a graduate of a two-year school, a state license (which requires passing the entry level examination). Duties include assignment to all areas of the hospital except the interhospital transport team and the extracorporeal membrane oxygenation team.

[iv]Oops, this is another obscure aged cultural reference. This is from that icon to late 20th century television art, Rowan and Martin's *Laugh-In*. Although somewhat uneven at times, it was simply the most consistently funny thing I ever saw on television.

[v]Latin for "no offense intended." The train is leaving the station, and with compassion and concern I suggest that you get on board and get your advanced practice credential, pronto.

- RT-II—Minimal requirements include an RRT credential, one year of pediatric/neonatal critical care experience, and membership on either the ECMO team or interhospital transport team. Membership in either of these teams requires Pediatric Advanced Life Support and/or Neonatal Resuscitation Program credentials.

Such a system is far from perfect, but it does offer a career path and thus incentives for people to do self-development. I have also always practiced "you pass, I pay." I have found a way to pay for the examination fees for staff members who passed the advanced practice examinations. I tell staff members not to bother asking for pay in advance or if they flunk. But if they passed, I paid. How did I achieve this? Well, I just did it. I did not ask permission, I just started cutting reimbursement checks from my miscellaneous expense account. So far I have gotten away with this. Often my miscellaneous expense account is over budget because of this. But this is usually coincidental with some other accounts being under budget. I often tend to overspend my travel and education account too, operating under the same principle of asking for forgiveness as opposed to permission. And the truth is that if the quality of your clinical staff improves, this will be noted by physicians and administrators, and allowances will often be made. Probably one of the reasons I have gotten away with sometimes overspending my travel and education accounts is the rate at which we have published and presented abstracts and research projects at conferences. This gets the hospital good press, improves your recruiting posture, and in the end is probably worth every penny of over spending, a fact that is not lost on most progressive administrators. If your administrator is not progressive in such matters, you may want to think about relocation.

Clinical ladders in general are controversial. This is because they are sometimes either not designed properly or used properly. As I stated earlier, just paying for the possession of an advanced practice credential rubs some people the wrong way. They want to see some difference in the way practitioners with different credentials are assigned work. Some clinical ladders sort of give lip service to this concept, but in the daily ebb and flow of staffing assignments, the clinicians on different levels of the clinical ladders are used the same way and given the same assignments. And thus you have the controversy: different pay for similar work. The best goal is to set a ladder that promotes professional development and uses the advanced practitioners in a different pattern of patient assignments and duties than those without advanced practice credentials.

HIRING

The turnover rate is typically defined as the number of respiratory therapy positions that were vacated during the year divided by the total number of therapists employed at the end of the year. The national turnover rate for full-time staff is 17%, and for part-time staff it is 25%.[16] There are probably a lot of good reasons and some not so good reasons for these findings. Women make up 60% of the RT workforce, and they enter and leave the workforce more for child bearing and rearing. I also believe that the nature of hospital schedules—working nights, weekends, and holidays—drives some people from the field. And finally, I believe these high turnover rates are in part contributed to by poor management practices. If department leadership does not create a good work environment, retention can be poor.

All this results in an endless cycle of recruitment and hiring. Unless you are very lucky, you will end up interviewing and hiring a lot of people in your career. I think this is one of the areas that is most lacking of training and skill at the department management level in the respiratory therapy community. I know I have struggled with it. I got a bachelors degree in health care management and a masters in business administration, and yet I got almost no practical training in the subtleties of interviewing and selecting candidates. I have hired some great candidates, and I have hired some bad ones. Once, my team and I reviewed all the hires in a department I was managing over a 4-year period. We looked at all the people we had hired and how well they worked out. We concluded that our good hiring rate was 0.75. In other words, about 75% of our hires worked out very well. It also means that, in retrospect, we wished we had not hired about 25% of the folks we did.

It is very challenging to hire people "cold." By this I mean clinicians who come to you from other hospitals or new graduates about whom you know very little. The cold part refers to the fact that I can get no meaningful first-hand information about them. When I call their previous supervisors, I am often referred to human resources departments, who are legendary in their reluctance to tell you anything important. They will typically only confirm dates of employment and eligibility for rehire (maybe). This is so pervasive it makes the hiring process very difficult. The conventional wisdom is that if you say anything negative about an employee when you are called for a reference, you can get sued, although I cannot say exactly what it is that you might be sued for. Slander I suppose. I must say that in my entire career I have never met anyone or heard of anyone who ever got sued for giving a bad reference. But I am sure there was some notorious lawsuit filed somewhere by someone that resulted in a big settlement. And, as is often the case, we over react. Now it is impossible to get formal, meaningful references from a hospital about a former employee.

There is of course an informal network of managers and supervisors who routinely call one another about staff they are thinking about hiring. I personally almost always give an honest appraisal of an employee if I am called for a reference. Where you can get into trouble is saying something about an employee that is untrue or that you cannot prove. If you say that an employee had crummy attendance but you never mentioned this in the performance reviews of that employee, you might get yourself in a jam if this information was then used to exclude this person from a job they were seeking.

Even though you may not get former employers to talk to you on the phone, I always try anyway. Sometimes you get lucky.

I will summarize my views on the hiring process.

- The application—Patti Gurza-Dully and Margaret Melaney from Stanford University Medical Center did some very interesting research on various things that can be known about an applicant before you hire them and how predictive these things are of the future quality of the employee.[17] I highly recommend that you study this report. It sort of confirms my intuitive conclusion that hiring new graduates is probably, on the whole, no riskier than hiring experienced therapists. Their data showed that the most significant predictors were "grade point average in respiratory therapy school, college education in addition to respiratory therapy training, and surprisingly, the neatness of the application form itself." Go figure. Now, of course, most applications are submitted online. But I have always asked about grade point average, at least for recent new graduates. And of course, additional college education is almost always a good thing.

- Work history—Carefully examine the work history on the application. Check for continuity to see if they have been continuously employed. If not it could be because they could not get hired in a given community or they had problems staying motivated to work or keep a job. Of course there are other good reasons for periods of unemployment, so just remember this might be a flag to direct you to probe carefully during the interview about their work history. Another important consideration is their longevity at jobs. If they have moved around every 2–3 years, it is not a good sign, and they might be someone who has trouble fitting in or is just never quite satisfied with their job or their chosen field.

- Technology history—By this I mean you should carefully examine the history of the kinds of equipment the person has worked with. Respiratory practice is very technology driven. Occasionally a candidate will over represent his or her skill or experience level, particularly with regard to his or her experience with given pieces of equipment. You must ask your questions about this in a manner that will draw out what they really know about the equipment they claim to have experience with.
- The interview—Interviews should be just that. They are not a chance for you to pontificate and share your vast wisdom with the applicant. The applicant should do most of the talking; a nice goal is 75%. You should have a standard list of questions you ask. They should be designed to test the applicant's communication skills and motivations. Here are mine:
  - Why did you choose respiratory therapy?
  - Why this hospital? (Or a variant: why pediatrics?)
  - Everyone has strengths and weaknesses. Please tell me your principal strength and principal weakness (with regard to whatever job they are applying for).
  - Tell me about a time when you dealt with a very emotionally charged situation at your previous job. How did you handle it? What, if anything, could you have done better?
  - What questions do you have about the job you are applying for?

- I also make a point of telling the applicant the strengths and weaknesses of the hospital and some basic expectations for standards of interpersonal behavior. If they are applying for their first night shift position, I make sure they understand the impact nights may have on their life and give some brief examples of how to manage the rigors of working nights. I almost never hire anyone without having them also be interviewed by other members of the leadership team in a separate interview. I usually ask another supervisor or manager to sit in on my interview too.
- Appearance—I am old school. I think you ought to dress up for interviews and dress professionally at work. Appearances matter. Of course I have been known to spend the entire weekend at home in my pajama bottoms and a T-shirt (in fact, the *same* pajama bottoms and T-shirt), but come Monday morning I am wearing a tie again. I know, I know, the whole tie thing is a bizarre cultural phenomenon based on irrational and outdated views of conformity. But for inexplicable reasons, it seems to matter and it seems to transmit a message to your patients, their

families, and your staff and colleagues that you take yourself and your
work seriously. I remember once taking my daughter (who was five at
the time) to a hospital to get blood drawn. The phlebotomist came in. He
was a tall young strapping figure of a man, resplendent in his denim
shorts, T-shirt, ponytail, and tasteful gym shoes, all topped off with a
dazzling white lab coat. I was pretty uncomfortable and wondered how
serious he was about his job. It turns out he was quite skilled in leech
craft and got her blood sample with a minimum of pain. But why did I
have to feel uncomfortable at all? Why could he not have dressed in an
outfit that conformed a little more with the norms of the community
being served?

- Persistence—I like applicants who call back or e-mail about once a week
  to see if the position has been filled. This tells me they are determined. I
  like that. However let's not get carried away here.

Finally, I do not tend to make hiring decisions in a vacuum. I ask all those
who conducted interviews to render a yes/no opinion. No waffling permitted. But even if you do it all properly, sometimes hires don't turn out so good.

Case Study 15: Steadily Depressing, Low Down Mind Messing, Working on the Night Shift Blues

Louis Wu, RRT was hired to work the night shift at St. Elsewhere Medical
Center. He had just gotten divorced and decided to relocate to another state for
a new start. He had 17 years of experience in a community hospital intensive
care unit. But he had never worked nights. He knew that he would have to take
a night shift job to get a position at a good hospital like St. Elsewhere, which
was renowned as a busy, academic medical center. So he took the plunge. He
was hired based on his years of experience and the excellent letters of reference that came with him. The department director, Teela Brown, RRT, was
pretty proud of landing Louis, and his hiring was broadly considered quite a
coup. But the euphoria was short lived. Louis oriented on day shift. There were
some concerns about the pace of his work, and he had a couple of technical
mistakes, but altogether it wasn't deemed enough to pull the plug during orientation. Then Louis moved to night shift. He started making a series of technical
mistakes, lapses, and oversights. Any one of them could have been ascribed to
any good RT, but all of them together started giving Teela a real bad feeling
about Louis. She met with him and reviewed his progress, and she shared
her concerns and put him on corrective discipline. She was convinced he was

profoundly sleep deprived and was having trouble adjusting to working nights. He initially denied this. But all was for naught. Things did not improve, and finally he resigned, knowing as he did, that he was about to be terminated.

Teela called her leadership team together and they debriefed about the hiring decision for Louis. They concluded the following: (1) his experience in a community based ICU did not turn out to prepare him well enough for the complexity of the academic medical center environment, and (2) he might have been able to learn, but the debilitating effects of night shift was not conducive to him learning much. They decided that the hiring decision was reasonable based on the information they had at the time.

RECRUITMENT

Of course, you won't have to make any tough hiring decisions if you get no applicants for your open positions. Don't laugh. In some parts of the country this is not uncommon. And if your department gets a bad reputation in town, your applicant pool will dry up faster than a West Texas lake in August. Recruitment activities in respiratory care are complicated by the calculus of the workforce. Demand for new respiratory therapists is outpacing the supply of new graduates each year by about 1000 therapists nationwide. Therefore, there is some pretty fierce competition for staff going on.

My view is that the very best long-term recruitment activity is to create a healthy workplace for respiratory therapists. If you do this, you won't have to recruit very hard. This is because word will get out on the street and your department will begin to get a steady stream of applicants. A healthy work environment consists of competitive compensation, fair treatment, good leadership, interesting work, a chance for professional development, and a sense of recognition for your work. But these things take time to develop. In the interim, you will have to try some of the more classical recruitment tools.

- Booths at national conferences—You can rent booths at conferences and try to recruit therapists that attend scientific and professional meetings. This is very pricey. Booths at national meetings will run you three large for the booth and then the travel expenses of the staff to run the booth. I have done this about five times in my career and have had very poor luck. Maybe I am no good at it. I have let the human resources folks run the booth sometimes, but other times I have made a point of running the booth myself. It didn't seem to make any difference. There are probably several reasons why this happens. First, the folks that go to conferences and meetings are generally the cream of the crop, and the reason they are there is because they work at hospitals that will support their attendance. Thus they are pretty happy at their jobs and not looking to change. And recruiting at national meetings means folks have to relocate to your hospital. Long distance relocations rarely happen for RTs in my experience.

- Booths at state conferences—These are probably a better bet for your recruiting dollar. But the hit rate from them has historically been low for me too, although slightly better than recruiting at national conferences. They certainly are cheaper, and because you *should* be going to the state meeting anyway, you might as well recruit while you are there.

- Advertising—I have had a mixed bag of success advertising. It has gotten somewhat better lately with the advent of online job posting Web sites. The sad truth is that trade journals are regularly reviewed by only a small portion of the RT community. Nevertheless I periodically advertise in journals like *Advance for Respiratory Care Practitioners, Focus, Respiratory Therapy* and the *AARC Times,* as well as online job postings on the major job sites. If you do advertise, give some careful thought to your ad copy. In some organizations, you can kick back and let the recruiters in human resources write your ad copy for you. This is probably not a good idea because they typically don't know a lot about respiratory therapists and may not understand what motivates respiratory therapists. You should write your own ad copy, and use your own intuition about what it is in a job that interests respiratory therapists.

- Job fairs—If you take the long view, the best way to improve the quantity and quality of candidates for respiratory therapy jobs is to get more people interested in being respiratory therapists. One way to do this is to participate in job fairs. These events give you a chance to tout the glories of respiratory therapy as a profession. They take many forms. Some are put on by local entities like employment agencies and high schools. Sometimes hospitals hold their own job fairs to encourage non-clinical employees to consider a career change into some of the difficult to recruit clinical disciplines like pharmacy, laboratory, or respiratory therapy. Whenever I am asked to participate in these, I agree. And we usually make a big deal about it. If possible I bring along the most exotic looking equipment and the most complex devices and turn them on so they are running. I take along oximeters and flow meters and offer to measure folks' lung health. I openly display our pay scales and typically bring along a staff member or two to give them the unvarnished, nonmanagement view. This is a great opportunity to recruit into the field, don't miss out on it.

Other things you must consider when developing your recruitment activities include the practices of offering sign-on bonuses and relocation allowance. Let's start with the least important one, relocation. In my experience I just haven't had much luck attracting people from outside the region of whatever hospital I was working in. It does happen but not very often. Typically hospitals have a standard relocation package that they offer. It is generally not available for all types of positions and sometimes not for respiratory therapists. You need to lobby to include therapists in the list of positions for which the hospital is willing to pay relocation allowances. Paying relocation and sign-on bonus is a lot cheaper in the long run than using agency or traveling staff.

Sign-on bonuses are a useful tool and probably help attract some people, especially because so many hospitals are offering them for respiratory therapists. I have seen them range from $2000 to $15,000. Yes, Pinky, I said $15,000. I saw this advertised in *Advance for Respiratory Care Practitioners*. I don't know the details, but I suspect it was not all paid out up front at the time of hiring. This is a growing trend. Departments (including mine) have been burned by paying sign-on bonuses up front only to have people leave in 9 months. Some organizations expressly state in their offer letters that sign-on bonuses come with an expectation of a certain minimum length of employment, but of course this is difficult to enforce. If the newly hired people leave before the proscribed period, they are supposed to refund a prorated amount of the sign-on bonus to the hospital, but this is difficult to enforce. One way to avoid this is to split up the bonus and pay part at the time of hire and the remainder at the end of the minimum required length of employment. I suspect that the $15,000 example was paid out in increments over a three-year period.

RETENTION

With turnover rates among respiratory therapists between 17% and 25%, it would seem that we should be very focused on retention. Turning over staff is very expensive. I estimate that the cost of training and orienting a new hire in my department currently ranges between $25,000 and $35,000, especially if he or she is a new graduate. This includes their total training costs from hiring to completion of ICU training, which can be a period spanning 18 months in our department. During this time they are not always in training and do spend a considerable time doing billable procedures. It has been estimated that turnover costs may exceed 5% of annual operating budgets in hospitals.[18] And yet there is not a lot of formal work being done on the department level to improve retention.

It is widely recognized that the causes of good retention rates are multifactorial. Here is my list of the factors that contribute to good retention of respiratory therapists.

Compensation

Money may not buy happiness, but it does buy a very exquisite brand of sorrow. Salary matters, but don't over estimate its role in staff satisfaction. I think that a good salary is not a staff satisfier but a noncompetitive salary is a staff *dissatisfier*. So you can have very well paid and yet very unhappy employees concomitantly. When you are thinking about the compensation of your staff, be sure to consider the entire benefits package. The hospital is paying for a lot of benefits for employees, and these are a form of compensation (fortunately they are not yet taxed). Typically, for every $1.00 spent in salaries there is $0.30 spent on benefits. So if your salary is $75,000 per year, your total compensation is approaching $100,000 per year. You should be talking about this with your staff. No, no, I don't mean *your* total compensation. I mean *their* total compensation.

Point out to them what the hospital spends on their benefits and how this really adds to their total compensation. I will discuss setting salaries in much more detail later. One aspect of salaries that can really be a powerful staff dissatisfier is poor internal equity. This term describes the comparative equity of salaries between employees. If Joe and Sharon have been working for you about the same length of time and perform at about the same level, they should be making about the same amount of money. If not, and they compare salaries, somebody is going to be a bit unhappy. You can try to get people to keep their mouths shut about their salaries, but good luck with that. More on this later.

Scheduling

Scheduling is a very big deal and is one of the main things that drive people out of the health care business and cause people to change jobs within and between employers. Working nights, weekends, and holidays pretty much sucks. This is a harsh reality of health care. But if you carefully administer a fair scheduling system, it will be greatly appreciated by your staff, even if it is not explicitly stated by them very often. A certain amount of grousing about the schedule is perfectly normal and can be a fun and healthy exercise. But keep your ear tuned to it and watch for any increase in the baseline. Schedulers are only human. They, like everyone, are prone to bias, both conscious and unconscious. They have some staff members they like more than others, and if they are not very careful they can slip into favoring those folks. The staff will pour over the schedule with a fine tooth comb and find any inequalities. For more information see the scheduling chapter.

Self-scheduling has been proposed as a method of improving staff satisfaction, and perhaps it might have a salutary effect on retention.[19] However it has also been reported as being difficult to implement and maintain.[20]

Working Conditions

The nature of the work your team does, the environments in which they do it, and your leadership style are huge determinants of the satisfaction and morale of your team. This has been shown in industry in general,[21] in health care,[22-26] and specifically for respiratory therapists.[27-30] When I talk to therapists all over the country a couple of frequent themes emerge from those who seem pretty negative about their jobs. First, they think a lot of what they do is pointless, mundane, routine, and unappreciated.[vi] I realize this is pretty dark and jaded, but trust me, there are a fair number of people in the respiratory therapy field who harbor this kind of resentment. Some of it is baggage they bring with them, but some of it we have taught them. They learn this when they find themselves giving lots of unnecessary or ineffective therapies every shift. They learn it when they are not listened to or respected by other members of the health care team. They learn it when they see ineffective leadership in their own department. They learn it when they perceive that no one is advocating for them. As a director–manager you may lapse into a sort of numbness about this, thinking there is not much you can do about these kinds of apparently intractable problems. I simply reject this kind of defeatism. To this I say, "If not us, whom?" "If not now, when?" This is

---

[vi]This reminds me of a patch I had sewn on my jeans when I was a corpsman with the Marines. It read, "We are the unwilling, led by the unqualified, to do the unnecessary, for the ungrateful." This is a frequent theme of the peace-time military and, while admittedly rather dark, sums up how some people feel in crummy work environments.

exactly what real leaders ought to do. You should be a leading advocate in the hospital for standardizing care through the use of evidence-based practice and therapist driven protocols. If done properly, this will equip the therapists with the tools they need to minimize the use of ineffective or unnecessary care and will eventually elevate them in the eyes of nurses and physicians, and they will gradually earn the respect they desire. They will begin to see that the work they do is highly valued. The value of this approach has been clearly demonstrated at the Cleveland Clinic where the respiratory therapy department was transformed over a decade into a very protocol driven service with "enhanced professionalism, communication, and participation" of the staff.

Of course, you will have to invest a lot in the training and development of your staff, but nothing good comes easy. Developing protocols and evidence-based practice is hard. And protocols and guidelines will fail if you don't set up systems to measure their progress and if someone doesn't own these projects and keep pushing them. You will have to work very hard, and you may fail the first time you try, to develop and implement a large therapist driven protocol. But learn from your failures, and "When the morning light comes streaming in, you'll get up and do it again" (Jackson Browne).

On a more mundane note, do what you can to keep respiratory therapy work spaces clean and neat. I have been in a lot of respiratory therapy departments and staff rooms that were pretty grubby, dirty, and cluttered. Yes, yes, I know this is mostly "their" fault. You're not their mother so why should you clean up after them? Well, this is all true. But if you want people to feel better about where they work, you might make efforts to keep these areas nicer. Keep your department clean. If housekeeping doesn't come often enough, push them to come more often. Go through once a week yourself and clean up. By the way, keep your own office cleaned up. I go through periods when I am doing a lot of scholarly work, and my office can begin to look like the front end of a paper recycling facility. I have come to realize that this is not the best message to send to the people who come to your office. You like to think it makes you look scholarly and academic. Mostly it makes you look disorganized and slovenly. Get the department repainted regularly too.

Recognition

It took me a long time to finally understand how vital it is to a respiratory therapy team to be recognized by their clinical colleagues and by management. This professional identity crisis that respiratory therapy suffers from is fueled in part by a perceived lack of recognition. Of course, I try to remind people that if they want respect they should try getting it the old-fashioned way, by earning it. By this I mean I encourage people to work on their self-development through continual learning, skills development, and advanced credentialing.

But the truth is that the path to professional recognition for respiratory therapists has been a long and winding road. You are not going to get the recognition that you want for the respiratory therapists by demanding it or by whining about it. The best thing you can do is start with yourself and your leadership team. You should encourage all managers and leaders to be positively effusive in praising and recognizing good work of the respiratory therapists when they see it. This needs to be done on a regular basis, and it needs to be genuine. Contrived, manipulative, unearned praise has a certain pungent aroma that most adults can quickly recognize. As I said earlier in this book, it is a very good idea to like and admire the people you work with. If you don't, you might want to consider another line of work.

Another important tool for you to use in your work to recognize the contributions of your staff is National Respiratory Therapy Week. Proclaimed by Ronald Reagan in 1982, this is a week devoted to acknowledgment of the contributions respiratory therapists make to the care of people with respiratory disease or dysfunction. I have had good success using this event to make my staff feel valued and appreciated. Here are some things we have done:

- Soirees—Once we rented a pavilion at a nearby park and had a steak fry. The hospital provided all the food and all the cooking was done by members of the leadership team. Families were invited. We have also had catered meals at restaurants. Warning: alcohol consumption at events like this is a bit of a risk issue. If an event is formally sponsored by the hospital and alcohol is consumed, there can be some risk to the organization if someone gets hurt driving or otherwise.
- Displays throughout the hospital—This included pictures of every member of the staff displayed in glass cases in high traffic areas of the hospital. Sometimes I would prominently display posters of research done by the department throughout the hospital.
- Banners—I have bought large (10 foot) banners proclaiming National Respiratory Therapy Week and had them displayed over the main entrance to the hospital or in the cafeteria.
- Letters—I have solicited open letters from the chief of the medical staff and the CEO or COO to the respiratory care staff acknowledging the contributions the RTs make to the quality of patient care.

- Meals in the hospital—We have had the leadership team come in for the morning change of shift and cook breakfast for everybody coming or going. We always invite our administrator and medical director.
- Pumping the vendors—I usually ask our larger vendors to come in and provide meals or snacks for the therapists at change of shift.
- Gifts—We have given various types of gifts to the staff such as sweatshirts, fleece vests, duffle bags, books, coffee mugs, and gift baskets. The clothing and mugs were imprinted with the hospital logo or a department logo that we created. Nowadays you have to be careful and check with your marketing department about any images associated with the hospital that might be worn by staff outside the hospital. They will most likely approve what you want to do, but be sure you run it by them.
- Funding—This stuff costs money. Sometimes I have spent as much as $3000 on employee recognition activities, but as far as I am concerned, it is worth every penny. Sometimes I have had luck getting vendors to kick in and help with these expenses.

It is pretty hard to overdo it in your efforts to communicate to your staff the value you place in them. And if you don't value them that much, what does that say about you as their leader?

Another effective technique for recognizing your staff is by displaying their credentials. In one department, I had all the staff credentials (RRT, NPS, CRT, etc.), bronzed, mounted, and displayed on a long wall in the department. At the time (15 years ago), I found a place to do it for $25 each. It was way cool and many people on staff really appreciated it. My belief is that it encouraged some to get their advanced practice credentials so they could have theirs displayed as well.

Some hospitals have well developed systems for recognizing years of service. As an example, I know one hospital that has a catered breakfast every quarter to recognize all employees who have 15 years of service or more (in 5 year increments). If your hospital doesn't have such a thing, you could develop your own in your department.

Collaboration

I tend to think of two major aspects of collaboration: clinical and managerial. Clinical collaboration can be thought of as the inclusion of respiratory therapists into the moment-to-moment deliberations and decisions regarding clinical care. Managerial collaboration is the degree to which your staff members are included in the management of the respiratory therapy department. It is clear that a lack of either of these collaboration aspects is an often cited reason for staff dissatisfaction. This theme has been prevalent in the field since I started, but in some aspects it has substantially improved in recent years. Do not underestimate the importance of collaboration to respiratory therapists. They need it to have a healthy view of themselves and their jobs.

Clinical collaboration is a complex phenomenon and involves medicine, nursing, pharmacy, and other clinical disciplines. You cannot force clinical collaboration to happen by demanding respect for the therapists, complaining about it at meetings, jumping up and down, and being generally whiny about this. Clinical collaboration comes when the other clinical disciplines perceive there is increased value to their patients or themselves when they involve respiratory therapists. This happens when therapists are highly trained, skilled, motivated, and supported by their leadership. This is where your focus should be. As I noted earlier, the best path to clinical collaboration is by standardizing clinical processes through finely crafted and executed therapist driven protocols, clinical practice guidelines, and all the other names for evidence-based practice.

Managerial collaboration is just another name for a whole series of practices generally referred to as participative management. Managerial styles run the gambit from autocratic to democratic. Neither end of this spectrum is really where you want to be. I believe in the principles of participative management but only up to a certain point. You cannot totally delegate your responsibility to make decisions to some committee or council. Your team wants to know that you can be decisive when you need to be. I tend to choose a management style or practice that fits the current state. In other words, if we are dealing with money, such as compensation, you really cannot use much group think to arrive at tough decisions. Adam Smith reminded us that folks tend to be driven by their own economic self-interest. I, yes even I, have never felt like I was paid enough. If you asked me to participate in setting my salary, I would not be particularly balanced about it. So when it comes to salary setting I tend to be somewhere between paternalistic and autocratic. But other topics might lend themselves very well to a participative management style, such as designing care models, equipment selection, and development of policies and procedures. There are some misconceptions out there about participative management styles. Some of them are listed in Table 9-2.

Table 9-2. Misconceptions About Participative Management

Misconception	Comment
One size fits all	Participative management cannot work for all decisions. It should only be used for certain kinds of decisions. Applying it to each and every decision will be slow and cumbersome, and it often will not bear any edible fruit.
Permissiveness	Some will interpret a participative management style as a sort of "culture of permissiveness." This will happen if you don't temper your participative approach with a continued commitment to accountability.
Weakness	Don't allow your participative style to be viewed as weakness or indecisiveness. You have to speak clearly and often tell your staff that their participation is essential and vital but that in the end the buck stops on somebody's desk, which of course would be *your* desk.
Giving up authority	See "weakness" above.
Postponement	Postponement has gotten a bad name. Do not rush into decisions. The deliberative process of participative management might be regarded by some as postponing tough decisions. I am all about postponing any tough decision that *can* be postponed. There is a time for decisiveness. But if possible, tough decisions should be postponed until they absolutely have to be made. You never know—new information might be forthcoming that makes the correct path more obvious.

Lately the toughest thing for me about a participative management style is getting staff members motivated to get involved. Meetings are tough to organize. People are busy, busier than ever, in fact it seems as if most of the world is insanely busy. Staff members are generally reluctant to make extra trips to the hospital. If you are not really pushing for participation, you might not get very much. You have to plan very carefully about *how* to get participation. Conference calls, e-mail threads, and net meetings are important tools that might improve the participation of your staff. I think we are still learning how to use these tools, but I believe they can be leveraged to really increase staff participation.

SETTING SALARIES

A common theme among respiratory therapists is how frustrating it is that they are not paid as much as nurses, or physical therapists, or ultrasonographers, or whoever else is on their radar screen. There is a suggestion in this complaint that they ought to make as much as nurses because, after all, they have the same number of years of schooling as most nurses and what they do for patients is equally as important as what nurses do for patients. This is a very emotionally satisfying argument, but unfortunately it belies a lack of understanding of the basic economics of one of the most immutable forces in nature: the market. Comparable worth is an artificial social construct that would suggest that there is something wrong when plumbers make more than teachers or football players make more than nurses. The theory goes that these salary differences are a social injustice based on someone's subjective view of what is best for society. As is the case with so many well intentioned worshippers at the first church of government, there is a genuine belief that something must be done about this injustice. This is a pleasant fiction, but it is completely impossible to carry out and potentially very dangerous. Who would decide what the salaries ought to be? What criteria would be used for these deliberations? What effect would these artificial adjustments have on the composition of the workforce?

What really sets salaries is the market. Employers pay what they need to pay to attract employees. They have a fiduciary responsibility to their companies not to pay any more than necessary. Thus what causes respiratory therapists to make less than nurses is the demand for nurses versus the supply of nurses. This gap between supply and demand drives what employers have to pay to get the employees they need. There is a gap between the demand and supply of respiratory therapists too, but the gap is not as large as it is for nursing. Thus nursing salaries are higher.

The gap between the supply and demand of respiratory therapists has caused their salaries to grow faster than the inflation rate over the last 13 years (see Table 9-3).

As further proof of the effect of the market on salaries, note that the growth of staff therapists' salaries has exceeded the growth of directors' salaries. That is because there is not much of a gap between the supply and demand for people wanting to be a department director.

The basic approach hospitals use for setting salaries is to look at what other hospitals are paying for similar positions and trying to set their salaries accordingly. Human resource departments typically buy market salary data

Table 9-3.   Changes in Respiratory Therapists' Salaries

	1992	2005	% change
Respiratory therapist hourly rate	$11.81	$21.87	85.2%
Director hourly rate	$19.20	$33.60	75.0%
% change in the Consumer Price Index from 1992 through 2005			50.8.0%

From the 2005 AARC Human Resources Manpower Study.
   Source: Data from American Association for Respiratory Care. Respiratory therapist: human resources study. American Association for Respiratory Care. Dallas. 2005.

from companies who survey the hospitals in a given region or city. These data will customarily reflect the entry level and top of the pay scale for respiratory therapists and/or the average hourly rate of all the incumbents. At this point there is a strategic decision to be made. Habitually hospitals say they want to attract the best people, but then they simultaneously announce that they want to be in the middle of the pack with regard to salaries. I have always found this conundrum to be perplexing. Generally the best people migrate to the best money. Admittedly it is not only money that makes a good work environment, but I would suggest that money does initially get a prospective employee's attention.

So if you have not seen any market salary data, ask your human resources department to produce it for you. If they don't have market salary data for other hospitals, suggest that they get it. You could also try to do your own survey of the five or 10 hospitals that are your chief competitors in recruiting. If you are having serious trouble recruiting, it may be that your salaries are not competitive.

If your respiratory therapists are unionized, salary setting becomes very simple. It will be dictated by the terms of the union contract. Typically people who come into your department are placed on the union scale according to their years of experience. Union pay scales usually have steps that reflect years of service, and as union members gain years of experience they move through the steps. A customary pay scale might have between 15 and 20 steps with differences between the steps usually being around 2–3%. Contracts will vary in the details, but the ones I have dealt with allowed you to place new employees on a step for each year of experience. In other words, if your newly hired employee has 10 years of experience he or she would be placed on the pay scale at step 10. Other contracts might dictate 2 years of experience for every step on the contract, so 10 years of experience would equate to placement on step 5. If you are having recruitment troubles and find yourself making salary offers to prospective employees that they turn down, you may be tempted to bump people up on the scale to fill your positions. This might be a short-term fix that could cause long-term trouble. If you have incumbent staff that discover that you are hiring new people with similar or less experience at a higher rate, you will find yourself answering a lot of tough questions. Your staff, through their union representative, may demand that you raise all incumbents up to the same extent that you brought in the new employee.

If you do not have a union, you can have a little more leeway in setting salaries, but you still need to have a systematic approach. Your human resources department will typically have a standardized approach that you can use. It will probably be similar to the union approach, although hospitals don't often have their nonunionized pay scales divided into so many discrete steps. Hiring new graduates is easy because they are typically hired at the entry level. My rule of thumb is that if you have 7 years of experience I would hire you at about midpoint on the salary scale, and if you have more than 15 years of experience I would hire you at or near the top of the scale.

Whatever your system, it needs to be as consistent and objective as possible. If you don't develop a consistent system you will create problems with internal equity where there are large differences in salary that cannot be explained by years of experience or performance differences.

Figure 9-1 describes a simple regression analysis tool that I use for checking internal equity among supervisors' salaries.

I construct a table of each person's total years of respiratory experience, years of experience at my hospital, years of supervisory experience, and hourly rate. From the various types of experience I then calculate what I call an "experience coefficient," which is a weighted coefficient of the different types of experience. My weightings reflect the value I place in the various kinds of experience. Your weightings might be different depending on your approach. The experience coefficient is then plotted against the hourly rate using a simple Excel x-y chart. To the chart you add a trend line and ask the program to display the regression equation and correlation coefficient on the chart. The R^2 in this example is the correlation coefficient, and it indicates that 90% of the differences in salary can be explained by differences in experience as expressed by the coefficient. There are no hard rules here about what the

	Sam	Merry	Pippin	Frodo	Gandalf	Aragorn	Boromir	Gimli
Years Total RT Experience	32	19	31	25	11	8	16	6
Years at Current Employer	12	14	15	4	2	2	2	6
Years Supervisory Experience	25	12	5	8	2	4	5	0
Current Hourly Salary	$34.25	$31.98	$31.93	$31.24	$25.45	$25.45	$25.00	$22.74
Experience Coefficient	25.9	15.9	20.0	15.6	6.6	5.7	9.9	4.2

Experience Coefficient =
(total years experience × 0.5) + (years at current employer × 0.2) + (years supervisory experience × 0.3)

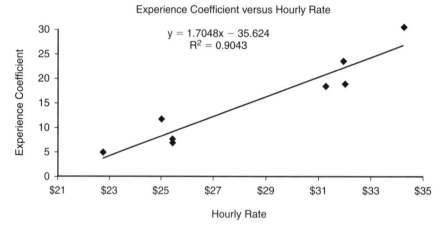

Figure 9-1. Regression Analysis Tool for Supervisor Salaries
Regression analysis of hourly rate versus experience coefficient. The experience coefficient is a weighted derivative of various types of experience. The weighting equation assigns a 50% weight to total years of experience, 20% to years at the current employer, and 30% to years of supervisory experience. The R^2 value (correlation coefficient) of 0.9043 indicates that 90% of the difference in salaries can be explained by differences in the experience coefficient.

correct percentage should be. I suggest that it ought to be about 75% or more with the remainder of the salary differences being attributable to other causes, presumably job performance or mysterious cosmic forces.

ORIENTATION

Historically the respiratory therapy community has not done the greatest job orienting new employees. People love nostalgia and long for the good old days. Sometimes I do too but not with regard to something as important as training and orientation. When I started in my first NICU oh so many years ago, I had no neonatal or pediatric experience. I had never worked with a neonatal ventilator. I started on night shift, and one of the supervisors from days (we had no night shift supervisors) came to nights to orient me for one week. He spent a couple of hours going over equipment and procedures with me and then he would go to bed and tell me to call him if something came up. There were no training documents or equipment manuals. I never saw a policy and procedure manual. Thank goodness those days are gone. At least I hope they are.

Orientation of new employees is a combination of training and competency verification. This is usually done by pairing the new staff member with an experienced therapist or with your clinical coordinator in what is sometimes called a mentor or preceptor relationship. This therapist then begins to show the new staff member the system guided by an orientation checklist. Appendix G is a series of documents and forms associated with orientation and training. Document G-1 is a single page from a multipage intensive care unit orientation checklist. Obviously orientation is a major component of ensuring patient safety. And as such, many departments have become very detailed and methodical about orientation. But this detail takes time and is costly. The alternative is to turn therapists who are not properly prepared loose to practice autonomously.

Every department should develop its own standards, and these will differ depending on the complexity of your processes of care and patient populations. For a complex critical care environment, I recommend 80–200 hours of one-on-one orientation for each type of unit (PICU, NICU, SICU, and CVICU). This is a large range and has to be customized to the individual depending on their level of experience and speed of assimilation.

Skills assessment and verification, which is also called competency assessment, is required by the JCAHO. I regard this as having two components: one is a cognitive component and the other is a skills review. Written testing or computer aided testing are tools for assessing cognitive competency, and a skills review is typically done with a return demonstration.[vii] There are several written tests in Appendix G. They are intended to test the cognitive skill of the therapist regarding working in a certain area or on a certain type of device. The mechanical ventilator cognitive competency (document G-2) was designed to be an overall assessment of the complex issues surrounding mechanical ventilation, in this case, of children. Note that it is quite long (120 questions). It came

---

[vii]Return demonstration is a method of verifying competency in which the clinician must actually do the procedure at hand in front of the evaluator. As an example a return demonstration of training to initiate mechanical ventilation would require that the student actually set up and start the ventilator in front of an evaluator.

with an accompanying 110 page training document that was written by a group of respiratory therapists including the clinical coordinator, supervisors, and staff members. Everyone who worked in critical care had to take and pass the examination with an 80% score or better. I allowed people to take the test home and paid 10 hours for completion of the examination. We applied for and got AARC Category I CEUs for the process (10 contact hours).

The acute care cognitive competency (Appedix H, Document H-4) is given to staff members who are completing their orientation to our nonintensive care areas. I have not included all of our cognitive assessments because they are very device specific and are focused on neonatal and pediatrics.

IN-SERVICE TRAINING AND EDUCATION

As you have by now appreciated, I am a big fan of training and training and more training. In-service training is customarily thought of as the ongoing training and teaching activities for your staff that are not really part of orientation or competency assessment, although obviously all of these activities are linked. For a director–manager it can be very challenging to keep the in-service training program vital, fresh, and interesting. Many departments do in-service training as a sort of afterthought. You can get caught up in the urgency of the moment and let the in-service training program slip.

I have had habitual trouble getting people to come to staff meetings. One solution is to use every staff meeting as an educational opportunity. When we started offering an in-service training class at every staff meeting, attendance improved. It did not hurt that most of these classes were approved for AARC Category I continuing education credits and that our state requires therapists to have continuing education units to renew their practice license. This requires some planning and filing forms with the AARC, but this is a small price to pay for what you get.

There are a variety of in-service and training tools to help you. The traditional lecture with slides is always good, but if that is all you do, it can get stale. There are a growing number of computer-aided training resources you can use. Joseph D. Limauro, MEd, RRT has developed an excellent series of computer interactive training modules for clinicians that include pulmonary waveform interpretation, oxygen therapy, and congenital cardiac defects.[viii] These self-guided tutorials are developed in hypertext markup language

[viii]http://www.jlenterprise.com/jl.html

(HTML) and come with animation and self-assessment features. They are reasonably priced, and we use them extensively.

Another example is the excellent computer interactive training program that comes with inhaled nitric oxide delivery systems from INO Therapeutics.[ix] The Web masters at Ventworld.com have put together a list of computer/Web-based training resources.[x]

To keep your in-service training program fresh and interesting, invite doctors and nurses to come and speak at your classes. This helps build better relationships between these disciplines. We have started videotaping all our classes and will soon be offering them as streaming video on our department Web page. I have had mixed luck in the past with videotaping in-service classes. The image quality is often weak, and the audio can be really crummy. Make sure you get some expert technical advice and assistance if you hope to record your in-service classes.

Records must be kept of your training programs. And they must be kept in such a fashion that you can readily recover the training history of each individual staff member.

PERFORMANCE APPRAISALS

Yearly performance appraisals of all staff members are done and there must be a signed copy of this appraisal in the employees' personnel files. There should also be a 90-day evaluation done for all newly hired employees. I am not a big fan of this system. It can become pretty perfunctory. It just becomes another paper chase if you don't work hard at it. In Appendix B you can find some examples of how hospitals design the job description (or work content description) so that it can also be used as a performance appraisal tool. For high performers it is easy. You write them a glowing performance review and have a nice talk and go about your merry way. But for marginal performers it gets more challenging. If you gloss over their performance issues in their review it can come back to haunt you. Later if their performance deteriorates to the point where you are considering corrective discipline for them, the performance appraisal will be reviewed to determine if this employee has ongoing problems. If you have not clearly documented the problems in the performance appraisal, it looks as if this person is a better employee than they really are.

[ix]http://www.inotherapeutics.com/aboutINO.htm
[x]http://www.ventworld.com/education/courses.asp

If employees are not performing very well, their yearly review generally should not be the first time they hear about it. If there are performance problems, coaching sessions should be happening throughout the year. Some departments actually have a midyear performance review for all staff that is done approximately 6 months into the performance review cycle. This is a good way of keeping staff members informed of issues and opportunities for improvement and development.

Coaching

Human nature being what it is, most people, including me, don't respond very well to criticism (initially). So performance reviews turn out to be pretty stressful for most people. I suggest that a performance review should be a coaching session. As you plan your coaching sessions, you should ponder the strengths and weaknesses of each employee. Make notes. Have a plan. When you talk with them, let them know what value they bring and the good things they do every day. If there are some problems with performance (or what some people like to describe as "growth opportunities"), wait to discuss these until the end of the coaching session. When you say something to someone that stings, many people just kind of shut down and stop listening. If you start your coaching sessions with criticisms, they won't hear much of the good you are saying to them.

As I noted in the chapter on department measurement, we try to build objective measurement systems so we can bring data on individual performance to the yearly performance review sessions. These include measures of billing accuracy, attendance, compliance with charting guidelines, and the status of training and development. These measures give staff members some objective numbers.

In many industries and in some hospital departments, each employee has a direct supervisor who is responsible for performance appraisals and coaching sessions. But the ebb and flow of 12-hour shift schedules and the design of leadership structures can make this difficult in 24/7 clinical operations like respiratory care. There may be two or three different supervisors who work with a given employee. That is the structure that I have the most experience with. To help ensure an objective assessment of staff performance under these circumstances, we do a team approach to evaluation performance. Our whole leadership team gathers, and we review each individual's performance for the year. We make a master list of strengths and weaknesses of each staff member, and these are used to structure the performance review/coaching session.

Finally, goal setting is an important part of the performance review cycle. People need goals. Continued growth and development can lapse if there are not some targets to shoot for. We sometimes use advanced practice credentials as one goal for staff members. We don't insist, but we urge members to get their advanced credentials. Other goals include improved understanding of complex technologies or disease processes or specialized advanced training like Pediatric Advanced Life Support or the Neonatal Resuscitation Program.

REFERENCES

1. Torrington KG. Protocol-driven respiratory therapy: closing in on appropriate utilization at comparable cost and patient outcomes. *Chest.* 1996;110(2):313–314.
2. Thaggard I, Stoller JK. Practical aspects of a respiratory care protocol service. *Respir Care.* 1999;44(5):532–534.
3. Stoller JK. The rationale for therapist-driven protocols. *Respir Care Clin N Am.* March 1996;2(1):1–14.
4. Wright J, Gordon J, Guidry H. Multi-modality patient assessment protocol. *Respir Care.* 1994;39:1096.
5. Stoller JK, Mascha EJ, Kester L, Haney D. Randomized controlled trial of physician-directed versus respiratory therapy consult service-directed respiratory care to adult non-ICU inpatients. *Am J Respir Crit Care Med.* 1998;158(4):1068–1075.
6. Stoller JK, Skibinski CI, Giles DK, Kester EL, Haney DJ. Physician-ordered respiratory care vs physician-ordered use of a respiratory therapy consult service. Results of a prospective observational study. *Chest.* 1996;110(2):422–429.
7. Lierl MB, et al. *Respir Care.* 1999;44(5):497–505.
8. Kollef MH, Shapiro SD, Clinkscale D, et al. The effect of respiratory therapist-initiated treatment protocols on patient outcomes and resource utilization. *Chest.* 2000;117(2):467–475.
9. Meredith RL, Pilbeam SB, MaCarthy K, Stoller JK. Proficiency among respiratory therapy educators, staff, and students in using algorithms for therapist-driven protocols. *Respir Care.* 1996;41(7):595–600.
10. Drucker PF. *An Introductory View of Management.* New York, NY: Harper's College Press; 1977.
11. Maxfield D, Grenny J, McMillan R, Patterson K, Switzler K. Silence kills: the seven crucial conversations in healthcare. VitalSmarts L.C. http://www.aacn.org/aacn/pubpolcy.nsf/Files/SilenceKillsExecSum/$file/SilenceKillsExecSum.pdf. 2005.
12. Cosby KS, Croskerry P. Profiles in patient safety: authority gradients in medical error. *Acad Emerg Med.* 2004;11(12):1341–1345.
13. Alkov RA, Borowsky MS, Williamson DW, Yacavone DW. The effect of trans-cockpit authority gradient on navy/marine helicopter mishaps. *Aviat Space Environ Med.* 1992;63:659–661.

14. Kosnik LK. The new paradigm of crew resource management: just what is needed to reengage the stalled collaborative movement? *Jt Comm J Qual Improv.* 2002;28:235–241.

15. Barden C, ed. AACN standards for establishing and sustaining healthy work environments: a journey to excellence. American Association of Critical Care Nurses. http://www.aacn.org/AACN/hwe.nsf/vwdoc/HWEHomePage. 2005.

16. American Association for Respiratory Care. Respiratory therapist: human resources study. American Association for Respiratory Care. Dallas. 2005.

17. Gurza-Dully P, Melaney M. Application form items as predictors of performance and longevity among respiratory therapists: a multiple regression analysis. *Respir Care.* 1992;37(2):137–143.

18. Waldman JD, Kelly F, Arora S, Smith HL. The shocking cost of turnover in health care. *Health Care Manage Rev.* 2004;29(1):2–7.

19. Teahan B. Implementation of a self-scheduling system: a solution to more than just schedules! *J Nurs Manag.* 1998;6(6):361–368.

20. Bailyn L, Collins R, Song Y. Self-scheduling for hospital nurses: an attempt and its difficulties. *J Nurs Manag.* 2007;15(1):72–77.

21. Hueslid MA. The impact of human resource management practices on turnover, productivity, and corporate financial performance. *Academy of Management Journal.* 1995;38:645.

22. Bratt MM, Broome M, Kelber S, Lostocco L. Influence of stress and nursing leadership on job satisfaction of pediatric intensive care unit nurses. *Am J Crit Care.* 2000;9(5):307–317.

23. DiMeglio K, Padula C, Piatek C, et al. Group cohesion and nurse satisfaction: examination of a team-building approach. *J Nurs Adm.* 2005;35(3):110–120.

24. Anthony MK, Standing TS, Glick J, et al. Leadership and nurse retention: the pivotal role of nurse managers. *J Nurs Adm.* 2005;35(3):146–155.

25. Shader K, Broome ME, Broome CD, West ME, Nash M. Factors influencing satisfaction and anticipated turnover for nurses in an academic medical center. *J Nurs Adm.* 2001;31(4):210–216.

26. Hayhurst A, Saylor C, Stuenkel D. Work environmental factors and retention of nurses. *J Nurs Care Qual.* 2005;20(3):283–288.

27. Blake SS, Kester L, Stoller JK. Respiratory therapists' attitudes about participative decision-making: relationship between managerial decision-making style and job satisfaction. *Respir Care.* 2004;49(8):917–925.

28. Orens DK, Kester L, Konrad DJ, Stoller JK. Changing patterns of inpatient respiratory care services over a decade at the Cleveland Clinic: challenges posed and proposed responses. *Respir Care.* 2005;50(8):1033–1039.

29. Rawlins TD. Attrition in respiratory care: the role of stress versus the role of intrinsic and extrinsic rewards. *Respir Care.* 1987;32(5):325–331.

30. Akroyd HD, Robertson R. Factors affecting the job satisfaction of respiratory therapists who work in adult general and critical care: a multivariate study. *Respir Care.* 1989;34(3):179–184.

Colleges and Universities Offering a Bachelor's Degree in Respiratory Therapy

Alegent/IMC Midland Lutheran College
6901 N. 72nd St.
Omaha, NE 68122-1799
Baccalaureate Degree
402-572-2314
Todd Klopfenstein
tklopfen@alegent.org
Jeff Dennis
Louis ADVioli

Armstrong Atlantic State University (LB)
Department of Respiratory Therapy
11935 Abercorn St.
Savannah, GA 31419
Baccalaureate Degree
912-921-7446
Ross L. Bowers, MHS, RRT
bowersro@mail.armstrong.com
William J. Smith, MHS, RRT
Robert J. DiBenedetto, MD
Stephen L. Morris, MD

Baptist College of Health Sciences
1003 Monroe Ave.
Memphis, TN 38104
Baccalaureate Degree of Health Sciences
901-227-6933
Andrew J. Mazzoli, PhD, RRT
andrew.mazzoli@bchs.edu
Gracie R. Knight, CRT
C. Michael Smith, MD

Bellarmine University (LB)
2001 Newburg Rd.
Louisville, KY 40205
Baccalaureate Degree
502-852-8280
Jerome F. Walker, EdD
jwalker@bellarmine.edu
Christy J. Kane, Med
Harvy L. Snider, MD

Boise State University (LB)
1910 University Dr.
Boise, ID 83725-1850

Associate Degree/Baccalaureate
   Degree
208-426-3670
Lonny Ashworth, MEd, RRT
lashwor@boisestate.edu
David Merrick, MD

East Tennessee State University
   1000 Jason Witten Way
   Elizabethton, TN 37643
   Baccalaureate Degree
   423-547-4916
   Douglas Eugene Masini, EdD,
      RRT-NPS, RPFT, AE-C, FAARC
   masini@etsu.edu
   Shane Keene, MS, MBA, CPFT,
      RRT-NPS
   Jeff R. Farrow, MD, FCCP

Florida A&M University (LB)
   Ware-Rhaney Building
   School of Allied Health Science
   Tallahassee, FL 32307-3500
   Baccalaureate Degree
   850-561-2027
   Alphonso Baldwin, PhD, RRT
   Michael Higginbotham, MEd,
      RRT
   David Saint, MD

Gannon University
   Respiratory Care Program
   109 University Square
   Erie, PA 16541-0001
   Associate Degree/Baccalaureate
      Degree
   814-871-5637
   Charles Stephen Cornfield, MS,
      RRT
   cornfield@gannon.edu

Robert David Tarkowski, MS, RRT
John T. Schaaf, MD

Georgia State University
   Cardiopulmonary Care Sciences
   C2 Kell Hall
   Atlanta, GA 30303-3083
   Baccalaureate Degree
   404-651-1490
   Joseph L. Rau, PhD, RRT
   resjlr@langate.gsu.edu
   Lynda T. Goodfellow, EdD, RRT
   Cindy Dawn Powell, MD

Indiana University of Pennsylvania,
The Western Pennsylvania Hospital
(LB)
   School of Respiratory Care
   4800 Friendship Ave.
   Pittsburgh, PA 15224
   Baccalaureate Degree
   412-578-7003
   William J. Malley, MS, RRT
   bmalley@wpahs.org
   Kathryn G. Kinderman, MS,
      RRT
   Paul C. Fiehler, MD

Indiana University School
of Medicine
   1140 West Michigan St.
   Coleman Hall 224
   Indianapolis, IN 46202-5119
   Baccalaureate Degree
   317-278-7381
   Deborah L. Cullen, EdD, RRT,
      FAARC
   dcullen@iupui.edu
   Joseph A. Koss, MS, RRT
   Simon Hillier, MD

Long Island University (LB)
  Division of Respiratory Care
  School of Health Professions
  1 University Plaza
  Brooklyn, NY 11201-9815
  Baccalaureate Degree
  718-488-1492
  Thomas J. Johnson, MS, RRT
  tjohnson@liu.edu
  James Knight, MS, RRT
  Albert Heurich, MD

Louisiana State University
Health Sciences Center
  1900 Gravier St.
  Department of Cardiopulmonary
    Science
  New Orleans, LA 70112-2262
  Baccalaureate Degree
  504-568-4235
  Jimmy M. Cairo, PhD, RRT
  jcairo@lsuhsc.edu
  Kim F. Simmons, MHS, RRT
  Mack Thomas, MD

Medical College of Georgia
(LB)
  Department of Respiratory
    Therapy
  HM-143
  Augusta, GA 30912-0850
  Baccalaureate Degree
  706-721-3554
  Shelley C. Mishoe, PhD, RRT,
    FAARC
  smishoe@mail.mcg.edu
  Arthur A. Taft, PhD, RRT
  Bashir A. Chaudhary, MD, FCCP,
    FACP

Midwestern State University (LB)
  3410 Taft Blvd.
  Wichita Falls, TX 76308-2099
  Baccalaureate Degree
  940-397-4653
  Annette O. Medford, MA, RRT
  ann.medford@mwsu.edu
  Tammy R. Kurszewski, BAAS,
    RRT
  Lowell L. Harvey, MD

Millersville University Program
in Respiratory Therapy
  Roddy Science Center
  Program in Respiratory Therapy
  P.O. Box 1002
  Millersville, PA 17551-0302
  Baccalaureate Degree
  717-290-5511 Ext. 7105
  John M. Hughes, RRT, MEd
  jhughes@marauder.millersville.
    edu
  Elaine Chrissos, BSEd, RRT
  Harshadkumar B. Patel, MD

Nebraska Methodist College
of Nursing and Allied Health (LB)
  8501 W. Dodge Rd.
  Omaha, NE 68114-3426
  Associate Degree/Baccalaureate
    Degree
  402-354-4913
  Christine A. Hamilton, MA, RRT
  chamil1@methodistcollege.edu
  John A. Jarosz, BS, RRT
  Patrick G. Meyers, MD

North Dakota State University (LB)
  MeritCare Hospital
  Respiratory Care Services

P.O. Box MC
Fargo, ND 58122-0118
Baccalaureate Degree
701-234-6147
Gary Lee Brown, BA, RRT
garybrown@meritcare.com
Michelle Lee Sele, BS, RRT
Patrick J. Stoy, MD

Ohio State University (LB), The
Respiratory Therapy Division
  1583 Perry St.
  Columbus, OH 43210-1234
  Baccalaureate Degree
  614-292-8445
  F. Herbert Douce, MS, RRT
  douce.2@osu.edu
  Phillip D. Hoberty, EdD, RRT
  Jeffrey E. Weiland, MD

Our Lady of Holy Cross College
  Oschner School of Allied Health
    Sciences
  1516 Jefferson Hwy.
  New Orleans, LA 70121-2484
  Baccalaureate Degree/Certificate
    of Completion
  504-842-3736
  Mary Nunez LaBiche, MEd,
    RRT
  Mlabiche@ochsner.org
  Erin Ellis Davis, MS, MEd, RRT
  Brad Burns, MD

Salisbury State University (LB)
  Respiratory Therapy Program
  1101 Camden Ave.
  Salisbury, MD 21801
  Baccalaureate Degree
  410-543-6409
  Sidney R. Schneider, PhD, RRT

srschneider@ssu.edu
Rodney Layton, MD
William J. Nagel, MD

Sistema Universitario Ana G.
Mendez
  Universidad Metropolitana
  Department of Respiratory
    Therapy
  P.O. Box 21150
  San Juan, PR 00928-1150
  Baccalaureate Degree
  787-766-1717 Ext. 6554
  Leyda Luz Torres-Lopez, MA,
    RRT
  um_ltorres@suagm.edu
  Yolanda Carromero, JD, RRT
  Juan Jimenez-Vega, MHSA, MD

Southwest Texas State University
  601 University Dr.
  San Marcos, TX 78666-4616
  Baccalaureate Degree
  512-245-8243
  Cade J. Harkins, MSHP, RRT
  ch03@swt.edu
  S. Gregory Marshall, PhD
  George J. Handley, MD

St. Alexius Medical Center/
University of Mary Respiratory
Therapy Program
  900 E. Broadway
  Bismarck, ND 58502
  Baccalaureate Degree/Certificate
    of Completion
  701-530-7757
  Will Beachey, PhD, RRT
  wbeachey@primecare.org
  Pamela Rangen, MEd, RRT
  James A. Hughes, MD, FACCP

State University of New York
at Stony Brook (LB)
   Respiratory Care Program
   School of Health Technology and
      Management/HSC
   Stony Brook University
   Stony Brook, NY 11794-8203
   Baccalaureate Degree
   631-444-3180
   James A. Ganetis, MS, RRT-NPS
   jganetis@notes.cc.sunysb.edu
   Lisa M. Johnson, MS, RRT-NPS
   Gerald Smaldone, MD, PhD

SUNY Upstate Medical University
(LB)
   750 E. Adams St.
   Syracuse, NY 13210
   Associate Degree/Baccalaureate
      Degree
   315-464-5580
   Joseph G. Sorbello, MSEd, RRT,
      RT
   Sorbellj@upstate.edu
   Sheila A. Young, MS, RRT, RT

Tennessee State University
   Cardio-Respiratory Care
   3500 John Merritt Blvd.
   Nashville, TN 37209-1561
   Baccalaureate Degree
   615-963-7420
   Thomas John, PhD, RRT
   tjohn@tnstate.edu
   Sharonda Hickman, MEd, RRT
   Michael Niedermeyer, MD

University of Alabama
at Birmingham, The
   Respiratory Therapy Program
   317 Learning Resource Center

   1714 Ninth Ave. South
   Birmingham, AL 35294-1270
   Baccalaureate Degree
   205-934-3783
   Wesley M. Granger, PhD, RRT
   grangerw@uab.edu
   Jonathan B. Waugh, PhD, RRT
   Manuel F. Carcelen, MD

University of Arkansas for Medical
Sciences
   4301 W. Markham
   Slot 704 (14B/NLR)
   Little Rock, AR 72205
   Baccalaureate Degree
   501-257-2343
   Erna L. Boone, MEd, RRT
   BooneErnaL@uams.edu
   Robert H. Warren, MD

University of Central Florida
   Cardiopulmonary Sciences
      Department
   P.O. Box 25000
   Orlando, FL 32816-2205
   Baccalaureate Degree
   407-823-2214
   L. Timothy Worrell, MPH, RRT
   worrell@pegasus.cc.ucf.edu
   Jeffery Ludy, MEd, RRT
   Lawrence Gilliard, MD

University of Charleston (LB), The
   2300 MacCorkle Ave.
   Charleston, WV 25304
   Baccalaureate Degree
   304-357-4837
   Anna W. Parkman, PhD, RRT
   aparkman@ucwv.edu
   Jean Fisher, MBA, RRT
   Dominic Gaziano, MD

University of Kansas Medical
Center (LB)
  Respiratory Care Education
  3901 Rainbow Blvd.
  Kansas City, KS 66160-7606
  Baccalaureate Degree
  913-588-4634
  Barbara A. Ludwig, MA, RRT
  bludwig@kumc.edu
  Hugh S. Mathewson, MD

University of Missouri-Columbia
(LB)
  HRP/Cardiopulmonary and
    Diagnostic Science Department
  Respiratory Therapy Program
  605 Lewis Hall
  Columbia, MO 65211-4230
  Baccalaureate Degree
  573-882-8423
  Michael W. Prewitt, PhD, RRT
  prewittm@health.missouri.edu
  Rosemary G. Hogan, Med, RRT
  Andrew McKibben, MD

University of South Alabama
  Department of Cardiorespiratory
    Care
  1504 Springhill Ave., Rm. 2545
  Mobile, AL 36604-3273
  Baccalaureate Degree
  334-434-3405
  William V. Wojciechowski, MS,
    RRT
  wwojciec@jaguar1.usouthal.edu
  H. Fred Hill, MA, RRT
  Ronald C. Allison, MD

University of Texas Health Science,
The Center at San Antonio
  Department of Respiratory Care
  Mail Code: 6248
  7703 Floyd Curl Dr.
  San Antonio, TX 78229-3900
  Baccalaureate Degree
  210-567-8850
  David C. Shelledy, PhD, RRT
  shelledy@uthscsa.edu
  Terry S. LeGrand, PhD, RRT
  Douglas M. Anderson, MD
  Jay I. Peters, MD

University of Texas Medical Branch
at Galveston, School of Allied
Health Sciences
  UTMB-SAHS
  Department of Respiratory Care
  301 University Blvd.
  Galveston, TX 77555-1028
  Baccalaureate Degree
  409-772-5693
  Jon O. Nilsestuen, PhD, RRT,
    FAARC
  jnilsest@utmb.edu
  Marilyn R. Childers, MEd,
    RRT
  Donald S. Prough, MD
  Mali Mathru, MD

University of Toledo
  2801 W. Bancroft St.
  Toledo, OH 43606-3390
  Baccalaureate Degree
  419-530-5308

Suzanne Spacek, MEd, RRT-NPS, CPFT
suzanne.spacek@utoledo.edu

Wheeling Jesuit University
316 Washington Ave.
Wheeling, WV 26003-6295
Baccalaureate Degree
304-243-2372
Allen H. Marangoni, MMSc, RRT
amaran@wju.edu
Marybeth M. Emmerth, MS, RRT
Michael Blatt, MD

York College of PA/York Hospital
School of Respiratory Care
1001 S. George St.
York, PA 17405-7198
Associate Degree/Baccalaureate
Degree

717-851-2464
Mark L. Simmons, MSEd, RRT
msimmons@wellspan.org
James I. Heindel, BS, RRT
Richard D. Keeports, MD

Youngstown State University
Respiratory Care Program
One University Plaza
Youngstown, OH 44555
Baccalaureate Degree
330-941-1764
Louis N. Harris, EdD, RRT
Lnharris.01@ysu.edu
Janet M. Boehm, MS, RRT
Tejinder S. Bal, MD

Respiratory Therapist Job Descriptions and Performance Evaluation Forms

The following is an example of a combined job description (sometimes called a work content description) and performance appraisal form.

DOCUMENT B-1: WORK CONTENT DESCRIPTION/PERFORMANCE EVALUATION FORM

Action Being Taken

☐ Annual Performance Evaluation	☐ New Position	☐ Position Reclassification	☐ Position Update	☐ 90 Day Review

Employee Information

Employee Name:					Employee ID #:		Date:

Job Class	Pos Code	Old Job #	**Job Title:**	**Respiratory Therapist I**		Working Tittle:	
RSP	**2720-001**	053					

Location: Hospital	Dept. #	12345	Dept. Title:	Respiratory Care	Reports To:	Clinical Supervisor

Position Purpose

Provide respiratory care to all patients in all intensive care units, ED, medical, surgical, heme/onc and rehab units. Applies the knowledge and skill necessary to provide appropriate interactions with staff, patients, and families of all ages.

(Continues)

Major Responsibilities, Activities, And End Results					
% of Time	Essential Functions/ Responsibilities/ Accountabilities	How Is It Done *(Activities)*	Outcomes/Measures	Perform Rating 1 or 2	Comments
80%	1) Provide Respiratory Care	• Understand and follow current policies and procedures for the respiratory care service and the areas of the hospital where respiratory care is administered including, but not limited to: intensive care units, during patient transport, in the acute care and emergency department areas, limited to the following: • Airway management and care • Ventilator management • Patient assessments • Airway clearance techniques • Respiratory monitoring • Administration of therapeutic gases • Administration of therapeutic aerosols • Intra-hospital transport of ventilated patients • Documentation and charging of all interactions with patients according to department and hospital guidelines • Participate in professional development • Complete annual competencies	• Patients are provided safe, age-appropriate, timely and coordinated care as measured by successful outcomes of the care plan, patient/ parent satisfaction, direct observation, and supervisory feedback • Policies, procedures, and guidelines are followed and documented in the medical record through annual chart review • Review annual CQI memos relating to individual practice • Participate in care planning with medical and nursing staff by attending patient rounds • Attend 66% of RT staff meetings per year • Participates in department QA program • Attend educational offerings related to neonatal and/or pediatric respiratory care • Attend in-services on new products or therapies • Attendance at annual skills fair • Be a trained preceptor		
15%	2) Provide Customer Service	• Communicate with patients, parents, team members, and all other customers	• Respectful, sensitive, and effective communications measured by substantiated feedback from any customer		

Major Responsibilities, Activities, And End Results					
% of Time	Essential Functions/ Responsibilities/ Accountabilities	How Is It Done *(Activities)*	Outcomes/Measures	Perform Rating 1 or 2	Comments
5%	3) Education of Others	• New employee orientation • New resident orientation • Ongoing RT education	• Precept new RTs and RT students as requested/ keep a list of who and dates precepted • Participate in RT education for RT, RN or new resident classes as requested/keep a list of who and dates educated		
In all work	Identifies and applies planning, care and/or intervention techniques appropriate to the physical, motor and sensory, cognitive, and psychosocial characteristics of each patient population served	Assesses and/or interprets data about the patient's status to identify each patient's needs and provide the appropriate care, including age-related care	Patients are provided safe, age-appropriate, timely, and coordinated care as measured by successful outcomes of the care plan, patient/parent satisfaction, direct observation, peer and supervisory feedback		

Work Requirements	
Education and Experience (Required)	• AS in respiratory care from an AMA approved school of respiratory care • RRT or registry eligible with the NBRC • Current Washington State license • Current CPR certification
Education and Experience (Preferred)	• One year current critical care experience: adult, pediatric, or neonatal • PALS, NRP and/or neonatal/pediatric specialty credential from the NBRC
Knowledge, Skills, and Abilities Required to Perform the Essential Functions of the Work	• Knowledge of human growth and development to modify care to the age and development status of the neonate, infant, toddler, preschool child, school-age child, or adolescent, according to the age/development focus of the assigned department • Good communication and interpersonal skills • Able to work independently and as a member of a multidisciplinary team • Frequently comes in contact with potentially hazardous materials to include compressed gases, aerosolized medications, and cleaning solutions • Requires attending to patients with infectious diseases • Exposure to blood borne pathogens, category "I" may occur • Frequently involves stressful and emotional situations dealing with severely ill and/or dying children and their families
Physical Requirements	• Visual acuity, depth perception, and color identification • Auditory acuity • Manual dexterity for operating and troubleshooting equipment • Computer usage • Physical mobility to walk up and down stairs, bend, push, pull, and lift moderately heavy equipment • Able to walk and/or stand for extended periods of time • Able to lift and turn patients of all sizes

(Continues)

Performance Improvement Plan—Required If Position Needs Improvement	
Specific Areas in Need of Improvement	Plan Description and Comments (actions to be taken; resources needed; monitoring and feedback processes; time frames, etc.)
1)	
2)	

Goal Setting Plan	
Specific Goals to be Achieved During Next Cycle	Plan Description and Comments (actions to be taken; resources needed; monitoring and feedback processes; time frames, etc.)
1)	
2)	

Overall Rating			
Overall Performance Rating: (Check one)	☐ (1) Work performance needs improvement	☐ (2) Meets work expectations	☐ (3) Exceeds work expectations

Evaluator Comments

Employee Comments

Manager Name (print and sign):	Employee Name (print and sign):
Date:	Date:

DOCUMENT B-2: WORK CONTENT DESCRIPTION/PERFORMANCE EVALUATION FORM

Action Being Taken

☐ Annual Performance Evaluation	☐ New Position	☐ Position Reclassification	☐ Position Update	☐ 90 Day Review

Employee Information

Employee Name:				Employee ID #:	Date:

Job Class	Pos Code	Old Job #	Job Title: Respiratory Therapist II	Working Tittle:
RSP	**2721-003**	372		

Location: Hospital	Dept. #	12651	Dept. Title: Respiratory Care	Reports To: Clinical Supervisor and ECMO Coordinator

Position Purpose

The respiratory therapist applies the knowledge and skills necessary to provide appropriate respiratory care for any age-related needs of the patients served on his or her assigned unit/department. Applies the knowledge and skill necessary to provide appropriate interactions with staff, patients, and families of all ages.

Major Responsibilities, Activities, And End Results

% of Time	Essential Functions/ Work Responsibilities/ Accountabilities	How Is It Done (Activities)	Outcomes/Measures	Rating 1 or 2	Comments
100%	1) Performs respiratory diagnostic and therapeutic interventions	• Patient status to identify each patient's needs and provide the appropriate care including age related care. • Understand and follow current policies and procedures for the assigned unit/ dept. to include but not limited to the following: • Airway management and care • Ventilator management • Patient assessments • Airway clearance techniques • Respiratory monitoring	• Patients are provided safe, age-appropriate, timely, and coordinated care as measured by successful outcomes of the care plan, patient/ parent satisfaction, direct observation, and supervisory feedback • Policies, procedures and guidelines are followed and documented in the medical record through annual chart review • Review annual CQI memos relating to individual practice • Participate in care planning with medical and nursing staff by attending patient rounds		

(Continues)

Major Responsibilities, Activities, And End Results					
	2) Performs duties associated with being a specialist on the extra corporeal membrane oxygenation team 3) Performs inter-hospital transport	• Administration of therapeutic gases • Administration of therapeutic aerosols • Intra-hospital transport of ventilated patients • Documentation and charging for all interactions with patients according to department and hospital guidelines • Participate in professional development • Perform annual competencies See WCD for ECMO specialist • Perform inter-hospital transport as member of the neonatal ground transport team • Complete annual competencies	• Attend 66% of RT staff meetings per year • Attend 66% of neonatal ground transport team meetings • Participates in department QA program • Attend educational offerings related to neonatal and/or pediatric respiratory care • Attend in-services on new products or therapies • Attendance at annual skills fair • Be a trained preceptor	Rating 1 or 2	
In all work	Identifies and applies planning, care and/or intervention techniques appropriate to the physical, motor and sensory, cognitive, and psychosocial characteristics of each patient population served	Assesses and/or interprets data about the patient's status to identify each patient's needs and provide the appropriate care, including age-related care	Patients are provided safe, age-appropriate, timely, and coordinated care as measured by successful outcomes of the care plan, patient/parent satisfaction, direct observation, peer, and supervisory feedback		

Education and Experience (Required)	**1. To Become an RT-II**
	1.1. AS in respiratory care from an AMA approved school of respiratory care
	1.2. Registered respiratory therapist by the National Board for Respiratory Care
	1.3. Current Washington State license
	1.4. Current CPR certification
	1.5. Either of the following:
	    1.5.1. Completion of ECMO specialist training and selection to be on the team of ECMO specialists
	    1.5.2. Completion of neonatal ground transport training and selection to be on the neonatal ground transport team				

Major Responsibilities, Activities, And End Results
2. To Maintain status as an RT-II 2.1. Accumulation of **100 points yearly** by combination of these factors listed below: (for more details on the items listed below, see department policy manual)   **Points** ECMO training/good standing on the ECMO specialist team . . . . .50 Neonatal Ground Transport team/good standing . . . . .50 Pediatric-neonatal specialist by the National Board for Respiratory Care . . . .25 Pediatric advance life support (PALS) certification .25 Neonatal resuscitation program (NRP) certification . . . . .25 Pediatric advance life support (PALS) instructor . . . . .40 Neonatal resuscitation program (NRP) instructor . . . . .40 Mentor . . . . .25 Department level in-service instructor . . . . .15 Research 20

Knowledge, Skills, and Abilities Required to Perform the Essential Functions of the Work	• Knowledge of human growth and development to modify care to the age and development status of the neonate, infant, toddler, preschool child, school-age child, or adolescent, according to the age/development focus of the assigned department • Knowledge of patient safety according to the assigned department • Good communication and interpersonal skills • Able to work independently and as a member of a multidisciplinary team • Frequently comes in contact with potentially hazardous materials to include compressed gases, aerosolized medications, and cleaning solutions • Requires attending to patients with infectious diseases • Exposure to bloodborne pathogens, category "I" may occur • Frequently involves stressful and emotional situations dealing with severely ill and/or dying children and their families
IV.D. Physical Requirements	• Visual acuity, depth perception, and color identification • Auditory acuity • Manual dexterity for operating and troubleshooting equipment • Computer usage • Physical mobility to walk up and down stairs, bend, push, pull, and lift moderately heavy equipment • Able to sit, stand, and kneel for extended periods of time • Able to lift and turn patients of all sizes

Requirements Checklist

	Training and Testing Requirements Checklist (check all that apply):
	Training and Testing Requirements Checklist (check all that apply):
☐	Age-Specific Category 1 position. Position with incidental contact.
☐	Age-Specific Category 2 position. Position with regular contact. Age-specific competency summary form is attached (required with performance evaluation).
☐	Age-Specific Category 3 position. Position with direct care contact. Age-specific competency summary form is attached (required with performance evaluation).
☐	Ergonomics (safe patient handling, materials handling, and office/computer work). Provide appropriate equipment, training, and demonstrates ability to perform job safely.
☐	Blood exposure (required annual bloodborne pathogens training has been completed).

(Continues)

Requirements Checklist

☐	TB exposure (required annual TB testing and education has been completed).
☐	Annually required training has been completed (see child/education and development tab/required training).
☐	Required compliance training has been completed.
☐	Required HIPAA/privacy training has been completed.
☐	Required diversity training has been completed.
☐	Performance improvement plan follows (required with performance evaluation if work performance needs improvement).
☐	Goal setting plan follows.

Performance Improvement Plan—Required If Position Needs Improvement

Specific Areas in Need of Improvement	Plan Description and Comments (actions to be taken; resources needed; monitoring and feedback processes; time frames, etc.)
1)	
2)	

Goal Setting Plan

Specific Goals to be Achieved During Next Cycle	Plan Description and Comments (actions to be taken; resources needed; monitoring and feedback processes; time frames, etc.)
1)	
2)	

Overall Rating

Overall Performance Rating: (Check one)	☐ (1) Work performance needs improvement	☐ (2) Meets work expectations	☐ (3) Exceeds work expectations

Evaluator Comments

Employee Comments

Manager Name (print and sign):	Employee Name (print and sign):
Date:	Date:

DOCUMENT B-3: NIGHT SHIFT SUPERVISOR JOB DESCRIPTION

General Hospital Job Description/Expectations Evaluation RT Night Clinical Supervisor		Ratings	
Job Title/Job Code: Respiratory Therapy Night Clinical Supervisor Department Name/#: Respiratory Therapy	**Commendable Performance**	**Successful and Solid Performance**	**Needs Improvement**
Sup. Title/Job Code: Respiratory Therapy Manager/ 937301 Person Being Evaluated: ——————————— Employee ID #: ——————————— ——————— Date: ——————————— ——————— Evaluator Signature: #: ——————————— ☐ Self Evaluation ☐ Supervisor Evaluation	Performance is of the highest caliber, achieving unique and exceptional accomplishments. ☐ Always ☐ Exceptional ☐ Goes above and beyond ☐ Initiative ☐ Invariable ☐ Inventive ☐ Role model ☐ Significant positive influence	Performance consistently meets all essential requirements and expectations. ☐ Accountable ☐ Achieves ☐ Adaptable ☐ Dependable ☐ Effective ☐ Focused ☐ Reliable ☐ Routinely	Performance inconsistently meets requirements and expectations with significant growth opportunities that require performance improvement plan. ☐ Indifferent ☐ Inflexible ☐ Infrequent ☐ Marginal ☐ Negative influence ☐ Occasionally ☐ Questionable ☐ Unsatisfactory
General Summary: The Respiratory Therapy (RT) Night Clinical Supervisor is a registered respiratory therapist who promotes/delivers quality care and maintains RT shift operational flow in collaboration with the respiratory therapy manager. The RT Night Clinical Supervisor functions as a leader/clinical representative of the health care team by acting as a facilitator, coach, mentor, and clinical/supervisory resource.			
Percentage of Time	**Essential Functions/Competencies**		
	Defines operational standards, organizes department-level activities to achieve optimum service delivery/systems/care/processes, setting high performance objectives for the department. Holds self and others accountable to meet stated objectives, outcomes, goals, timetables and commitments, adhering to standards even in the face of unforeseen circumstances.		

(Continues)

Percentage of Time	Essential Functions/Competencies
40%	Synthesizes all available information to make informed decisions. Fosters creativity, innovation, and divergent thinking in self and others. Manages complex situations using multiple sources of information and advice. Prioritizes, proposes, and leads operational projects/system changes based on careful analysis of current processes.
30%	The RT Night Clinical Supervisor has the authority/accountability as the supervisory representative to provide direction, system expertise, decisions, resource, and leadership to ensure uninterrupted department operations. This is accomplished through direct communication with all departments and other disciplines as appropriate.
25%	Creates an environment that fosters high individual and team engagement by demonstrating service excellence, effective conflict resolution, leading by example, and developing staff through clinical and supervisory expertise.
5%	Demonstrates professional development and leadership related to the role and the role's direct/indirect impact within the RT department and hospital wide.
100%	**Secondary Functions/Competencies** Performs other related duties as assigned.

☐ Commendable performance
☐ Successful/solid performance
☐ Needs improvement

Comments (strengths, growth opportunities):

---

1. Leads staff in achieving department/organization outcomes by clearly communicating the expectations and vision.
Patient Satisfaction
- Identifies, facilitates, and leads performance improvement projects that enhance patient care delivery systems and/or family/customer satisfaction.
- Meets department/organization patient satisfaction goals.
- Department specific:
  - Ensures that RTs implement therapies in accordance with the patient/family plan of care and patient's condition/needs.

2. Takes personal responsibility in leading staff to adhere to department/organization policies and procedures, compliance and regulatory agency requirements.
- Leads staff in emergency situations (i.e., CPR, internal/external disaster, disruptive individuals, Code Adam).
- Develops, reviews, revises, and implements policies and procedures on an ongoing basis to assure department's consistency and compliance with hospital standards and accrediting bodies including: JCAHO, OSHA, HIPAA, Infection Control, Environment of Care, National Patient Safety Goals.

3. Fosters and supports a work environment that focuses on staff, customer, patient/families through safe practices and effective communication.
- Demonstrates and supports staff/visitor/patient/vendor identification policy.
- Directs the utilization of the variance reporting system to enhance safety and identifies, implements changes for best practice.
- Ensures that privacy and confidentiality is protected in patient relationships and all other appropriate work-related areas.
- Delegates responsibilities to others, giving staff the authority, resources, and guidance to make decisions and accomplish tasks independently.

Financial
- Develops annual department budget and monitors/analyzes budget and fiscal performance monthly.
- Makes decisions that demonstrate sound stewardship of financial resources. Oversees the implementation of identified systems/processes to improve efficiency and reduce expenses without compromising quality of services/mission.
- Meets department/organization financial goals.
- Department specific:
  - Coordinates shift operational activities of the department by providing quality patient care and promoting efficient use of resources. This would include but not be limited to staffing, patient flow, equipment, supplies, communication inside and outside of the department, concern reports, department standards, safety.

Quality
- Directs performance measurement to improve patient/customer outcomes.
- Exhibits conceptual vision/forward momentum, evaluating new opportunities objectively and with an eye toward innovative ideas.
- Adjusts to unforeseen situations and overcomes obstacles and setbacks.
- Coordinates department workload and maintains optimal staff to provide quality services.
- Department specific:
- Ensures quality patient care, through:
  a. Coordinating assignments by matching patient needs to staff competencies through ongoing assessment of patient and department needs.
  b. Serving as a clinical expert and systems resource to facilitate patient care delivery.

- Manages staff in addressing noncompliance with standards and develops an action plan as necessary.
- Administers policies, performance evaluations, and disciplinary actions with consistency and without regard to personal agendas or beliefs.
- Ensures self and staff meet department/organization job requirements within established time frames (i.e., licensure/certification, CPR for direct care providers, physicals, annual mandatory reviews, participates and physically attends 75% of required staff meetings).
- Keeps abreast of department/organization policies/regulations, as well as industry knowledge through technical publications, newsletters, personal networks, and professional affiliations.
- Department specific:
  - Understands the hospital's mission, vision, values, culture and policies. Supports the performance improvement process.
  - Adheres to department policies/standards, rules and regulations as outlined by Children's Hospital based on JCAHO and other external regulatory agencies.
  - Participates in compliance program to prevent illegal and unethical conduct.

- Effectively recruits, hires, evaluates, develops, and coaches staff to achieve desired outcomes.
- Collaborates with other departments to maintain effective communication channels by gathering and exchanging information, obtaining solutions to problems, and coordinating services to ensure optimal outcomes are achieved.
- Drives changes with an enthusiastic "can-do" attitude for department/organization initiatives. Sets an example that inspires superior performance while instilling confidence and trust in others.
- Effectively uses a variety of communication skills in achieving positive/optimum outcomes, to include confronting issues with tact and diplomacy.
- Creates an environment for raising concerns and ideas on providing constructive feedback.
- Leads and/or participates in appropriate committees and workgroups, managing effective group/team meetings.
- Department specific:
  - Provides a safe work environment.
  - Establishes a culture of clinical safety.
  - Uses work practices and engineering controls appropriately to reduce the risk of exposure to blood and body fluids.

(Continues)

c. Providing continuous and annual feedback on staff performance and quality patient care in conjunction with the Respiratory Therapy Manager. d. Acting as a liaison between patients, families, and the health care team to provide excellent care.		
☐ Commendable performance ☐ Successful/solid performance ☐ Needs improvement	☐ Commendable performance ☐ Successful/solid performance ☐ Needs improvement	☐ Commendable performance ☐ Successful/solid performance ☐ Needs improvement
Comments (strengths, growth opportunities): _____	Comments (strengths, growth opportunities): _____	Comments (strengths, growth opportunities): _____

Additional summary/evaluator comments: _____

_____

Overall Evaluation Rating: _____ **Commendable Performance** _____ **Successful/Solid Performance**
_____ **Needs Improvement**

Knowledge, Skills and Abilities:
- Must have a current valid Nebraska license and be a registered respiratory therapist.
- Must possess leadership skills including communication, organizational skills, time management, coping skills, motivation, problem solving, autonomy, and supporting the team.
- Must be certified in basic cardiac life support.
- Required NRP and PALS certification within 6 months of employment.
- Department specific certification preferred, required within 3 years of accepting position to include neonatal/pediatric RT certification and asthma certification.

Education And Experience:
- Bachelors degree in respiratory care or related field preferred with recommendation of pursuit of masters degree in health related field.
- A minimum of 5 years experience as an RT with minimum of 3 years in pediatrics.
- A minimum of 1 year supervisory experience preferred.

Physical Requirements/Working Conditions:

	N/A	Less than 10%	11% to 49%	Greater than 50%	Work Environment	N/A	Less than 10%	11% to 49%	Greater than 50%
Stand				X	Blood and body fluid exposure*				X
Walk				X	Sharps, needles, etc.			X	
Sit		X			Wet, humid conditions (nonweather)	X			
Talk or hear				X	Work near moving mechanical parts		X		
Displays manual dexterity				X	Fumes or airborne particles			X	
Climb or balance		X			Toxic or caustic chemicals		X		
Stoop, kneel, crouch, or crawl			X		Outdoor weather conditions	X			
Reach with hands and arms				X	Extreme cold (nonweather)	X			
Taste or smell		X			Extreme hot (nonweather)	X			
Lifting/pulling/pushing				X	Risk of electrical shock		X		
Visual: Looking at computer screen				X	Hand power tools		X		
Other: Running		X			Risk of radiation		X		
Weight Demands					Vibration			X	
Up to 10 pounds				X	Loud noise		X		
Up to 20 pounds			X		Quiet environment		X		
Up to 40 pounds			X		Other: Environmental noise				X
Up to 100 pounds			X						
More than 100 pounds			X						

*Please refer to the Infection Control Manual for a listing of job classifications that may be at risk of occupational exposure.

DOCUMENT B-4: CLINICAL EDUCATOR JOB DESCRIPTION

General Hospital Job Description/Expectations Evaluation RT Clinical Educator		Ratings	
Job Title/Job Code: Rt Clinical Educator Department Name/#: Respiratory Therapy	**Commendable Performance**	**Successful and Solid Performance**	**Needs Improvement**
Sup. Title/Job Code: Respiratory Therapy Manager/ 973301 Person Being Evaluated: _____ Employee ID #: _____ _____ Date: _____ _____ Evaluator Signature: #: _____ ☐Self Evaluation ☐ Supervisor Evaluation	Performance is of the highest caliber, achieving unique and exceptional accomplishments. ☐ Always ☐ Exceptional ☐ Goes above and beyond ☐ Initiative ☐ Invariable ☐ Inventive ☐ Role model ☐ Significant positive ☐ influence	Performance consistently meets all essential requirements and expectations. ☐ Accountable ☐ Achieves ☐ Adaptable ☐ Dependable ☐ Effective ☐ Focused ☐ Reliable ☐ Routinely	Performance inconsistently meets requirements and expectations with significant growth opportunities that require performance improvement plan. ☐ Indifferent ☐ Inflexible ☐ Infrequent ☐ Marginal ☐ Negative influence ☐ Occasionally ☐ Questionable ☐ Unsatisfactory

General Summary: The Inpatient Respiratory Therapy Educator works with the RT management/staff team to promote competent, quality respiratory care at Children's Hospital. The Educator promotes the delivery of quality respiratory care through clinical practice, education, collaboration, continuous quality improvement, evaluation of products/ equipment, leadership, and the utilization of benchmarking/research. The Educator oversees the orientation and ongoing education of the respiratory therapy department staff. The RT Clinical Educator works in partnership with physicians and other health care disciplines to ensure the established RT standards of care and expected outcomes are achieved with patient care.

Percentage of Time	Essential Functions/Competencies
	Defines operational standards, organizes department-level activities to achieve optimum service delivery/systems/care/processes, setting high performance objectives for the department. Holds self and others accountable to meet stated objectives, outcomes, goals, timetables and commitments, adhering to standards even in the face of unforeseen circumstances.

Percentage of Time	Essential Functions/Competencies
30%	Synthesizes all available information to make informed decisions. Fosters creativity, innovation, and divergent thinking in self and others. Manages complex situations using multiple sources of information and advice. Prioritizes, proposes, and leads operational projects/system changes based on careful analysis of current processes.
20%	Collaborates with departmental manager, medical director, and RT staff regarding development, implementation, and evaluation of respiratory care practices, systems, and education programs (staff and/or patient/family) ensuring that the practice at Children's meets established national RT clinical standards for pediatric patients.
20%	Assumes daily accountability and responsibility for the clinical/unit orientation program of new RT employees assigned to the Inpatient Department.
15%	Coordinates the identification, development, and implementation of educational programs for both clinical and professional development of RT staff and other health care disciplines regarding respiratory care practices.
5%	Assumes responsibilities associated with the role of staff RT as needed.
100%	**Secondary Functions/Competencies** Performs other duties as assigned.

☐ Commendable performance
☐ Successful/solid performance
☐ Needs improvement

Comments (strengths, growth opportunities):

---

1. Leads staff in achieving department/organization outcomes by clearly communicating the expectations and vision.
Patient Satisfaction
- Identifies, facilitates, and leads performance improvement projects that enhance patient care delivery systems and/or family/customer satisfaction.
- Meets department/organization patient satisfaction goals.
- Department specific:
  - Ensures that RTs implement therapies in accordance with the patient/family plan of care and patient's condition/needs.
Financial
- Develops annual department budget and monitors/analyzes budget and fiscal performance monthly.

2. Takes personal responsibility in leading staff to adhere to department/organization policies and procedures, compliance and regulatory agency requirements.
- Leads staff in emergency situations (i.e., CPR, internal/external disaster, disruptive individuals, Code Adam).
- Develops, reviews, revises, and implements policies and procedures on an ongoing basis to assure department's consistency and compliance with hospital standards and accrediting bodies including: JCAHO, OSHA, HIPAA, Infection Control, Environment of Care, National Patient Safety Goals.
- Manages staff in addressing noncompliance with standards and develops an action plan as necessary.

3. Fosters and supports a work environment that focuses on staff, customer, patient/families through safe practices and effective communication.
- Demonstrates and supports staff/visitor/patient/vendor identification policy.
- Directs the utilization of the variance reporting system to enhance safety and identifies, implements changes for best practice.
- Ensures that privacy and confidentiality is protected in patient relationships and all other appropriate work-related areas.
- Delegates responsibilities to others, giving staff the authority, resources, and guidance to make decisions and accomplish tasks independently.

(Continues)

- Makes decisions that demonstrate sound stewardship of financial resources. Oversees the implementation of identified systems/processes to improve efficiency and reduce expenses without compromising quality of services/mission.
- Meets department/organization financial goals.
- Department specific:
  - Informs manager of education costs as necessary.
  - Informs manager of any known cost variances, especially with respect to education.
  - Communicates financial goals to staff as needed.

Quality
- Directs performance measurement to improve patient/customer outcomes.
- Exhibits conceptual vision/forward momentum, evaluating new opportunities objectively and with an eye toward innovative ideas.
- Adjusts to unforeseen situations and overcomes obstacles and setbacks.
- Coordinates department workload and maintains optimal staff to provide quality services.
- Department specific:
  - Understands the hospital's mission, vision, values, culture, and policies. Supports the Quality Initiative, which is based on continuous quality improvement.

- Administers policies, performance evaluations, and disciplinary actions with consistency and without regard to personal agendas or beliefs.
- Ensures self and staff meet department/organization job requirements within established time frames (i.e., licensure/certification, CPR for direct care providers, physicals, annual mandatory reviews, participates and physically attends 75% of required staff meetings).
- Keeps abreast of department/organization policies/regulations, as well as industry knowledge through technical publications, newsletters, personal networks, and professional affiliations.
- Department specific:
  - Participates in mandatory inservices and continuing education programs as mandated by policies and procedure, external agencies, and as directed by supervisor.

- Effectively recruits, hires, evaluates, develops, and coaches staff to achieve desired outcomes.
- Collaborates with other departments to maintain effective communication channels by gathering and exchanging information, obtaining solutions to problems, and coordinating services to ensure optimal outcomes are achieved.
- Drives changes with an enthusiastic "can-do" attitude for department/organization initiatives. Sets an example that inspires superior performance while instilling confidence and trust in others.
- Effectively uses a variety of communication skills in achieving positive/optimum outcomes, to include confronting issues with tact and diplomacy.
- Creates an environment for raising concerns and ideas on providing constructive feedback.
- Leads and/or participates in appropriate committees and workgroups, managing effective group/team meetings.
- Department specific:
  - Provides clinical/system/consultation leadership to the healthcare team members and patients/families in the utilization of established protocols, care standards, and teaching education of respiratory patients.
  - Uses work practices and engineering controls appropriately to reduce the risk of exposure to blood and body fluids.
  - Promotes service to the patient and family with consideration to the patient's age cognitive level.

☐ Commendable performance ☐ Successful/solid performance ☐ Needs improvement	☐ Commendable performance ☐ Successful/solid performance ☐ Needs improvement	☐ Commendable performance ☐ Successful/solid performance ☐ Needs improvement
Comments (strengths, growth opportunities): _____ _____ _____ _____ _____ _____ _____ _____	Comments (strengths, growth opportunities): _____ _____ _____ _____ _____ _____ _____ _____	Comments (strengths, growth opportunities): _____ _____ _____ _____ _____ _____ _____ _____

Additional summary/evaluator comments: _____

_____

Overall Evaluation Rating: _____ **Commendable Performance** _____ **Successful/Solid Performance**
_____ **Needs Improvement**

Additional comments: _____

_____

Knowledge, Skills and Abilities:
- Licensed as a Registered Respiratory Therapist. CPR, NRP, and PALS instructor certification required. Neonatal, pediatric, and asthma certification required or obtained within 3 years of job acceptance. Must be vested in the RT clinical focus of the role. Possess leadership skills to include: effective communication style, teaching/mentoring skills, organizational skills and detail oriented, time management, creative planner/developer, systems thinker, motivator, and team oriented. Experience with program, project, and protocol development.

Education And Experience:
- Graduate of an accredited program for respiratory therapy with a bachelor's of science degree in respiratory care or related field. Master's degree in health care/education related field required. Will consider individual with career plan that includes pursuit of master's degree.
- Minimum of 5 years experience in pediatric respiratory care required.

(Continues)

Physical Requirements/Working Conditions:

	N/A	Less than 10%	11% to 49%	Greater than 50%	Work Environment	N/A	Less than 10%	11% to 49%	Greater than 50%
Stand				X	Blood and body fluid exposure*				X
Walk				X	Sharps, needles, etc.			X	
Sit		X			Wet, humid conditions (nonweather)	X			
Talk or hear				X	Work near moving mechanical parts		X		
Displays manual dexterity				X	Fumes or airborne particles			X	
Climb or balance		X			Toxic or caustic chemicals		X		
Stoop, kneel, crouch, or crawl			X		Outdoor weather conditions	X			
Reach with hands and arms				X	Extreme cold (nonweather)	X			
Taste or smell		X			Extreme hot (nonweather)	X			
Lifting/pulling/pushing				X	Risk of electrical shock		X		
Visual: Looking at computer screen				X	Hand power tools		X		
Other: Running		X			Risk of radiation		X		
Weight Demands					Vibration			X	
Up to 10 pounds				X	Loud noise		X		
Up to 20 pounds			X		Quiet environment		X		
Up to 40 pounds			X		Other: Environmental noise				X
Up to 100 pounds			X						
More than 100 pounds			X						

*Please refer to the Infection Control Manual for a listing of job classifications that may be at risk of occupational exposure.

DOCUMENT B-5: CLINICAL SPECIALIST JOB DESCRIPTION

Job Competency Description and Assessment

Description Detail Section I			
Title: Clinicical Specialist RCP	Job Code: 70-666	FLSA: Non-Ex	Originating Date: 8/2001
Department Name:	Cost Center #: 107180		Revision Date: 6\2002
Reports to (Title): Clinical Director, Respiratory Care Services	Approval:		
Print Incumbent's Name:	Incumbent's Signature:		

Primary Purpose:

Provides preventative, supportive, and corrective interventions related to the cardio-pulmonary system in assigned patient care areas in accordance with established hospital and departmental policies, procedures, and all applicable regulations and standards.

Minimum Qualifications:

1. Current State of Arizona license as a Respiratory Care Practitioner. Registered Respiratory Therapist preferred.
2. Current BLS certification or ability to obtain within 30 days of hire; certification in either NRP or PALS required based on work area.
3. Must have at least 1 year previous experience in general pediatric and/or neonatal respiratory care.
4. Six months prior experience with Windows-based PC applications preferred.

Work Environment:

Work activities are performed in an environmentally controlled nursing unit subject to extended periods of walking, standing, pushing/pulling equipment up to 180 pounds; lifting equipment/supplies up to 25 pounds; potentially frequent exposure to blood and other high risk body fluids, communicable diseases, hazardous materials, chemicals, and waste. Regularly required to lift and position infant, toddler, school age, adolescent, and adult patients in the delivery of therapeutic care. Regularly required to use fine motor skills to manipulate and/or maintain equipment.

Supervision Received/Given:

This position receives regular supervision of completed tasks by the Clinical Director, Respiratory Care Services, or delegate. This position does not supervise any other position.

Essential Functions and Outcomes	Values and Competency Criteria	Proficiency Level				Comments
		1	2	3	4	
1. Provides assessment and intervention for cardio-pulmonary system function to patients by applying age appropriate methods in accordance with established policies and procedures and safety and quality standards.	• Demonstrates ability to apply knowledge and understanding of the principles, practices, methods, and techniques of cardio-pulmonary treatment (Family Centered Care). • Demonstrates ability to modify approach and communication style to accommodate different developmental levels of children and families (Family Centered Care and Caring). • Demonstrates ability to perform a variety of complex diagnostic and therapeutic procedures according to established standards and training under supervision of appropriate health care professional (Family Centered Care). • Demonstrates expended skill and emergent intervention skills by applying and utilizing appropriate judgment and critical thinking for problem resolution considering all aspects of the whole. • Demonstrates understanding and knowledge of the methods and techniques of infection control, safe/ergonomically correct body mechanics and all applicable regulations, standards, and licensing requirements.	☐	☐	☐	☐	
2. Interprets evaluations and test results to determine appropriate treatment plan(s) in consultation with interdisciplinary healthcare team.	• Demonstrates ability to accurately and reliably interpret data. • Demonstrates ability to work effectively and foster collaborative team efforts by developing mutually beneficial relationships including reporting deviations from expected outcomes to appropriate professional(s) (collaboration and accountability). • Demonstrates ability to apply critical thinking skills for problem identification, resolution, and/or escalation/triage to proper health care professional (accountability).	☐	☐	☐	☐	

Essential Functions and Outcomes	Values and Competency Criteria	Proficiency Level				Comments
		1	2	3	4	
3. Documents patient care service(s) by charting in patient and department records to provide timely and complete information.	• Demonstrates ability to foster and instill trust in others through consistency in work methods, behaviors, and follow through (leadership). • Demonstrates ability to effectively manage multiple priorities through application of effective and efficient time and work methods (accountability). • Consistently demonstrates personal responsibility for completion of all tasks through timely, thorough, clear, and concise communication and documentation of outcomes (accountability and collaboration).	☐	☐	☐	☐	
4. Maintains professional and technical competency through constantly pursuing knowledge and self-improvement by remaining apprised of current respiratory care, management, and health care delivery trends and developments including awareness of latest technology and practices to improve patient outcomes.	• Demonstrates commitment to continuous skill improvement and development by identifying appropriate learning experiences and opportunities (innovation/excellence). • Demonstrates ability to apply professionally accepted standards or practice to assess own learning and skill needs (innovation/excellence and accountability).	☐	☐	☐	☐	
5. Participates in hospital and department operational and quality improvement initiative; proactively evaluates systems, practices and assists creating and implementing changes to increase and enhance the effectiveness of care delivery methods/coordination.	• Demonstrates understanding of the principles, practices, methods, and techniques of quality and performance improvement (accountability and innovation/excellence). • Demonstrates understanding of hospital and departmental operations, programs, goals, and initiatives.	☐	☐	☐	☐	
6. Reviews and reinforces with patient/family education of basic procedures and therapies to ensure understanding of proper/safe techniques and methods.	• Demonstrates understanding of verbal and nonverbal communication styles (caring).	☐	☐	☐	☐	

(Continues)

Essential Functions and Outcomes	Values and Competency Criteria	Proficiency Level				Comments
		1	2	3	4	
7. Completes preventive maintenance requirements of equipment in accordance with established instructions; identifies and troubleshoots malfunctions to ensure continuous proper operations.	• Demonstrates ability to perform routine assembly and troubleshooting of complex equipment (accountability). • Demonstrates understanding and knowledge of the proper and safe use of equipment (accountability).	☐	☐	☐	☐	
8. Assists Respiratory Educator by providing staff orientation and ongoing educational programs as needed; provides feedback and assists to identify educational needs and opportunities.	• Demonstrates ability to apply knowledge and understanding of the methods and techniques of adult learning (innovation/excellence).	☐	☐	☐	☐	

Values Defined

Family Centered Care—A culture of family centered care ensures family empowerment and guides facility design, work design, program development, and policy decisions that focus on the needs of children and families first.

Leadership—By instilling confidence, loyalty, trust, and support in others, PCH team members help establish the desired culture and set the standard for child health within the organization and the community.

Innovation/excellence—A culture of innovation and excellence allows the individual and the organization to openly report, discuss, learn from, and seek optimal solutions; always striving to enhance performance and quality now and in the future.

Caring—A culture of caring recognizes and respects the differences in others and empowers team members to do the right thing at the right time to help others feel valued.

Collaboration—A culture of collaboration drives the achievement of organizational mission and goals through effective teamwork, cooperation, and exchange of information in an environment of mutual respect and trust.

Accountability—A culture in which each team member takes responsibility for his/her own actions to support and safeguard the organization's mission, vision, values, and resources.

DOCUMENT B-6: RT DEPARTMENT DIRECTOR JOB DESCRIPTION

Job Competency Description and Assessment

Description Detail Section			
Title: Respiratory Care Equipment Manager	Job Code:	FLSA: Exempt	Originating Date: Oct 2005
Department Name: Respiratory Care Services	Cost Center #: 10-7180		Revision Date:
Reports to (Title): Admin. Director, Respiratory Care	Approval:		
Print Incumbent's Name:	Incumbent's Signature:		

Primary Purpose:

Manages, evaluates, and assumes responsibility for respiratory equipment oversight inclusive of budgetary fiscal management relative to capital assets, consumable supplies, rentals, and medical gases. Supervises operational activities relative to equipment related practices including but not limited to staff education, ongoing safety, and service delivery. Acts as a liaison with other departments to facilitate quick resolution of issues to ensure excellence in a family centered care environment.

Minimum Qualifications:

1. Must have a minimum of 4 years of clinical experience in respiratory care; pediatric/neonatal experience preferred.
2. Requires a minimum of 2 years in a leadership position.
3. Graduation from an accredited institution for respiratory care services; associate's degree in respiratory care. Bachelor's degree is preferred.
4. Requires RRT certification and current Arizona licensure.
5. BLS certification required within introductory period.
6. Must be able to effectively utilize PC-based standard office software such as Word and Excel.
7. AARC membership is preferred.
8. Must demonstrate behaviors consistent with those identified as PCH core values behaviors.
9. Must be able to work in a high demand, stressful environment and apply sound judgment and critical thinking skills.
10. Must be able to communicate, collaborate, delegate, and manage crisis situations.
11. Must be able to develop documents and spreadsheets, such as data tracking tools, inventory spreadsheets, policies, and procedures.
12. Must have the ability to educate, coach, and mentor people.

Work Environment:

Activities are performed in an environmentally controlled hospital setting subject to frequent long periods of standing and walking; frequent physical demands including, but not limited to: stooping, bending, reaching, pulling, climbing, lifting, and pushing objects of varying weights up to and including 40 pounds. Regularly works in an environment subject to high stress levels and exposure to fumes, chemicals and noise; frequently changing priorities. Ability to clearly communicate in English, reads, writes, sees, and hears to perform essential duties.

Supervision Received/Given:

This position receives supervision and direction from the Administrative Director, Respiratory Care Services.

This position provides management of a vital program relative to operational functions along with providing direction to staff members to ensure achievement of service delivery and quality standards.

Essential Functions and Outcomes	Values and Competency Criteria	Proficiency Level				Comments
		1	2	3	4	
1. Manages and assumes responsibility to provide oversight for respiratory care capital assets and consumable supplies to ensure the achievement of safe, optimal service delivery.	• Effectively maintains capital equipment inventory and ensures equipment availability and functionality. • Demonstrates the ability to work in conjunction with Material Services to assure consumable supplies inventory levels are appropriate based on patient care needs. • Effectively works with Material Services to define critical par levels and determine processes and/or acceptable substitute products in the event of supply backorders.	☐	☐	☐	☐	
2. Partners with Material Services to review contract compliance/opportunities and ensure supply expenses are appropriately allocated.	• Utilizes the Material Services contract experts as a resource when evaluating equipment supplies. • Effectively represents the department on committees and action teams relative to product reviews and new equipment evaluations.	☐	☐	☐	☐	

Essential Functions and Outcomes	Values and Competency Criteria	Proficiency Level				Comments
		1	2	3	4	
	• Effectively tracks and monitors staff members' compliance in utilizing supply dispensing systems correctly. • Educates as necessary and addresses compliance deviations as necessary.	☐	☐	☐	☐	
3. Evaluates the respiratory equipment program on an ongoing basis; suggests and implements changes as necessary that result in measurable outcomes toward enhancement of service and opportunities to decrease expenses.	• Evaluates equipment/supplies utilized and looks for opportunities to decrease expenses while maintaining quality patient care. • Enacts procedures and processes to keep equipment breakage and loss to an absolute minimum.	☐	☐	☐	☐	
4. Collaborates with Biomedical Engineering to ensure performance of timely equipment maintenance and investigation into equipment related occurrences and events.	• Demonstrates the ability to effectively troubleshoot respiratory care equipment and recreate patient scenarios to analyze factors that may have contributed to equipment related occurrences. • Understands and follows safety and risk management processes when analyzing equipment related issues and events. • Effectively and accurately tracks respiratory equipment downtime and monitoring of timeliness in equipment repair turnaround.	☐	☐	☐	☐	
5. Assists in ensuring that daily operational functions are met through the management of the rental equipment program.	• Demonstrates the ability to proactively determine rental equipment needs, rents equipment as necessary, and follows equipment policies that support timely and safe patient care delivery. • Effectively demonstrates financial responsibility by ensuring rental equipment is returned in a timely fashion when no longer needed. • Effectively tracks arrival and departure times of rental equipment and maintains a detailed and accurate database of all rental activities.	☐	☐	☐	☐	

(Continues)

Essential Functions and Outcomes	Values and Competency Criteria	Proficiency Level				Comments
		1	2	3	4	
6. Provides direction, guidance, and support to staff members for equipment related practices and collaborates with department educator, supervisors and clinical coordinator staff members when competency related issues are identified.	• Demonstrates the ability to identify equipment related competency issues; acts appropriately to ensure patient safety and assists in educating staff members relative to competency needs. • Able to help evaluate staff members' performance, provide effective and timely feedback, and share information relative to performance strengths and weaknesses to the appropriate members of the respiratory care team.	☐	☐	☐	☐	
7. Acts as a department liaison and collaborates with others to facilitate quick resolution to issues and troubleshoot processes toward the goal of performance improvement and service excellence.	• Demonstrates the ability to work effectively in a team-based work environment applying critical thinking and problem solving skills. • Demonstrates the ability to work effectively in stressful situations involving quickly changing priorities and display appropriate leadership skills to instill trust and credibility.	☐	☐	☐	☐	
8. Stays up to date on regulatory agencies, policies, safety guidelines, and standards of care and ensures the equipment program practices comply with all outlined standards.	• Effectively represents the department on committees and action teams relative to safety and emergency preparedness initiatives. • Assists with the review, revision, and implementation of emergency related policies and procedures relative to respiratory care medical gas safety. • Demonstrates knowledge and stays current on JCAHO standards and National Patient Safety Goal information.	☐	☐	☐	☐	

Essential Functions and Outcomes	Values and Competency Criteria	Proficiency Level				Comments
		1	2	3	4	
9. Understands and participates in identifying opportunities for improvement and implementing performance improvement initiatives for the Respiratory Care Services Department and PCH.	• Able to identify system and process issues that impact work flows and the ability of staff members to provide excellent care and service. • Able to collect, interpret, and present measurement information to identify changes that result in improvements. • Effectively represents Respiratory Care on performance improvement work teams. • Acts as a change agent, displays a positive attitude, and influences staff members' understanding and acceptance of change in the work environment.	☐	☐	☐	☐	
10. Manages multiple projects and priorities, demonstrates personal responsibility for project completion through timely, clear communication and documentation of outcomes.	• Demonstrates the ability to keep track of multiple priorities and the status of projects over time. • Demonstrates the ability to effectively and efficiently manage personal work time and schedules. • Able to meet established deadlines.	☐	☐	☐	☐	
11. Stays up to date on current respiratory care practices, industry trends, national standards in pediatric/ neonatal respiratory care, literature, and equipment technology advancements that optimize patient outcomes and departmental efficiency.	• Maintains technical competence relative to respiratory care equipment procedures. • Demonstrates commitment to continuous skill improvement and development by identifying ongoing learning experiences and following through with ongoing educational opportunities.	☐	☐	☐	☐	
12. Supports and assists in the implementation of the hospital's strategic plan, mission, and values along with the departmental goals and improvement initiatives.	• Demonstrates an understanding of the hospital's strategic plan along with the department goals and improvement initiatives. • Actively participates and supports goals and initiatives. • Influences others to become involved in operational initiatives.	☐	☐	☐	☐	

Values Defined

Family Centered Care—A culture of family centered care ensures family empowerment and guides facility design, work design, program development, and policy decisions that focus on the needs of children and families first.

Leadership—By instilling confidence, loyalty, trust, and support in others, PCH team members help establish the desired culture and set the standard for child health within the organization and the community.

Innovation/excellence—A culture of innovation and excellence allows the individual and the organization to openly report, discuss, learn from, and seek optimal solutions; always striving to enhance performance and quality now and in the future.

Caring—A culture of caring recognizes and respects the differences in others and empowers team members to do the right thing at the right time to help others feel valued.

Collaboration—A culture of collaboration drives the achievement of organizational mission and goals through effective teamwork, cooperation, and exchange of information in an environment of mutual respect and trust.

Accountability—A culture in which each team member takes responsibility for his/her own actions to support and safeguard the organization's mission, vision, values, and resources.

DOCUMENT B-7: RT DEPARTMENT DIRECTOR JOB DESCRIPTION

Management Work Content Description/Performance Evaluation Form

Action Being Taken

☐ Annual Performance Evaluation	☐ New Position	☐ Position Reclassification	☐ Position Update	☐ 90 Day Review

Position Information

Employee Name:				Employee ID #:	Date:	
Job Class **MGT**	Pos Code	Position Title:	**Director, Respiratory Care**	Working Title:	Location:	Hospital
Dept. #		Dept Title:	Respiratory Care	Reports To:	Administrator, Clinical Systems and Logistics	

I. Position Purpose
Direct respiratory care operations for General Hospital and Regional Medical Center. Coordinate and facilitate patient services with Home Care Services. Lead and participate in scholarly activity to advance the knowledge of respiratory care practice. Assure emergency systems are in place within the facility to support patient needs.

II. Major Responsibilities, Activities, And End Results

% of Time	Essential Functions	Responsibilities and Accountabilities	Outcomes/ Measures	Rating 1, 2, or 3	Comments
25%	1. Develop and implement systems and policies that provide for the delivery of quality respiratory care services.	• Provide infrastructure for quality respiratory care services to patients and families. • Provide systems that are responsive to patient and family expectations. • Develop and/or use internal systems to leverage, collect, and respond to data and trends affecting patients and families. • Provide readily visible data identifying key performance measures and actions taken to continuously improve. • Assure that policies are current. • Assure that staff participate on intra-department and inter-department improvement teams. • Document improvement.	• Services to patients and families are: • Timely • Effective • Efficient • Equitable • Safe • Patient centered • As evidenced by family satisfaction surveys and defined metrics • Patient privacy and confidential information is strictly managed		
25%	2. Recruit, develop, and retain highly engaged and competent staff.	• Meet service standards. • Provide training and development aimed at improvement opportunities. • Lead impact planning activities targeting high staff engagement. • Provide staff with leadership development that supports a succession plan.	• Gallup engagement scores demonstrate effort to further engage staff as evidenced by ratings above the 75th percentile and/or statistically significant improvement over time. • Participation rate in survey is at least 85%.		

(Continues)

II. Major Responsibilities, Activities, And End Results					
% of Time	Essential Functions	Responsibilities and Accountabilities	Outcomes/ Measures	Rating 1, 2, or 3	Comments
			• Performance reviews demonstrate customer oriented, technical, and age specific competencies. • Emergency response demonstrates safe and thorough system design. • Low voluntary staff turnover. • Diversity of staff contributes to culturally competent service provided by the division.		
20%	3. Coordinate and direct financial planning, budgeting, and procurement.	• Use activity benchmarks and demonstrate actions taken to improve performance against appropriate benchmarks. • Use evidence-based, thorough, and objective practices in assessment and recommendations for respiratory care products and equipment. • Analyze revenue or cost reduction opportunities consistently. Present and act upon. • Know, report, and act upon unfavorable budget variances.	• Effective internal controls are consistently maintained. • Annual budgets are comprehensive, accurate, and timely. • Resources are at or below the budgeted level adjusted for new services and patient volumes. • Procurement practices demonstrate competency in planning, selection, acquisition, and inventory management.		
10%	4. Develop and implement the strategic plan for the department in partnership with the medical director for respiratory care.	• Develop vision for services to be provided in alignment with the organization's vision, mission, and strategic plan. • Develop and implement plans for new services, expanded, retracted, additional, or alternative sites of service.	• Respiratory care services are well aligned with patient needs and organizational vision. • Information systems are leveraged to achieve strategic objectives. • Staff articulate aligned goals and service expectations.		

II. Major Responsibilities, Activities, And End Results

% of Time	Essential Functions	Responsibilities and Accountabilities	Outcomes/ Measures	Rating 1, 2, or 3	Comments
		• Develop and lead system integration with other services to achieve vision. • Plan, communicate, and implement department priorities aligned with the goals of the organization. • Involve department staff in strategic planning and assessment to continuously improve services. • Utilize CPI as your management system.			
10%	5. Assure compliance with regulatory requirements.	• Demonstrate regulatory and standards compliance for respiratory care practice consistently in the division. This includes, but is not limited to hospital policy, JCAHO, OSHA, CMS, WAC, DOH, CDC, and other appropriate agencies.	• External survey results and audits demonstrate compliance. • Internal feedback mechanisms such as e-FeedbackNOW, compliance audits, internal control audits, and JCAHO readiness audits all consistently represent compliance.		
10%	6. Provide leadership to organizational initiatives outside of area of primary responsibility within the institution. Participate in leadership forums within the industry.	• Participate and/or lead broad hospital initiatives. • Attend leadership meetings. • Share perspectives and practices with other leaders. • Develop appropriate relationships with colleagues throughout the organization. • Develop appropriate relationships with colleagues across the industry. • Publish scholarly work.	• Participatory leader. • Approach demonstrates CPI knowledge and continuous application. • Leading practices are adopted by others. • New practices are evaluated and implemented as appropriate. • Director is knowledgeable and can consistently speak to industry practice. • Peer reviewed journals accept scholarly submissions.		

(Continues)

II. Major Responsibilities, Activities, And End Results

% of Time	Essential Functions	Responsibilities and Accountabilities	Outcomes/ Measures	Rating 1, 2, or 3	Comments
			• Posters, presentations, and abstracts are accepted by and presented to national organizations. • All of the above are measured through formal and informal feedback from patients, families, and peers. • Direct observation. • Outcome measurements.		
100% Total	Performance Rating: (1) Needs Improvement (2) Meets Expectation (3) Exceeds Expectation				

III. CPI Leadership Competencies

Our continuous performance improvement (CPI) philosophy promotes a culture of never-ending improvement at all levels in the organization. Children's management system is designed to ensure the ultimate goal of patient and family satisfaction, based on continuous improvement in **quality, cost, delivery, safety,** and **engagement** (QCDSE). As leaders, management staff must demonstrate competency in each of these areas. The following are examples of observable behaviors and performance indicators that demonstrate the relevant CPI leadership competency. CPI competencies should be integrated with the above essential function described in Section II when evaluating an individual manager's overall performance.

Leadership Competency	Desired Qualities/Behaviors	Comments
Quality: **Customer Service** Develops and maintains systems and practices that are consistently responsive to the needs of patients, families, and coworkers.	• Where applicable, executes essential functions in a manner consistent with the practice of Family Centered Care. • Ensures employees' adherence to Children's Customer Service Standards; models these standards and holds staff accountable for similar behaviors. • Demonstrates continuous improvement in customer service indicators, such as FES scores where applicable, or other internal customer service survey scores. • Identifies customer needs and delivers quality and timely solutions to meet them. • Responds in a timely and thorough manner to customer complaints and concerns, as measured by eFeedback indicators and other customer service indicators.	

Leadership Competency	Desired Qualities/Behaviors	Comments
	• Adjusts systems as needed to deliver best possible internal and/or external customer service. • Maintains patient privacy and other work-related confidentiality; does not discuss patients, other staff members, or hospital business inappropriately or in public places.	
Cost: **Financial Stewardship** Manages organization's assets (including its human resources) and/or budget in a manner that derives maximum value from resources.	• Develops and uses work methods that reduce complexity, errors, steps, and cost. • Develops and monitors effective system of internal controls that safeguard hospital assets and accuracy of financial reporting. • Where applicable, ensures proper pricing and coding of services in compliance with federal and state regulations. • Translates financial data into useful information for decision making. • Manages department financial resources at or below budgeted FTEs and other expense categories. • Quantifies savings from waste reduction activities. • Appropriately monitors and oversees staff productivity, position control, time reporting, and adherence to all applicable federal, state, and local regulatory requirements with respect to compensation (FLSA) and benefits (FMLA/ADA).	
Delivery: **Operations Management** Provides leadership and management oversight to ensure that operational outcomes achieve measurable results in support of hospital goals and business objectives.	• Acts strategically; organizes and prioritizes resources in areas most likely to impact hospital goals/business objectives. • Manages multiple projects efficiently and in compliance with all relevant regulatory requirements. • Anticipates trends in areas of responsibility and makes recommendations to senior management to address those issues in a proactive manner. • Proactively implements operational improvements. • Makes sound decisions in a timely manner.	

(Continues)

Leadership Competency	Desired Qualities/Behaviors	Comments
	• Ensures continuous readiness for all accreditation surveys, including 100% compliance with mandatory training and certification. • Utilizes 5S tools to organize work areas; sustains progress as measured by 3rd party 5S audit. • Builds and maintains cooperative working relationships with individual, inter-disciplinary, and group stakeholders.	
Change Management Ensures that improvement objectives are achieved and are implemented in a planned, controlled, and sensitive fashion with minimal negative impact on individuals, the work team's productivity, and overall morale.	• Implements strategies to align departmental operations and activities with changing hospital goals and initiatives. • Mobilizes energy and commitment to change by communicating rationale, vision, progress, and results. • Monitors and adjusts strategies in response to problems in the change process. • Understands and responds appropriately to employees' reactions to change.	
Safety: Continuously improves patient and staff safety within areas of responsibility, and as applicable, ensures all staff in area of responsibility understands and complies with all National Patient Safety Goals.	• Provides leadership and support for safe work environment, including compliance with all regulatory requirements and hospital policies for employee safety. • Staff is trained to perform duties in a safe manner, and their compliance with safe work environment practices is evaluated. • Systems are introduced to reduce errors and defects in work and care delivery practices. • Patient and staff safety incidents are investigated in a timely and thorough manner. • Patient and staff safety trends are monitored, and appropriate action is initiated in response to data about risks in the environment. • Staff are provided the materials and equipment they need to perform their jobs safely, as demonstrated by continuous improvement in safety indicators such as lost time due to on the job injuries, number of safety incidents in department, etc.	

Leadership Competency	Desired Qualities/Behaviors	Comments
Engagement: **Performance Management** Develops and maintains a work environment that enables individuals and teams to fully optimize their performance toward departmental and organizational goal achievement.	• Recruits and hires qualified, engaged employees. • Actively seeks to build a diverse staff; acts in a nondiscriminatory manner in hiring, promotion, and other personnel decisions. • Ensures adequate orientation, training, and developmental opportunities. • Ensures that employees have the tools and information they need to succeed in their jobs. • Demonstrates continuous improvement in staff engagement indicators, including workplace survey scores, turnover statistics, and employee absenteeism. • Provides timely and honest confirming and corrective performance feedback. • Conducts thorough and timely performance evaluations.	
ARTful Management Personally models accountability, respect and teamwork; displays leadership attributes that stimulate employee engagement.	• Delegates appropriately to share responsibility and authority; credits others' contributions and achievements. • Rewards appropriate risk-taking by employees despite results. • Applies HR and other policies, regulatory requirements, and management practices of the hospital fairly and consistently. • Takes accountability for own decisions regardless of results. • Makes ethical choices and exhibits sound judgment. • Communicates consistently, frequently, and clearly, especially regarding organizational mission, vision, and initiatives. • Values and promotes diversity of perspective, opinion, and approach. • Facilitates conflict resolution in a positive and productive manner. • Honors and seeks to better understand individual differences based on nationality, gender, race, sexual orientation, age, etc. (i.e., is culturally competent). • Confronts problems in a timely and effective manner; does not allow uncomfortable or unproductive situations to linger in an unresolved fashion. • Assumes responsibility for own learning and career growth.	

(Continues)

IV. Work Requirement	
Education and Experience (Required minimum)	• Baccalaureate degree in respiratory care or related field • Registered (RRT) with the National Board of Respiratory Care • Licensed by the State of Washington as a Certified Respiratory Care Practitioner • Five years experience in respiratory care management • Pediatric clinical experience
Education and Experience (Preferred)	• Academic experience including peer reviewed publications • Regional or national clinical or management presentation experience • MBA, MHA, or equivalent education • Bilingual or multilingual in common patient and/or workforce second language(s)
Knowledge, Skills and Abilities Required to Perform the Essential Functions of the Work	• Leadership competencies in change management, strategic innovation, people development, and teamwork • Commitment to diversity • Knowledge and proficiency with clinical, financial, and operational information systems and systems integration • Knowledge of state and federal regulatory and accrediting agency standards and guidelines for quality management and billing compliance
	If a clinical position: • Knowledge of human growth and development to modify care to the age and development status of the patient population served • Knowledge of patient safety according to the assigned department • Ability to identify and apply planning, care, and/or intervention techniques appropriate to the physical, motor and sensory, cognitive, and psychosocial characteristics of each patient population served
Physical Requirements	• Ability to perform essential job functions with or without accommodation.

V. Requirements Checklist

☐	Age-Specific Category 2 or 3 position (position with regular or direct care contact). Age-Specific Competency Summary Form, required with performance evaluation, is attached.
☐	All required training has been completed (see child/education and development tab/guide to required training for clinical and non-clinical employees).

VI. Goal Setting/Development Plan

Specific Goals to be Achieved During Next Cycle	Plan Description and Comments (actions to be taken; resources needed; monitoring and feedback processes; time frames, etc.)
1.	
2.	

VII. Overall Performance Rating			
Overall Performance Rating:(Check one)	☐ (1) Work performance needs improvement (Performance Improvement Plan is attached)	☐ (2) Meets work expectations	☐ (3) Exceeds work expectations
Evaluator Comments:			

Employee Comments:

Manager Name (print and sign):

Date:

Employee Name (print and sign):

Date:

Glossary of Reimbursement Terminology

Caution: 400 mg of ibuprofen recommended prior to consumption.

Beneficiary	A person certified as eligible for health care services. A beneficiary may be a dependent or a subscriber.
Capitation	A fixed amount of money paid per person for covered services for a specific time; usually expressed in units of per member per month (pm/pm).
Carve-in	A generic term that refers to any of a continuum of joint efforts between clinicians and service providers; also used specifically to refer to health care delivery and financing arrangements in which all covered benefits (e.g., behavioral and general health care) are administered and funded by an integrated system.
Carve-out	A health care delivery and financing arrangement in which certain specific health care services that are covered benefits (e.g., behavioral health care) are administered and funded separately from general health care services. The carve-out is typically done through separate contracting or subcontracting for services to the special population.
Case management	A system requiring that a single individual in the provider organization is responsible for arranging and approving all devices needed under the contract embraced by employers, health authorities, and insurance companies to ensure that individuals receive appropriate, reasonable health care services.

(Continues)

Claim	A request by an individual (or his or her provider) to that individual's insurance company to pay for services obtained from a health care professional.
Consolidated Omnibus Budget Reconciliation Act (COBRA)	An act that allows workers and their families to continue their employer-sponsored health insurance for a certain amount of time after terminating employment. COBRA imposes different restrictions on individuals who leave their jobs voluntarily versus involuntarily (Department of Labor, 2002).
Consumer	Any individual who does or could receive health care or services. Includes other more specialized terms, such as beneficiary, client, customer, eligible member, recipient, or patient.
Continuous quality improvement (CQI)	An approach to health care quality management borrowed from the manufacturing sector. It builds on traditional quality assurance methods by putting in place a management structure that continuously gathers and assesses data that are then used to improve performance and design more efficient systems of care. Also known as total quality management (TQM).
Cost-sharing	A health insurance policy provision that requires the insured party to pay a portion of the costs of covered services. Deductibles, coinsurance, and co-payment are types of cost sharing.
Creditable coverage	Any prior health insurance coverage that a person has received. Creditable coverage is used to decrease exclusion periods for preexisting conditions when an individual switches insurance plans. Insurers cannot exclude coverage of preexisting conditions, but may impose an exclusion period (no more than 12 months) before covering such conditions (Department of Labor, 2002). (See also Health Insurance Portability and Accountability Act.)
Deductible	The amount an individual must pay for health care expenses before insurance (or a self-insured company) begins to pay its contract share. Often insurance plans are based on yearly deductible amounts.

Drug formulary	The list of prescription drugs for which a particular employer or State Medicaid program will pay. Formularies are either "closed," including only certain drugs or "open," including all drugs. Both types of formularies typically impose a cost scale requiring consumers to pay more for certain brands or types of drugs.
Emergency Medical Treatment and Labor Act (EMTALA), also referred to as the Federal Anti-patient Dumping Law	An act pertaining to emergency medical situations. EMTALA requires hospitals to provide emergency treatment to individuals, regardless of insurance status and ability to pay (EMTALA, 2002).
Employee assistance plan (EAP)	Resources provided by employers either as part of, or separate from, employer-sponsored health plans. EAPs typically provide preventive care measures, various health care screenings, and/or wellness activities (Center for Mental Health Services, 2000).
Employment Retirement Income Security Act (ERISA)	Health plans that are self-insured are exempt from state regulation under this 1974 act.
Enrollee	A person eligible for services from a managed care plan.
Enrollment	The total number of covered people in a health plan. Also refers to the process by which a health plan enrolls groups and individuals for membership or the number of enrollees who sign up in any one group.
Fee for service	A type of health care plan under which health care providers are paid for individual medical services rendered.
Gatekeeper	Primary care physician or local agency responsible for coordinating and managing the health care needs of members. Generally, for specialty services such as mental health and hospital care to be covered, the gatekeeper must first approve the referral.

(Continues)

Group-model Health Maintenance Organization (HMO)	A health care model involving contracts with physicians organized as a partnership, professional corporation, or other association. The health plan compensates the medical group for contracted services at a negotiated rate, and that group is responsible for compensating its physicians and contracting with hospitals for care of their patients.
Health Employer Data and Information Set (HEDIS)	A set of HMO performance measures that are maintained by the National Committee for Quality Assurance. HEDIS data is collected annually and provides an informational resource for the public on issues of health plan quality (National Committee for Quality Assurance, 2002).
Health Insurance Portability and Accountability Act (HIPAA)	This 1996 act provides protections for consumers in group health insurance plans. HIPAA prevents health plans from excluding health coverage of preexisting conditions and discriminating on the basis of health status (Department of Labor, 2002).
Health Maintenance Organization (HMO)	A type of managed care plan that acts as both insurer and provider of a comprehensive set of health care services to an enrolled population. Services are furnished through a network of providers.
Horizontal consolidation	When local health plans (or local hospitals) merge. This practice was popular in the late 1990s and was used to expand regional business presence (Academy for Health Services Research and Policy, 2001).
Indemnity plan	Indemnity insurance plans are an alternative to managed care plans. These plans charge consumers a set amount for coverage and reimburse (fully or partially) consumers for most medical services (Insurance Finder, 2001).
Intensive case management	Intensive community services for individuals with severe and persistent mental illness that are designed to improve planning for their service needs. Services include outreach, evaluation, and support.
Length of stay	The duration of an episode of care for a covered person. The number of days an individual stays in a hospital or inpatient facility.

Local mental health authority	Local organizational entity (usually with some statutory authority) that centrally maintains administrative, clinical, and fiscal authority for a geographically specific and organized system of health care.
Managed care	An organized system for delivering comprehensive mental health services that allows the managed care entity to determine what services will be provided to an individual in return for a prearranged financial payment. Generally managed care controls health care costs and discourages unnecessary hospitalization and overuse of specialists, and the health plan operates under contract to a payer.
Medicaid	Medicaid is a health insurance assistance program funded by Federal, State, and local monies. It is run by State guidelines and assists low-income people by paying for most medical expenses (Centers for Medicare and Medicaid Services, 2002).
Medical group practice	A number of physicians working in a systematic association with the joint use of equipment and technical personnel and with centralized administration and financial organization.
Medical review criteria	Screening criteria used by third-party payers and review organizations as the underlying basis for reviewing the quality and appropriateness of care provided to selected cases.
Medically necessary	Health insurers often specify that, to be covered, a treatment or drug must be medically necessary for the consumer. Anything that falls outside of the realm of medical necessity is usually not covered. The plan will use prior authorization and utilization management procedures to determine whether or not the term "medically necessary" is applicable (Bazelon Center for Mental Health Law, 1997).
Medicare	Medicare is a Federal insurance program serving the disabled and people over the age of 65. Most costs are paid via trust funds that beneficiaries have paid into throughout the courses of their lives; small deductibles and some co-payments are required (Centers for Medicare and Medicaid Services, 2002).

(Continues)

MediGap	MediGap plans are supplements to Medicare insurance. MediGap plans vary from state to state; standardized MediGap plans also may be known as Medicare Select plans (Centers for Medicare and Medicaid Services, 2002).
Member	Used synonymously with the terms enrollee and insured. A member is any individual or dependent who is enrolled in and covered by a managed health care plan.
Network	The system of participating providers and institutions in a managed care plan.
Network adequacy	Many states have laws defining network adequacy, the number and distribution of health care providers required to operate a health plan. Also known as provider adequacy of a network.
Outcomes	The results of a specific health care service or benefit package.
Outcomes measure	A tool to assess the impact of health services in terms of improved quality and/or longevity of life and functioning.
Outcomes research	Studies that measure the effects of care or services.
Payer	The public or private organization that is responsible for payment for health care expenses.
Performance measure	A measure that describes the health care being provided. Current performance measures indicate whether a health plan or provider has appropriately provided certain services expected to lead to desirable outcomes.
Pharmacy benefit manager (PBM)	PBMs are third party administrators of prescription drug benefits.
Point-of-service plan (POS)	A modified managed care plan under which members do not have to choose how to receive services until they need them. Members receive coverage at a reduced level if they choose to use a non-network provider.

Practice guidelines	Systematically developed statements to standardize care and to assist in practitioner and patient decisions about the appropriate health care for specific circumstances. Practice guidelines are usually developed through a process that combines scientific evidence of effectiveness with expert opinion. Practice guidelines are also referred to as clinical criteria, protocols, algorithms, review criteria, and guidelines.
Preexisting condition	A medical condition that is excluded from coverage by an insurance company because the condition was believed to exist prior to the individual obtaining a policy from the insurance company. Many insurance companies now impose waiting periods for coverage of preexisting conditions. Insurers will cover the condition after the waiting period (of no more than 12 months) has expired. (See also HIPAA.)
Preferred provider organization (PPO)	A health plan in which consumers may use any health care provider on a fee-for-service basis. Consumers will be charged more for visiting providers outside of the PPO network than for visiting providers in the network (American Association of Preferred Provider Organizations).
Primary care physician (PCP)	Physicians with the following specialties: group practice, family practice, internal medicine, obstetrics/gynecology, and pediatrics. The PCP is usually responsible for monitoring an individual's overall medical care and referring the individual to more specialized physicians for additional care.
Prior authorization	The approval a provider must obtain from an insurer or other entity before furnishing certain health services, particularly inpatient hospital care, for the service to be covered under the plan.
Quality assurance	An approach to improving the quality and appropriateness of medical care and other services. Includes a formal set of activities to review, assess, and monitor care to ensure that identified problems are addressed.

(Continues)

Report card	An accounting of the quality of services compared among providers over time. The report card grades providers on predetermined, measurable quality and outcome indicators. Generally consumers use report cards to choose a health plan or provider, while policy makers may use report card results to determine overall program effectiveness, efficiency, and financial stability.
Risk	Possibility that the revenue of the insurer will not be sufficient to cover expenditures incurred in the delivery of contractual services. A managed care provider is at risk if actual expenses exceed the payment amount.
Risk adjustment	The adjustment of premiums to compensate health plans for the risks associated with individuals who are more likely to require costly treatment. Risk adjustment takes into account the health status and risk profile of patients.
Risk sharing	Situation in which the managed care entity assumes responsibility for services for a specific group but is protected against unexpected high costs by a prearranged agreement for higher payments for those individuals who need significantly more costly services. Risk is usually shared by the managed care entity and the State.
Section 1115 Waiver	A statutory provision that allows a State to operate its system of care for Medicaid enrollees in a manner different from that proscribed by the Centers for Medicare and Medicaid Services (CMS) in an attempt to demonstrate the efficacy and cost-effectiveness of an alternative delivery system through research and evaluation.
Section 1915(b) Waiver	A statutory provision that allows a State to partially limit the choice of providers for Medicaid enrollees; for example, under the waiver, a State can limit the number of times per year that enrollees can choose to drop out of an HMO.
Single-stream funding	The consolidation of multiple sources of funding into a single stream. This is a key approach used in progressive mental health systems to ensure that "funds follow consumers."

Staff-model HMO	An HMO that directly employs, on a salaried basis, the doctors and other providers who furnish care.
State Children's Health Insurance Plan (SCHIP)	Under Title XXI of the Balanced Budget Act of 1997, the availability of health insurance for children with no insurance or for children from low-income families was expanded by the creation of SCHIP. SCHIPs operate as part of a State's Medicaid program (Centers for Medicare and Medicaid Services, 2002).
State mental health authority or agency	State government agency charged with administering and funding its State's public mental health services.
Subcapitation	An arrangement whereby a capitated health plan pays its contracted providers on a capitated basis.
Subscriber	Employment group or individual that contracts with an insurer for medical services.
Third party payer	A public or private organization that is responsible for the health care expenses of another entity.
Underwriting	The review of prospective or renewing cases to determine their risk and their potential costs.
Utilization	The level of use of a particular service over time.
Utilization management (UM)	A system of procedures designed to ensure that the services provided to a specific client at a given time are cost-effective, appropriate, and least restrictive.
Utilization review	Retrospective analysis of the patterns of service usage to determine means for optimizing the value of services provided (minimize cost and maximize effectiveness/appropriateness).
Utilization risk	The risk that actual service utilization might differ from utilization projections.
Vertical disintegration	A practice of selling off health plan subsidiaries or provider activities. Vertical disintegration was a trend in the late 1990s (Academy for Health Services Research and Health Policy, 2001).

Source: Adapted from the U.S. Department of Health and Human Services Publication Mc98-70.

Samples of Capital Budgeting Forms

DOCUMENT D-1: EXAMPLE OF A MASTER PROCUREMENT AGREEMENT (ALSO KNOWN AS A SALES AGREEMENT)

Master Procurement Agreement

This Master Procurement Agreement (the "Agreement"), effective as of either _____, 2007 (if a date has been inserted in this sentence) or the latest date set forth on the signature page of this Agreement (if a date has not been inserted in this sentence) (the "Effective Date") is made between St. Elsewhere Medical Center ("Hospital") and Acme Ventilator, Inc. ("Vendor").

In consideration of the mutual promises, covenants and agreements herein and for other good and valuable consideration, the receipt and sufficiency of which are hereby acknowledged, the parties, intending to be legally bound, agree as follows:

1. **SCHEDULES AND APPENDICES.** This Agreement will include a different *Schedule* for each distinct Purchase Order that Hospital elects to issue hereunder. The first Purchase Order will be subject to *Schedule 1*, and if there are subsequent purchases, each subsequent Purchase Order will be subject to separate *Schedules* (i.e., *Schedule 2*, *Schedule 3*, etc.). Each separate *Schedule* will contain *Appendices A* and *B*:
   1.1 *Appendix A*—Products and Fees
   1.2 *Appendix B*—Documentation

2. **DEFINITIONS.**
   2.1 "**Accept**" or "**Acceptance**" means the acceptance of the Products by Hospital under the terms of this Agreement.
   2.2 "**Affiliate**" means an entity that is controlled by or is under common control with Hospital.

2.3 "**Defect**" means any failure of the Products, in whole or in part, to: (i) operate in accordance with and fully conform to the Documentation and as represented to Hospital; (ii) be free from defects in workmanship and material.

2.4 "**Documentation**" means: (i) the specifications set forth in *Appendix B* of the applicable *Schedule*; (ii) any other documentation made available by Vendor, whether in printed or electronic form, that describes the operation, functionality, or performance of the Products, including without limitation user manuals, operator instructions, training materials, interface capabilities and requirements, and customization capabilities and requirements; (iii) all correspondence from Vendor to Hospital describing the operation, functionality or performance of the Products; and (iv) any proposals, bids, quotes, and written responses to any request for proposal or quote regarding the Products, provided by Vendor to Hospital.

2.5 "**Equipment**" means Products that are not Software, that are set forth in *Appendix A* of the applicable *Schedule*.

2.6 "**Fee(s)**" means the fees for Equipment, and the license fees for Software, that are set forth on *Appendix A* of the applicable *Schedule*.

2.7 "**Intellectual Property Rights**" means any rights in any jurisdiction in the world under any patents (including any application, registration, extension, reexamination, reissue, continuation, or renewal patents, and any enhancements or improvements thereto), utility models, copyrights (including any applications, registrations or renewals thereof), mask work rights, trade secrets, trademarks (including any applications, registrations and the goodwill associated therewith), moral rights, or foreign equivalents of the foregoing, and any other proprietary rights of any nature.

2.8 "**Marks**" means logos, brands or other trademarks or service marks.

2.9 "**Material Breach**" will have the meaning set forth in Section 3 (TERM AND TERMINATION) of this Agreement.

2.10 "**Notice**" means any notice or demand, which under the terms of this Agreement or under any statute, must be given or made by Vendor or Hospital, and which is given by one party to the other in writing.

2.11 "**Products**" means the Equipment and Software.

2.12 "**Software**" means any computer software technology (and associated documentation) that is set forth in *Appendix A* of the applicable

Schedule and as described in the Documentation, including without limitation all Updates, all Upgrades, and all enhancements, modifications, and corrections to Defects performed or supplied by Vendor thereto, whether owned by Vendor or licensed to Vendor by a third-party which has authorized Vendor to sublicense such computer programs.

2.13 **"Updates"** means any minor enhancements, modifications, bug patches, fixes, or the like, to the Products (e.g., from version 1.1.a to version 1.1.b, or from version 1.1 to version 1.2).

2.14 **"Upgrades"** means any major version releases to the Products with materially enhanced and/or additional functionality and/or new features (e.g., from release 1.0 to release 2.0).

3. TERM AND TERMINATION.

3.1 Term. The term of this Agreement will commence on the Effective Date and will terminate pursuant to this Section.

3.2 Termination for Cause

a. Either Hospital or Vendor may terminate this Agreement upon the other party's Material Breach of this Agreement, provided that the party intending to terminate: (i) provides Notice to the other party describing the Material Breach in reasonable detail and demanding that it be cured; (ii) the party who receives such Notice does not cure the Material Breach within 30 days following its receipt of such Notice; and (iii) following the expiration of the thirty-day cure period, the party intending to terminate sends a second Notice to the other party indicating that this Agreement is terminated. The following will be considered a "Material Breach" of this Agreement:

  i. the execution of any assignment for the benefit of creditors or the filing for relief by either party under any applicable bankruptcy, reorganization, or similar debtor relief laws;

  ii. the appointment of a receiver for Vendor or Hospital, or for substantially all of their respective assets or properties;

  iii. the failure of either party to perform or observe any material term or condition to be performed by it under this Agreement; or

  iv. an unauthorized assignment of this Agreement.

b. Hospital may terminate any *Schedule* for cause without liability or cost if it does not Accept the Products under the *Schedule* pursuant to Section 7 (ACCEPTANCE).

3.3 Termination for Convenience. Hospital may terminate this Agreement at any time for any reason upon 30 days Notice to Vendor.

4. ORDERING AND DELIVERY.

4.1 Purchase Orders. Hospital will place orders for Products under this Agreement by executing a *Schedule* (or a series of *Schedules*, as appropriate) as set forth in Section 1, and issuing a purchase order (a "P.O.") (or a series of P.O.(s), as appropriate) to Vendor, pursuant to such *Schedule(s)*.

4.2 Delivery. Delivery will be F.O.B. Destination, Hospital's receiving dock (unless a different location is specified in the P.O. or applicable *Schedule*). Vendor will deliver the Products described in the P.O. or applicable *Schedule* in the manner and to the location specified in the P.O. or applicable *Schedule*. To the extent being transferred pursuant to this Agreement, title to the Products and risk of loss or damage thereto will pass to Hospital only upon Hospital's receipt of the Products at its receiving dock. If Vendor fails, for any reason, to deliver Products within five days of the delivery date set forth in the P.O. or applicable *Schedule*, Hospital may cancel and terminate the applicable P.O. and applicable *Schedule* without penalty and receive a full refund for all amounts prepaid hereunder.

5. PURCHASE AND LICENSE TERMS, AND INTELLECTUAL PROPERTY RIGHTS.

5.1 Equipment. Vendor agrees to sell to Hospital, and Hospital agrees to purchase from Vendor, the Equipment set forth in *Appendix A* of the applicable *Schedule*.

5.2 License Grant for the Software or other Intellectual Property Rights. If any Products include any Software or other Intellectual Property Rights, Vendor hereby grants to Hospital, its Affiliates, employees and agents a non-exclusive, worldwide, perpetual, irrevocable, transferable, royalty-free, fully-paid license, under the Intellectual Property Rights of Vendor, to install, copy, modify, test and use the Software and derivative works thereof, on computer equipment used by Hospital, its Affiliates, employees and agents. The foregoing license grant includes a license under any current and future patents owned or licensable by Vendor to the extent necessary (i) to exercise any license right granted herein, and (ii) to combine the Products or derivative works thereof with any hardware and software.

5.3 **Ownership Rights in the Software.** The Software is protected by copyright owned by Vendor. Hospital acknowledges that the license grant hereunder gives Hospital the right to use the Software but does not give Hospital any ownership of the Software, and Hospital will not reverse engineer or decompile the Software.

5.4 **Hospital Information and Materials.** All information or materials provided to Vendor by Hospital, or to which Vendor may gain access in connection with this Agreement (including without limitation goods, products, equipment, hardware, software, materials, texts, drawings, specifications, designs, algorithms, data and other recorded information, know-how, ideas, concepts, techniques, processes, procedures, methods, and tools, Hospital confidential information and trade secrets, provided by Hospital or its suppliers to Vendor for purposes of Vendor performing under this Agreement, on any media whatsoever) will remain solely and exclusively owned by Hospital, and Vendor is granted no rights whatsoever with respect thereto except the limited right to use it solely as necessary to perform its obligations to Hospital under this Agreement.

6. **FEES AND PAYMENT.** Subject to Vendor performing its obligations under this Agreement, Hospital will pay all of Fees (and any other fees) in accordance with the terms of this Agreement, and *Appendix A* of the applicable *Schedule*. No other costs, expenses, charges, fees or allocations of any kind whatsoever will be included in (or calculated as part of) any Fees. Travel expenses that are reasonable and necessary, and any other special or unusual expenses actually incurred (without markup) must be pre-approved in writing by Hospital, or Hospital will not be obligated to reimburse Vendor. Hospital will pay all correct invoices in full, or portions thereof which are not subject to a good faith dispute, within 30 days of receipt.

7. ACCEPTANCE.

7.1 Testing. Hospital will have the right to review and test the Products for 45 days after first patient use.

7.2 Acceptance or Rejection. Hospital will Accept the Products if they have no Defects during the initial Acceptance test period. If the Products have any Defects during the Acceptance test period, Hospital may reject the Products, and will provide Vendor with Notice setting forth in reasonable detail the specific aspects of the Products that contain Defects. Vendor will have 30 days from such Notice, at Vendor's sole cost, to cure the Defects and resubmit the Products to Hospital for a subsequent **[30]** day Acceptance test period.

7.3 Remedies. If Vendor fails to resubmit to Hospital the Products without Defects within such **[30]** day period, Hospital will have the right, at its sole option, to either: (i) extend the cure period for a duration to be set by Hospital; (ii) cancel the applicable P.O.(s) under which the Products were ordered, and terminate the applicable *Schedule(s)* for the Products, with no cost or liability to Hospital whatsoever, and Vendor will refund all Fees and other consideration previously provided to Vendor under the applicable P.O.(s) and *Schedule(s)*; (iii) retain just those Products under the applicable P.O.(s) and *Schedule(s)* that contain no Defects, and pay Vendor a lesser amount if such amount can be mutually agreed by Vendor and Hospital (and so long as Vendor agrees that the Products retained will be subject to the same warranties as they otherwise would have been if all Products had been Accepted); or (iv) retain all of the Products under the applicable P.O.(s) and *Schedule(s)* and pay Vendor a lesser amount due to such Defects, if such amount can be mutually agreed by Vendor and Hospital (and so long as Vendor agrees that the Products as retained will be subject to the same warranties as they otherwise would have been if it had been Accepted).

7.4 Deemed Acceptance. If Hospital fails to either Accept or reject the Products in writing within the initial or subsequent Acceptance test period (as applicable), then the Products will be deemed Accepted.

8. REPRESENTATIONS AND WARRANTIES.

8.1 Products Representations and Warranties.

    a. Vendor represents and warrants that for a period of 12 months following Acceptance, the hardware components of the Products will not have any Defects, and for a period of 24 months following Acceptance, all electrode and cable components of the Products will not have any Defects.

b. Vendor represents and warrants that the Products will not contain, as a result of Vendor's actions or inaction, any undisclosed software code, mechanisms, techniques, or devices (including without limitation viruses, worms, and software locks) intended to either now or in the future: (i) disrupt or prevent the Products from performing fully in accordance with the Documentation, or interfere in any manner with the license grants made to Hospital in this Agreement; (ii) alter, damage, destroy, or render inaccessible any data, software code, firmware, hardware, or the Products themselves; or (iii) intercept, mine, audit or expropriate any software code or data.

c. Vendor represents and warrants that neither the Products, the related documentation, nor the exercise by Hospital of its rights hereunder with respect thereto, in whole or in part, whether alone or in combination with other products and services of Hospital, will infringe or misappropriate any Intellectual Property Right or license of any person or entity.

d. Vendor represents and warrants that it has full authority and sufficient right, title, and interest in and to the Products to grant and convey the rights accorded to Hospital under this Agreement, and that for any part of the Products for which Vendor does not solely own all Intellectual Property Rights, Vendor has full right, power and authority to license such parts of the Products to Hospital as provided in this Agreement.

e. To the extent that Vendor is conveying ownership rights from Vendor to Hospital for any aspect of any Products, Vendor represents and warrants that the Products have been and will be created by employees of Vendor within the scope of their employment under obligation to assign inventions to Vendor, or by independent contractors under written obligations to assign all rights in the Products to Vendor.

8.2 General Representations and Warranties.

a. Vendor represents and warrants that in performing its obligations under this Agreement it and its employees and agents will: (i) adhere to the highest ethical and business standards; (ii) have all necessary training, skills, tools, and equipment; and (iii) perform all obligations under this Agreement in a timely, professional, and high quality manner, as required under any *Schedule*, and in accordance with applicable professional standards, if any.

b. Vendor represents and warrants that Vendor, in the performance of its obligations under this Agreement, and the Products and their use as contemplated by this Agreement, will comply with all applicable laws, ordinances, regulations and orders.

c. Vendor represents and warrants that Vendor's execution of and performance under this Agreement will not violate any employment, nondisclosure, confidentiality, consulting or other agreement to which Vendor is a party or by which it may be bound.

d. Vendor represents and warrants that: (i) no litigation proceeding (mediation, arbitration, court, administrative or otherwise), investigation, or controversy related to Vendor or the Products and that would jeopardize Vendor's ability to perform its obligations to Hospital under this Agreement, is pending before any mediator, arbitrator, court or governmental agency; (ii) to the best of Vendor's knowledge, no such mediation, arbitration, litigation, proceeding, investigation, or controversy is threatened or anticipated; (iii) Vendor is not in default with respect to any judgment, order, writ, injunction, or decree of any court or governmental agency related to the Products; and (iv) there are no unsatisfied judgments against Vendor related to the Products.

e. Vendor represents and warrants that the information that has been furnished by Vendor to Hospital in connection with the transactions contemplated under this Agreement does not include any untrue statement of a material fact and does not omit to state any material fact necessary to make the statements therein not misleading.

8.3 Remedies. If any Products do not comply with the warranties in this Section, Vendor will promptly repair or replace the Products at no cost to Hospital.

a. If within 30 days of receipt of Notice from Hospital Vendor has not repaired or replaced, in a manner acceptable to Hospital, any hardware components of the Products so that they comply with the warranties in this Section, then for each day after the 30th day, Vendor will extend the warranty period for such hardware components of the Products for an additional week. If within six weeks of receipt of Notice from Hospital Vendor has not repaired or replaced, in a manner acceptable to Hospital, any hardware components of the Products so that they comply with the warranties in this Section, then Hospital may at its sole option return to Vendor the Products with Defects in the hardware components, with no cost or liability to Hospital whatsoever, and Vendor will refund all Fees and other consideration previously provided to Vendor for such Products.

   b. If within 14 days of receipt of Notice from Hospital Vendor has not repaired or replaced, in a manner acceptable to Hospital, any electrode or cable components of the Products so that they comply with the warranties in this Section, then for each day after the 14th day, Vendor will extend the warranty period for such electrode or cable components of the Products for an additional week. If within six weeks of receipt of Notice from Hospital Vendor has not repaired or replaced, in a manner acceptable to Hospital, any electrode or cable components of the Products so that they comply with the warranties in this Section, then Hospital may at its sole option return to Vendor the Products with Defects in the electrode or cable components, with no cost or liability to Hospital whatsoever, and Vendor will refund all Fees and other consideration previously provided to Vendor for such Products.

9. MARKS.

   9.1 Use of Marks. Hospital agrees not to publish or use any advertising, sales promotions, press releases or other publicity matters relating to this Agreement, or where the name or Marks of Hospital or any of its Affiliates is mentioned, without Hospital's prior written approval after Vendor has submitted to Hospital for review copies of such advertising, sales promotion, press releases or other publicity matters.

   9.2 Rights in Marks. The Marks of either party will remain the exclusive property of that party and the other party has and will have no right to such Marks. All use of the Marks of either party will be deemed to inure only to the benefit of the owner of such Mark. Neither party without the express written consent of the other party will have the right to use any of the other party's Marks.

10. **VENDOR RESPONSIBILITY.** All services performed by Vendor's employees will be performed under the general direction, supervision and control of Vendor. Vendor will select, train and assign to Hospital employees of Vendor who, in Vendor's judgment, are best qualified to perform services required under this Agreement. Vendor agrees that it will be solely responsible for: (a) the conduct of its employees, agents, and subcontractors in the performance of Vendor's obligations under this Agreement; (b) complying with all federal, state and local laws governing access to, and use, of information obtained through general background checks obtained for Vendor's employees; and (c) any loss of, or damage to, other than ordinary wear and tear, Hospital's property in Vendor's possession or control. If there is any such loss or damage, Vendor will pay Hospital the full current replacement cost of such property within 30 days after Hospital has been made aware of the loss or damage.

11. **INDEMNIFICATION.**

    11.1 Vendor Indemnification Obligations. Vendor will defend, indemnify and hold harmless Hospital, its Affiliates, and their respective directors, officers, employees, agents, successors and assigns from and against any and all losses, costs, damages, expenses, liabilities, liens, taxes, demands, claims, arbitrations, lawsuits, and any other legal actions (including without limitation interest, penalties, and reasonable consultant, attorney and other legal fees incurred in connection with any of the foregoing) that may be asserted against, incurred or suffered by, imposed on, or awarded against any of them arising out of or in connection with, in whole or in part:

    a. any allegation, threat, demand or claim that the Products, or the related documentation, or the exercise by Hospital of its rights hereunder with respect thereto, in whole or in part, whether alone or in combination with other products and services of Hospital, infringes or misappropriates any Intellectual Property Rights or license of any person or entity.

       i. If any aspect of the Products or portion thereof is in any action held to constitute infringement or misappropriation and its use is enjoined, or at Hospital's option, at any time following the assertion of a claim described in the preceding paragraph, Vendor will promptly and at its expense either: (i) procure the right for Hospital to continue using such Products or portion thereof; (ii) modify the affected Products or portions thereof as necessary to cure the infringement; or (iii) if neither option (i) or option (ii) under this Section are possible, then replace the affected Products or portion thereof with an alternative product that is functionally equivalent, complies with the Documentation, and is acceptable to Hospital.

ii. If Vendor is unable to provide Hospital with one of the forms of relief described in the preceding sentence, Vendor will refund to Hospital the total Fees and any other consideration paid to Vendor for the Products under this Agreement;

b. any negligent acts or omissions or any willful misconduct by Vendor or its employees, agents, or subcontractors, or any Defects or errors in the Products, that result in any personal injury, death, or damage to any tangible or intangible property, or loss of use thereof; and any violation of any applicable laws, ordinances, regulations or orders.

11.2 Hospital Indemnification Obligations. Hospital will defend, indemnify and hold harmless Vendor, and its respective directors, officers, employees, agents, successors and assigns from and against any and all losses, costs, damages, expenses, liabilities, liens, taxes, demands, claims, arbitrations, lawsuits, and any other legal actions (including without limitation interest, penalties, and reasonable consultant, attorney and other legal fees incurred in connection with any of the foregoing) that may be asserted against, incurred or suffered by, imposed on, or awarded against any of them arising out of or in connection with, in whole or in part, any negligent acts or omissions or any willful misconduct by Hospital or its employees, agents, or subcontractors in their use of the Products, that result in any personal injury, death, or damage to any tangible or intangible property, or loss of use thereof.

11.3 Procedures. Each party will, upon becoming aware of a written claim made against it or an indemnified party above, to which the foregoing indemnification applies, promptly notify the indemnifying party of said claim and, at its own expense, provide reasonable cooperation with indemnifying party in the indemnifying party's defense of said claim. If the indemnified party wishes, however, it may employ separate counsel and participate in the defense thereof without diminishing its indemnification rights under this Section, but the indemnified party must bear any additional costs it itself incurs through that choice of participation. If there are any claims or actions, and in the absence of an injunction or other judicial action regarding the indemnified party's obligations under this Section, then if the indemnifying party desires to settle or compromise such claims or actions and such settlement or compromise would in any manner involve any action or forbearance by the indemnified party, or its Affiliates, or their respective directors, officers, employees, agents, successors and assigns, prior to agreeing to any such settlement or compromise the indemnifying party will obtain the written consent of the indemnified party, which may be withheld in the indemnified party's sole discretion. If the indemnified party withholds such consent, the indemnifying party will not be relieved of its indemnification obligations under this Section. If any claims or actions regarding the indemnifying party's obligations under this Section are to be settled or satisfied solely by the payment of money by the indemnifying party, the indemnifying party may control such settlement or satisfaction. The indemnification obligations contained in this Agreement continue in full force and effect after the termination of this Agreement.

12. LIABILITY DISCLAIMERS AND LIMITATION OF LIABILITY.

12.1 EXCEPT FOR INDEMNIFICATION OBLIGATIONS UNDER SECTION 12 (INDEMNIFICATION), IN NO EVENT WILL EITHER PARTY BE LIABLE TO THE OTHER PARTY FOR ANY INDIRECT, SPECIAL OR CONSEQUENTIAL DAMAGES (INCLUDING WITHOUT LIMITATION LOST PROFITS) ARISING OUT OF THIS AGREEMENT, WHETHER OR NOT SUCH PARTY HAS BEEN ADVISED OF THE POSSIBILITY OF SUCH DAMAGES.

12.2 EXCEPT FOR INDEMNIFICATION OBLIGATIONS UNDER SECTION 12 (INDEMNIFICATION), IN NO EVENT WILL EITHER PARTY BE LIABLE TO THE OTHER PARTY FOR MORE THAN TWICE THE AMOUNTS PAYABLE BY HOSPITAL TO VENDOR UNDER THIS AGREEMENT.

13. INSURANCE. Prior to furnishing any Products to Hospital, Vendor will procure and maintain at Vendor's expense insurance of at least the following types of coverage and limits of liability:

13.1 Comprehensive Commercial General Liability Insurance. This must include coverage for premises, operations, independent contractors, personal injury, broad form property damage, products and completed operations, and liability assumed under contract, including tort liability of another assumed in a business contract, annual limits of at least $3,000,000 per occurrence and in the aggregate.

13.2 Primary Coverage. All coverages must be maintained without interruption from the effective date of the Contract until the date of termination of the Contract. The insurance policies providing such coverage will specifically refer to, and provide insurance coverage for Vendor's indemnity obligations under the Contract. If Vendor carries limits in excess of the limits required in the Contract, the additional limits will be made available to Hospital as though those excess limits were required in the Contract. The insuring company must be reputable, admitted to do business in Washington State, and have a rating by A.M. Best of at least A-VII.

14. MISCELLANEOUS PROVISIONS.

14.1 Amendment or Modification. This Agreement will not be modified, either by amendment, waiver or discharge of any provision of this Agreement, except by a written agreement which specifically identifies this Agreement and the provision intended to be amended, is dated subsequent to the date of this Agreement, and is signed on behalf of a duly authorized representative of Vendor and Hospital. Each such amendment, waiver or discharge will be effective only in the specific instance and for the specific purpose for which given.

14.2 Applicable Law and Venue. This Agreement will be governed by and construed in accordance with the laws of the State of _____ without regard to any rules governing conflicts of laws. The parties agree that Bloom County in the State of Ohio will be the exclusive venue for any action brought under the Agreement, and Vendor consents to jurisdiction and venue in the state and federal courts sitting in _____ County, State of _____. Vendor agrees to waive all defenses of lack of personal jurisdiction and forum non conveniens.

14.3 Assignment and Subcontracting. Vendor may not assign or subcontract its rights or delegate its duties hereunder, in whole or in part, directly or indirectly, by merger or sale of stock or assets, or by any other form of transfer whether by operation of law or otherwise, without Hospital's prior written consent. Hospital may assign its rights or delegate its duties hereunder to: (i) any corporation resulting from any merger, consolidation or other reorganization to which Hospital is a party; (ii) any corporation, partnership, association or other entity or person to which Hospital may transfer all or substantially all of the assets and business of Hospital existing at such time; or (iii) any Affiliate of Hospital. All the terms and provisions of this Agreement will be binding upon and inure to the benefit of and be enforceable by the parties hereto and their respective successors and permitted assigns. Any attempted assignment or transfer in contravention of this Section will be null and void.

14.4 Bankruptcy. Vendor agrees that a failure by Hospital to assert its rights to "retain its benefits" to any of the Intellectual Property Rights that are part of the Products, pursuant to Sec. 365(n)(1)(B) of the Bankruptcy Code, 11 U.S.C., under an executory contract rejected by the trustee in bankruptcy, will not be construed by the courts as a termination of the Agreement by Hospital under Sec. 365(n)(1)(A) of the Bankruptcy Code.

14.5 Delays and Waiver. No delay or failure of either party at any time to exercise or enforce any right or remedy available to it under this Agreement, and no course of dealing or performance with respect thereto, will constitute a waiver of any such right or remedy with respect to any other breach or failure by the other party. The express waiver by a party of any right or remedy in a particular instance will not constitute a waiver of any such right or remedy in any other instance.

14.6 Dispute Resolution. Vendor and Hospital will attempt to settle any claim or controversy between them through consultation and negotiation in good faith and with a spirit of mutual cooperation. After attempts to resolve a dispute by Vendor and Hospital have failed, either party may, upon Notice to the other, request that such controversy or claim be referred to the appropriate management personnel of each party for negotiation and resolution. If such a request is made, the applicable and appropriate management-level personnel of the parties will meet in person or by telephone within seven days after such request and will review and attempt to negotiate a mutually acceptable resolution of the controversy or claim in dispute.

14.7 Entire Agreement. This Agreement and all of its *Appendices, Schedules,* and P.O.(s) (incorporated herein by this reference) constitute the entire agreement between Hospital and Vendor with respect to their subject matters, and all prior or contemporaneous oral or written communications, understandings or agreements between Hospital and Vendor with respect to such subject matters are hereby superseded in their entireties.

14.8 Force Majeure. If the performance by a party of any of its obligations under this Agreement are interfered with by reason of any unforeseeable circumstances beyond the reasonable control of that party, including without limitation, fire, explosion, acts of God, war, terrorism, revolution, or civil commotion, then that party will be excused from such performance for a period equal to the delay resulting from the applicable circumstances and such additional period as may be reasonably necessary to allow that party to resume its performance.

14.9 Headings. All headings used herein are for index and reference purposes only, and will not be given any substantive effect.

14.10 Legal Fees, Costs, and Expenses. In any dispute or legal proceedings (whether for damages and/or equitable relief) arising out of or related to this Agreement, the substantially prevailing party will be entitled to recover from the other party its reasonable legal fees, costs, and related expenses, including through appeal or arbitration. In connection therewith, the court or arbitrator will be entitled to exercise its reasonable discretion to determine which party should be deemed the "substantially prevailing party" based on the nature of any claims, counterclaims or other demands asserted, the amount or amounts demanded thereon and the nature and amount of the relief, judgment or award granted. For purposes of this Section, the services of in-house attorneys and their staff will be valued at rates for independent counsel prevailing in the metropolitan area in which such counsel and staff practice.

14.11 Notices. Any Notice given under this Agreement must be in writing and will be effective when addressed to the representatives set forth below upon either: (i) receipt if delivered in person or by facsimile; (ii) three days after deposit prepaid for overnight delivery with a national overnight express delivery service; or (iii) six days after deposit in the United States Postal Service that is registered or certified mail, postage prepaid, return receipt requested. Notices must be provided to the following representatives at the addresses below listed:

| **St. Elsewhere Medical Center** |
| Attn:
 (Insert Department Directors Name)

 Fax: |
| With a copy to:

 A. Einstein
 St. Elsewhere Medical Center
 Chief Technology Counsel &
 Dir. of Technology Acquisition
 10 North Downing Street
 Bismarck , ND
 Fax: 123-456-7890

 W. E. Kaiyote
 Acme Ventilator Company
 100 North Dallas Forty
 Irvine TX
 Fax: 321-7654-098 |

The above addresses may be changed at any time by giving prior Notice as above provided.

14.12 Relationship of the Parties. The provisions of this Agreement will not be construed to establish any form of partnership, agency or other joint venture of any kind between Vendor and Hospital, nor to constitute either party as the agent, employee or legal representative of the other. All persons furnished by either party to accomplish the intent of this Agreement will be considered solely as the furnishing party's employees or agents and the furnishing party will be solely responsible for compliance with all laws, rules and regulations involving, but not limited to, employment of labor, hours of labor, working conditions, workers' compensation, payment of wages, and withholding and payment of applicable taxes, including, but not limited to income taxes, unemployment taxes, and social security taxes.

14.13 **Remedies.** Unless and only to the extent expressly set forth to the contrary in this Agreement, no remedy conferred by any of the specific provisions of this Agreement is intended to be exclusive of any other remedy, and each and every remedy will be cumulative and will be in addition to every other remedy given hereunder, now or hereafter existing at law in equity or otherwise. The election of any one or more remedies by either party will not constitute a waiver of the right to pursue other available remedies.

14.14 **Severable Provisions.** If any provision in this Agreement is found to be illegal, invalid or unenforceable in any jurisdiction, for any reason, then, to the full extent permitted by law: (i) all other provisions will remain in full force and effect in such jurisdiction and will be liberally construed in order to carry out the intent of the parties hereto as nearly as possible; (ii) such invalidity, illegality or unenforceability will not affect the validity, legality or enforceability of any other such provisions hereof; and (iii) any court or arbitrator having jurisdiction thereover will have the power to reform such provisions to the extent necessary for such provision to be enforceable under applicable law.

14.15 **Survival.** The terms and conditions within the Sections of this Agreement entitled "PURCHASE AND LICENSE TERMS, AND INTELLECTUAL PROPERTY RIGHTS," "USE OF MARKS," "INDEMNIFICATION," and "LIABILITY DISCLAIMERS AND LIMITATION OF LIABILITY," together with all other provisions of this Agreement that may reasonably be interpreted or construed as surviving termination, will survive termination of this Agreement.

IN WITNESS WHEREOF, the parties hereto have executed this Agreement as of the Effective Date.

St. Elsewhere Medical Center   **Acme Ventilator Inc.**

Signature: _____   Signature: _____

Printed Name: _____   Printed Name: _____

Title: _____   Title: _____

Date: _____   Date: _____

Schedule 1
Appendix A
Products & Fees

PAYMENT SCHEDULE. Vendor will invoice Hospital for the Fees according to the following *Schedule*:

Upon execution of this Agreement:	15% of the total software Equipment and/or License Fees
Upon successful installation/ implementation of the Products:	55% of the total software Equipment and/or License Fees
Upon Acceptance of the Products:	30% of the total software Equipment and/or License Fees

DOCUMENT D-2: EXAMPLE OF A CAPITAL BUDGET QUESTIONNAIRE

ACME Medical Center Capital Equipment Process

CAPITAL PURCHASE QUESTIONNAIRE

Required for Items/Purchases of $25,000 and Up

Department		Phone	
Date Submitted		E-Mail	
Prepared By		Fax	

Select One:

Select One:

	Medical Equipment		New
	Information Technology		Replacement/Upgrade
	Facility/Renovation		Regulatory Requirement
	Non-Medical		Recruitment

Note: If "Regulatory Requirement" explain compliance issues in Section #1 below.

1. EQUIPMENT DESCRIPTION

Equipment Name	
Description of Function	

2. LIST THREE AVAILABLE MANUFACTURER ALTERNATIVES FOR THIS EQUIPMENT, PREFERRED MANUFACTURER FIRST

Manufacturer	Model	Cost	Qty	Shipping Cost	Cost Total	Install Cost

3. BUILDING/ROOM WHERE EQUIPMENT WILL BE LOCATED

4. SITE PREPARATION REQUIREMENTS: Check YES/NO as appropriate.

	YES	NO
Requires emergency power?		
Requires building modifications?		
Requires water, drainage, or steam?		
Requires gas, air, oxygen, or vacuum?		
Emits radiation, microwaves, laser, radio waves, or has radioactive components?		
Weight of equipment may require facility modification?		
Size may not be able to move through existing hallways/doorways/elevators.		
Requires special cooling, heating or ventilation?		
Requires installation: vendor or in-house?		
Additional services required? If so, please identify:		

5. HOSPITAL AND DEPARTMENTAL GOALS:

Please describe how this equipment purchase will support the hospital's or department goals:

6. EQUIPMENT EFFICIENCIES

Please explain any efficiency that will be gained with this piece of equipment (e.g., staff time):

7. SUPPORT DEPARTMENT REVIEWS

Biomedical or Building Engineering Support
1. Who will support the equipment?
2. Indicate cost if supplied by vendor: Annual Service Contract Cost: Training Cost for Acme's Biomedical and/or Building Engineering staff: Test/Support Equipment:
Information Services Support
1. Will Information Services connections/interfaces be required? If yes, please explain:
2. Indicate cost of the following (if required): Annual Service Contract Cost: Training Cost for the information technology staff: Test/Support Equipment:

8. FINANCIAL CONSIDERATIONS

- Describe the ANNUAL cost and revenue impact of the acquisition of this equipment.
- Year 0 numbers should reflect the IMMEDIATE cost impact of the acquisition.
- Year 1–3 numbers should reflect the ONGOING operational impact of the acquisition.
- *COSTS* refers to INCREMENTAL expense increases related to this acquisition.
- *REVENUES* refers to INCREMENTAL revenue increases related to this acquisition.

	Year 0	Year 1	Year 2	Year 3
COSTS				
Additional FTEs (salaries and benefits)				
Supplies				
Maintenance				
Renovation and Installation				
Other, Please Specify:				
Total Costs				
COST SAVINGS				
Reduced FTEs (salaries and benefits)				
Supplies				
Maintenance				
Other, Please Specify:				
Total Cost Savings				

	Year 0	Year 1	Year 2	Year 3
REVENUES				
Additional Units of Service				
Additional Patient Revenues				
Other Additional Revenues Please Specify:				
Total Revenues				

Please identify the title, salary, and number of the proposed additional FTEs or reduced FTEs in the table below. Assume one FTE is equal to 2080 hours per year.

Title	Salary and Benefits	Number of FTEs

9. REVIEW

Reviewed with Department Director?	YES	NO	Date: _____
Reviewed with Administrator?	YES	NO	Date: _____

DOCUMENT D-3: CAPITAL EQUIPMENT PAYBACK FORM

St. Elsewhere Hospital Schedule for Capital Equipment Payback

Department Name	Respiratory Therapy							
Equipment Description	Acme Hyperpulmonastic Contiguous Logomorphic Ventilator with Flux Capacitor™							
New (N) or Replacement (R)	Brand spanking new			Acquisition Costs $181,000				
	1st Year	2nd Year	3rd Year	4th Year	5th Year	6th Year	7th Year	8th Year
Statistical units of service for item	200	250	300	300	300	325	325	350
Gross revenue produced by item	$120,000	$150,000	$180,000	$180,000	$180,000	$195,000	$195,000	$210,000
Deductions from revenue	$42,000	$52,500	$63,000	$63,000	$63,000	$68,250	$68,250	$73,500
NET REVENUE	$78,000	$97,500	$117,000	$117,000	$117,000	$126,750	$126,750	$136,500
Salaries associated with item	$35,000	$50,000	$50,000	$50,000	$50,000	$50,000	$50,000	$50,000
28%	$9,800	$14,000	$14,000	$14,000	$14,000	$14,000	$14,000	$14,000
Supplies associated with item	$5,000	$5,500	$6,000	$6,000	$6,000	$6,500	$6,500	$7,000
Maintenance costs of equipment	$1,500	$2,000	$2,000	$2,000	$2,000	$3,000	$3,000	$3,000
Other incremental direct expenses	$3,500	$4,250	$4,250	$4,250	$4,250	$4,250	$4,250	$4,250
Incremental indirect expenses	$1,500	$1,500	$1,500	$1,500	$1,500	$1,500	$1,500	$1,500
TOTAL EXPENSES	$56,300	$77,250	$77,750	$77,750	$77,750	$79,250	$79,250	$79,750
Total incremental cash flow	$21,700	$20,250	$39,250	$39,250	$39,250	$47,500	$47,500	$56,750
Discount factor 7.0%	0.935	0.873	0.817	0.764	0.714	0.668	0.624	0.584
Discounted cash flow	20,283	17,692	32,055	29,971	28,025	31,711	29,654	33,136
Cumulative Discounted cash flow		$37,975	$70,031	$100,002	$128,027	$159,738	$189,392	222,528

Notes:

Payback period—The payback period is in the seventh year of this proposal, when the cumulative discounted cash flow exceeds the original acquisition costs, which is also sometimes called the depreciation expense.

Deductions from revenue—Those contractual discounts offered voluntarily or involuntarily to payers.

Incremental indirect expenses—Typically, these are the costs of running the hospital, for example the costs of running other departments and the facilities costs that are allocated to all departments. This is usually distributed according to some mystical formulation conjured by the finance department, having something to do with the proportion of the revenue that your department will generate compared to total hospital revenue. Your safest bet is to check with finance.

Discount factor—This will be assigned by finance and will be what they estimate to be the future cost of money combined with the relative risk of your proposal. The number in these cells is obtained as follows: 1st year = $1 \div 1.07$, 2nd year = $(1 \div 1.07) \div 1.07$, 3rd year = $((1 \div 1.07) \div 1.07) \div 1.07$ and so on.

Discount cash flow—Total incremental cash flow multiplied by the discount factor. This represents the current value of the future cash flows.

Common Mistakes Made by Directors–Managers

This list is highly credible. I ought to know. I have made every one of these mistakes.

1. *Being too authoritarian*—There are times when you have to run a sort of brutal, Stalinist regime, but these are very rare indeed. Ask people politely and respectfully to do things, just the way you like to be asked. The golden rule works very well here indeed.

2. *Not being authoritarian enough*—Of course being too mealy mouthed and "Casper-Wimpy-Milk Toast" is not good either. Chester Nimitz used to say, "When you are in command . . . command." There are times when your team can be paralyzed by a lack of leadership. Sometimes you must be decisive and in command. But even in these times you should work very, very hard to be respectful and appreciative.

3. *Getting too isolated*—This is very common and hard to avoid. It is also called "officeitis." The 1980s gave us an over used, hackneyed platitude: "Management by Walking Around " (MBWA). It was over used because it represented a great truth. It seems so obvious and yet it is hard to do, hard to maintain, and not nearly as widely practiced as you might hope. It goes under many names. The latest trendy management terminology for this is "Going to Gemba" (Gemba being the Japanese word for where the work is done). I do a lot of analytical work and writing which places me in my office a lot, and sometimes I slip into the isolation. I can usually sense it and then make an effort to reconnect.

4. *Getting too close to the people who work for you*—This is a tremendous challenge for some (including me). When you work closely with people for long periods of time in emotionally charged situations, it is unavoidable that you develop emotional attachments. And if your staff are the excellent therapists that you have helped them to become, you will have respect and admiration for them. This can lead to becoming close

friends with the people you supervise. This can make it very hard for you if circumstances require you to discipline them or assign them unpleasant or difficult duties. Save yourself the trouble. Be close to your staff, but not too close. Me personally, I rarely do things with people I supervise outside of work with the exception of activities sponsored by the hospital or attendance at conferences and educational activities.

5. *Not following up*—Man oh man have I gotten in trouble so many times for not following up. You can easily be overwhelmed by the volume of details that can assault you every day in a leadership position in a hospital. Everybody I know who has ever been effective as a director–manager develops a system to help them keep track of details they need to follow up on. Some folks use notebooks to keep lists. Others festoon their offices with sticky notes. Still others use some of the advanced functions in programs like Microsoft Outlook that allow you to develop to-do lists and tasks that you need to schedule and keep track of. Whatever you find that works for you, find something. Develop a system. Stick with it. One method that can help is programmed time for chasing details. Block out time on your schedule that is devoted to following up on details.

6. *Lip service*—Disingenuousness is tempting. You can use it to try to manipulate people, and in the short term it might bear fruit for you. But in the long run, folks will soon figure you out. If you regularly spout a lot of stuff you don't really believe, your staff will soon realize this (they are way smarter than you might think) and eventually you will lose credibility. You will find yourself sometimes having to represent positions from the administrative suite that you don't totally agree with. My suggestion is that you find a way to philosophically align yourself with the leadership of the hospital. If you often find yourself at variance with administration, perhaps you should move on to a hospital where you and administration are more properly aligned. You know, it just might be possible that the administrators know what they are doing and have more information than you do. If you want your staff to trust you, you should consider trusting your bosses too. One of the worst things you can do is let your staff think you don't really agree with administration. "Well, I don't really agree with this, but we have to do it," ought to never cross your lips when you are talking to your staff. If you don't like some plan that has been brought forth by administration, go meet with your bosses and be frank and direct about your concerns. Tell

them you don't agree with them. Try to understand what decision drivers led them to this plan. But after you leave their offices, you are expected to represent the hospital's goals and plans to the best of your ability. Don't bad-mouth administration.

7. *Failure to have a vision*—If you want to be a real leader, you must have a vision for your team. You need to see clearly where your department is heading. You should have an agenda of your own. This is what people want. They want leaders with a vision. *Where there is no vision, the people perish. (Proverbs 29:18, King James Version.)* Devote some careful thought and considerable time to developing your vision. Share it often.

8. *Setting the bar too low*—People tend to live up or down to whatever expectations you have for them. And I believe that most people can achieve more than they thought they could. I am not suggesting some of those awful statements people make about how "you can do anything you set your mind to." This is, of course, preposterously stupid. I will never be able to slam dunk, ever. If I had obsessively devoted myself to aerobic exercise, weight lifting, diet, and anabolic steroids from the time I was 15 until I was 25 I still would never have been able to slam dunk. But I do have a respectable 18-foot set shot. You should push people. Set the bar high. Expect a lot in terms of professional development and you will almost certainly be pleasantly surprised.

9. *Not helping people to save face*—People desperately need dignity and respect. You should always keep this in mind. Indeed folks screw up and sometimes need some remedial instruction in how to keep their jobs, but this should always be done with care not to embarrass folks in front of others. I made this mistake early in my career and paid for it. Try very hard to avoid correcting subordinates in front of others. You are not in the military. If you have to correct or reprove someone, give careful thought to doing it in some way that helps them to save face.

10. *Not liking the people you work with*—Every person brings something to the equation. Admittedly some contribute significantly less than others. But you should try to avoid dwelling on the negatives people have. If you don't find something to like about the people who work for you, you will not be a very happy camper. And your staff will pick up on this. I had a director once who would occasionally sit in his office and call the therapists who worked for him a wide variety of nasty things, many of which would cause a Marine Corps drill instructor to blush. To

some degree it was part of his shtick and it made for good comedic material when us managers would sit around and complain about him. But it belied an underlying disrespect he had for the people who worked for him. And although he tried hard to cover it up when he communicated with front line staff, they picked it up.

Resources

INTERNET RESOURCES

Below is a list of Internet resources for respiratory therapists and hospital managers.

American Association for Respiratory Care: United States based professional organization promoting the interests of respiratory therapists and respiratory health. The premier site for information and resources for respiratory therapists. While you are there, join up if you are not already a member.	http://www.aarc.org
National Board for Respiratory Care: The body that issues national credentials for respiratory therapists in the United States.	http://www.nbrc.org
VentWorld: A source of ventilator product and supplier information, news, discussion, education, tools, and resources for the respiratory and critical care community. Some way cool stuff here.	http://www.ventworld.com
RC_World: The gateway to a large closed and moderated Internet forum for respiratory therapists. There are hundreds and hundreds of clinicians and managers from all over the world. This is definitely worth signing up for, although sometimes it has a low signal to noise ratio.	http://ourworld.compuserve.com/homepages/hannigan/
NICU-NET: A closed and moderated forum for issues related to neonatal intensive care.	http://www.neonatology.org/nicu-net/join.html
CCM-L: An interdisciplinary Internet forum for topics related to the practice of critical care medicine.	http://www.ccm-l.org

Peds-CCM: An interdisciplinary Internet forum for topics related to pediatric critical care. Contains an excellent list of lots of other Internet based e-mail forums.	http://pedsccm.org/Piculist.php
Bureau of Labor Statistics information on the employment of respiratory therapists in the United States.	http://www.bls.gov/oco/ocos084.htm
The Canadian Society of Respiratory Therapists for our friends to the North.	http://www.csrt.com/
RT, a trade journal for respiratory therapists.	http://www.rtmagazine.com/
RT Corner 2.0: a Web site run by respiratory therapists for respiratory therapists.	http://www.rtcorner.net/
American Association of Cardiovascular and Pulmonary Rehabilitation	http://www.aacvpr.org/
National Association for Medical Direction of Respiratory Care	http://www.namdrc.org/
Neonatal Resuscitation Program	http://www.aap.org/nrp/nrpmain.html
Joint Commission on Accreditation for Healthcare Organizations	http://www.jointcommission.org
The FOCUS Journal for Respiratory Care & Sleep Medicine: This is the best trade journal out there, and Bob Miglino and his staff put on an outstanding conference every year for respiratory and sleep professionals.	http://www.foocus.com
Oximetry.org is a Web site devoted to pulse oximetry, oxygenation monitoring, and transport.	http://www.oximetry.org
Advance for Respiratory Care Practitioners: Another trade journal with some of the best job listings in the business.	http://respiratory-care.advanceweb.com/main.aspx
American Heart Association	http://www.americanheart.org

Abstracts from respiratory care since 1995 posted on the **Cardinal Health Web** site. Every abstract since 1995 is here. This is an invaluable resource, especially if you are looking for information on testing of particular products.	http://www.cardinal.com/mps/focus/respiratory/abstracts/
Respiratory Care: The Science Journal of the American Association for Respiratory Care: The premier respiratory science journal.	http://www.rcjournal.com
European Respiratory Care Association	http://www.eurorespicare.com/links.php
Respiratory Associates of Texas: This is a respiratory staffing agency whose Web site has an excellent list of Web sites of respiratory vendors and is also a provider of continuing respiratory care education.	http://www.respiratorycareonline.com/
Virtual Naval Hospital: Not really a respiratory Web site, but so totally cool, I just had to include it. Military medicine tour de force. Remember, everything we learned about trauma came from military medicine.	http://www.vnh.org
Medical Information Systems: An online provider of continuing respiratory education.	http://www.mededsys-rcp.com
American Association for Respiratory Care continuing respiratory education Web site.	http://www.aarc.org/crce_online
University of Medicine and Dentistry of New Jersey continuing respiratory education Web site.	http://www.umdnj.edu/rspthweb/ce.htm
Department of Respiratory Care at The University of Texas Health Science Center at San Antonio respiratory continuing education Web site.	http://www.uthscsa.edu/respiratorycare/onlinece.html

University of Missouri-Columbia School of Health Professions continuing respiratory education Web site.	http://www.umshp.org/rt/crce/index.htm
The Texas Society for Respiratory Care continuing respiratory education Web site.	http://www.tsrc.org/onlinece.html
JL Enterprise: Simply the best medical software tutorials for nurses and respiratory therapists I have seen, including pulmonary graphics interpretation, congenital cardiac disease, and neonatal respiratory care. They are HTML based interactive courses with excellent animation.	http://www.jlenterprise.com/jl.html
Critical Care Medicine Tutorials: Online training in critical care topics. This was posted by a physician at University of Pennsylvania but is not officially affiliated with the school.	http://www.ccmtutorials.com/index.htm
Oregon Health Sciences University PICU mechanical ventilation simulator. Very cool. Enter settings, out pop blood gases.	http://www.ohsu.edu/academic/picu/medialab/vent/index.html
C&S Solutions: Online respiratory training software.	http://www.cssolutions.biz/

BOOKS

Here is a list of written resources that have been important in my professional life:

Management Books

- *The One Minute Manager* by Kenneth Blanchard
- *In Search of Excellence* by Thomas Peters and Robert Waterman
- *The Goal* by Eliyahu Goldratt and Jeff Cox
- *Why We Do What We Do: Understanding Self-Motivation* by Edward Deci and Richard Flaste
- *Only the Paranoid Survive* by Andrew S. Grove

- *Hardwiring Excellence: Purpose, Worthwhile Work, Making a Difference* by Quint Studer
- *Zap, The Lightening of Empowerment* by William Byham and Jeff Cox
- *The Force* by David Dorsey
- *Six Thinking Hats* by Edward de Bono
- *Seven Habits of Highly Effective People* by Stephen Covey
- *The Toyota Way* by Jeffery Liker
- *Now Discover Your Strengths* by Marcus Buckingham and Donald Clifton
- *The 100-mile Walk: A Father And Son on a Quest to Find the Essence of Leadership* by Jonathon Sander and Mechele Flaum
- *Managing the Risks of Organizational Accidents* by James Reason
- *Human Error* by James Reason
- *The Respiratory Therapist's Legal Answer Book* by Anthony Dewitt
- *To Err is Human* by The Institute of Medicine

Nonmanagement Professional Books

- *Breathing for a Living* by Laura Rothenberg
- *Risk Adjustment for Measuring Health Outcomes* by Lisa Iezzoni
- *Sorry, Wrong Number* by John Brignell
- *Zen and the Art of Motorcycle Maintenance* by Robert M. Pirsig
- *Fundamentals of Respiratory Care Research* by Robert Chatburn
- *Understanding Variation: The Key to Managing Chaos* by Donald Wheeler
- *The Dartmouth Atlas of Healthcare* by Dartmouth Medical School
- *The Man Who Mistook His Wife for a Hat* by Oliver Saks
- *Confessions of a Medical Heretic* by Robert Mendelsohn
- *Biostatistics: The Bare Essentials* by Geoffrey Norman and David Streiner
- *The Spirit Catches You and You Fall Down* by Anne Fadiman

Respiratory Therapy Clinical Books (my all time favorites)

- *Clinical Monitoring* by Carol Lake
- *History of Blood Gases, Acids and Bases* by John Severinghous and Poul Astrup
- *Monitoring in Respiratory Care* by Robert Kacmarek, Dean Hess, and James Stoller
- *Essential of Respiratory Care* by Robert Kacmarek, Craig Mack, and Steven Dimas
- *Principles and Practices of Intensive Care Monitoring* by Martin Tobin
- *Pathophysiology: The Biologic Basis for Disease in Adults and Children* by Kathryn McCance and Sue Heuther

- *Respiratory Care: Principles and Practice* by Dean Hess, et al.
- *Neonatal Respiratory Care* by Carlo Waldemar and Robert Chatburn
- *Assisted Ventilation of the Neonate* by Jay Goldsmith and Edward Karotkin
- *Handbook of Respiratory Care* by Robert Chatburn
- *Perinatal and Pediatric Respiratory Care* by Michael Cservinske and Sherry Barnhart
- *Principles and Practices of Mechanical Ventilation* by Martin Tobin
- *Ventilators: Theory and Clinical Application* by Yvon G. Dupuis
- *Respiratory Care Pharmacology* by Joseph Rau

Important Nonprofessional Books

- *One Flew Over the Cuckoo's Nest* by Ken Kesey
- *House of God* by Samuel Shem
- *Man's Search for Meaning* by Victor Frankel
- *Sand Pebbles* by Richard McKenna
- *The Book of Ecclesiastes* by King Solomon
- *Flight from Science and Reason* by Paul R. Gross, Norman Levitt, and Martin W. Lewis
- *Higher Superstition: The Academic Left and Its Quarrels with Science* by Paul R. Gross and Norman Levitt
- *Undaunted Courage* by Stephen Ambrose
- *I Claudius, & Claudius the God* by Robert Graves
- *The Tao of Pooh* by Benjamin Hoff and E.H. Shepard
- *History of Western Civilization* by Will and Ariel Durant (all eleven volumes)
- *The Right Stuff* by Tom Wolfe
- *Two Years before the Mast* by Richard Henry Dana
- *Creation and Times* by Hugh Ross
- *A Brief History of Time* by Stephen Hawking
- *One Day in the Life of Ivan Denisovich* by Alexander Solzhenitsyn
- *Atlas Shrugged* by Ayn Rand
- *Stranger in a Strange Land* by Robert Heinlein
- *Longitude* by Dava Sobel
- *Freakonomics* by Steven Levitt and Stephen Dubner
- *The Quest for Cosmic Justice* by Thomas Sowell
- *Darwin's Black Box* by Michael Behe
- *Boyd* by Robert Coram

- *Reason in the Balance* by Phillip Johnson
- *Ringworld and Ringworld Engineers* by Larry Niven

ORGANIZATIONS THAT PUBLISH GUIDELINES OF CARE

- Society of Critical Care Medicine (www.sccm.org)
- American Thoracic Society (www.thoracic.org)
- American Academy of Pediatrics (www.aap.org)
- National Guideline Clearinghouse (www.guideline.gov)
- The Cochrane Collaboration (www.cochrane.org)
- Scottish Intercollegiate Guidelines Network (www.sign.ac.uk)
- Agency for Healthcare Research and Quality (www.ahrq.gov)
- National Heart, Lung, and Blood Institute (www.nhlbi.nih.gov/guidelines)
- American College of Chest Physicians (www.chestnet.org/education/guidelines)
- British National Library for Health (www.library.nhs.uk/pathways)
- Canadian Medical Association (http://mdm.ca/cpgsnew/cpgs/index.asp)
- Canadian Medical Association Journal (www.cmaj.ca/misc/service/guidelines.shtml)
- Medical Journal of Australia (www.mja.com.au/public/guides/guides.html)
- Royal Children's Hospital Melbourne (www.rch.org.au/rchcpg/index.cfm)

PEER REVIEWED JOURNALS

- *Respiratory Care*
- *Critical Care Medicine*
- *Pediatric Critical Care Medicine*
- *Chest*
- *American Journal of Respiratory and Critical Care Medicine*
- *Pediatrics*
- *Journal of Pediatrics*
- *Anesthesia*
- *Anesthesia and Analgesia*
- *Anaesthesia and Intensive Care*

- *Pediatric Pulmonology*
- *Thorax*
- *Journal of Trauma*
- *Archives of Disease in Childhood, Fetal and Neonatal Edition*
- *New England Journal of Medicine*
- *Journal of the American Medical Association*
- *Journal of Clinical Monitoring and Computing*

Documents Used in an Evaluation and Selection of Mechanical Ventilators

DOCUMENT G-1: EARLY PLANNING DOCUMENT

This document was used in the early planning stages of a ventilator evaluation, in this case a neonatal and pediatric ventilator. It represents the evaluation team's list of hoped for features and weighting factors for selecting new mechanical ventilators. The team was looking for a single device that could be used to ventilate any size patient.

Decision Modeling for Selection of Neonatal and Pediatric Mechanical Ventilators

1. This decision making process will be designed using a weighted factor model.
2. Factors will include:

Factor	Weighting
2.1. Available features	10%
2.2. Performance	25%
2.3. User interface design	20%
2.4. Maintenance	10%
2.5. Financial analysis	5%
2.6. Usable on all sized patients	30%

3. Each factor will be weighted.

   3.1. These weights will be assigned by a work group that includes neonatal and pediatric ICU respiratory therapists, physicians, and nurses.

4. Details

4.1. Available Features (factor = 10%)

Sub-Factor	Weight
Physical Features-Design	20%

- Overall size
  - Footprint
  - Mobility
  - Likelihood of tipping
  - Drawer/basket
  - Battery capability
  - Compressors
    - Costs
    - Weight
- Gas consumption
- Range of gas operating pressures-input
- Computer interface

Sub-Factor	Weight
Modes:	25%

- Volume control (limiting)
- Pressure control (limiting)
- Pressure support
- SIMV
- Assist control
- Combined modes: Ability to do volume targeted ventilation using decelerating flow profiles
  - Selection of flow profiles
  - With and without a set rate
  - Response to apnea
- Airway pressure release
- CPAP
- PEEP
- Noninvasive capabilities

Sub-Factor	Weight
Triggering capability	20%

- Flow
- Pressure
- Performance in the presence of a leak

Sub-Factor	Weight
Alarms	25%

- Overall volume and distinctiveness
- Remote
- Disconnect
- High and low airway pressure
- Minute ventilation
- F_1O_2
  - Lower limits below 0.21 for patients receiving sub-ambient oxygen therapy
- Max inspiratory time
- Apnea
- Alarm history
- High and low source gas alarms
  - Actual pressure readings
- Nuisance factors

Sub-Factor	Weight
Special gas delivery (heliox)	10%

4.2. Performance: Bench Testing Results (factor = 25%)

Sub-Factor	Weight
Accuracy of displayed parameters	40%

- Under adverse clinical conditions
  - V_T in all the ranges including neonatal
  - Pressure
  - Flow

Sub-Factors	Weight
V_T variation in V_T targeted decelerating flow modes	20%
Response time	20%
Performance with a leak (compensation)	20%

- Triggering
- Alarms
- Targeted tidal volumes

4.3. User Interface (factor = 20)

Sub-Factor	Weight
Ease of training/use	40%

- Simplicity, limitation of hierarchical drill down to find menus
- Terminology/nomenclature
- Clear labeling of controls
- Measured parameters available
  - Compliance
  - Resistance
  - Autopeep
  - V_D-V_T ratio
  - Rapid shallow breathing index

Sub-Factor	Weight
Reduced likelihood of errors	40%
Sub-Factor	Weight
On-screen graphics display	20%

- Visibility-readability of displays
  - Low and high light environments

4.4. Maintenance (factor = 10%)

- Upgradeability
- Company history-strength
- Local sales and service support
- Turnaround time
  - Cleaning and calibration requirements

4.5. Financial Analysis

- Purchasing costs
- Operating costs
- Maintenance costs
  - Supplies
  - Frequency
    - Routine
    - Periodic
  - Clinical Engineering training

5. Clinical Testing

5.1. Clinical testing will require manufacturers to produce at least three ventilators. One will be kept available for training, and two will be used on patients.

5.2. The goal is to give as many properly trained respiratory therapists the opportunity to work with the ventilator and use it on as many different kinds of patients as possible.

5.3. Training

- All respiratory staff working in the NICU and PICU would be trained on operation of the two instruments to be tested. Only those staff with 1 or more years of intensive care experience would be assigned a patient being ventilated with one of the instruments being tested.
- No respiratory therapist who has not completed the required training on the new instrument and completed the basic competency return demonstration on the device will use the device on a patient.
- Medical and nursing staff will receive training approved by the medical and nursing leadership of the pediatric and neonatal ICUs.

5.4. We will attempt to ventilate ≈ 50 patients on each device, attempting to ensure that patients from all weight ranges are ventilated.

- Target 15 patients in each group
  - neonates ≤ 1200 grams
  - Infants > 1200 grams ≤ 10 Kg
  - Children = > 10 Kg
- Only test in one unit at a time

5.5. Copies of all ventilator flow sheets used during these clinical trials will be kept for later analysis.

5.6. A structured evaluation instrument will be developed for each ventilator.

- All staff who have worked at least 3 shifts with an instrument will complete an evaluation.
- Evaluations will be compiled and results entered into the decision modeling software.

DOCUMENT G-2: PROTOCOL FOR BENCH TESTING

This was the protocol that was developed for bench testing.

Ventilator Testing Protocol

1. Bench Testing

   1.1. Purposes
      1.1.1. Determine the accuracy of displayed tidal volumes.
      1.1.2. Determine the variability of delivered tidal volumes during volume targeted, decelerating flow mode(s) in an erratic, spontaneously breathing lung model.

   1.2. Devices
      1.2.1. Ventilators tested
         1.2.1.1. Siemens Servo 300
         1.2.1.2. Siemens Servo-*i*
         1.2.1.3. Viasys Avea
         1.2.1.4. Drager Baby Log
         1.2.1.5. Drager Evita XL
         1.2.1.6. Hamilton Gallileo
         1.2.1.7. Puritan Bennet 840
      1.2.2. All instruments tested will be equipped with the latest neonatal software from the manufacturers.
      1.2.3. Representatives from the manufacturers are invited to be present during testing.

   1.3. Phase 1: Accuracy of displayed tidal volumes
      1.3.1. Volume will be measured independently at the proximal airway with a differential pneumotachometer (Novametrix CO_2SMO).
      1.3.2. All measurements will be made on a heated humidified system.
         1.3.2.1. Heated wire system
         1.3.2.2. Proximal airway temperature set at 37° C.
      1.3.3. Accuracy of the Cosmo will be determined before each run of data acquisition using Hans-Rudolf calibration syringe.
      1.3.4. Ventilator will be equipped with disposable infant ventilator circuit.

1.3.5. Test lung used will be a rigid container with compliance of 0.4 mL/cm.

1.3.6. Ventilating pressures used will be 35/5 and rate of 20.

    1.3.6.1. Inspiratory and exhaled tidal volumes displayed by the Cosmo and the ventilator being tested will be recorded, as well as values for compliance, resistance.

    1.3.6.2. Volume lost due to compressible loss will be calculated based on the compliance factor of the circuit and humidifier, which will be directly determined for any circuit used.

    1.3.6.3. Mean values of these tidal volumes will be determined and compared. The percentage difference between the mean values displayed by the ventilators and the CO_2SMO will be determined both corrected and uncorrected for compressible volume loss.

    1.3.6.4. Runs will consist of at least 50 breaths for each device tested.

    1.3.6.5. Devices will be tested in both constant flow and decelerating flow modes. Settings will be adjusted to achieve ventilating pressures of 35/5.

1.4. Phase II: Accuracy and variability of delivered tidal volumes during volume targeted decelerating flow modes

1.4.1. Test lung used, IngMar ALS 5000.

1.4.2. Test lung settings used will mimic an erratically breathing infant, with periods of tachypnea, eupnea, and apnea, superimposed on periods of small and large spontaneous tidal volumes.

1.4.3. This erratic breathing pattern is being programmed into the ASL and is reproducible for all tests. Each instrument will be operated in volume targeted decelerating flow mode for a minimum of 3 minutes.

1.4.4. Tidal volume will be measured independently at the patient airway with a computerized pneumotachometer (CO_2SMO).

1.4.5. Coefficient of variation of delivered tidal volume will be calculated for each device.

     1.5. At the end of this cycle of testing, we would select the two best devices to test clinically. The best being defined as a combination of the most accurate tidal volume display and lowest coefficient of variation in delivered tidal volumes.

2. Clinical Testing
     2.1. All respiratory staff working in the NICU and PICU would be trained on operation of the two instruments to be tested. Only those staff with 2 or more years of intensive care experience would be assigned a patient being ventilated with one of the instruments being tested.
     2.2. Nursing staff would also be trained in alarm management and F_1O_2 adjustment.
     2.3. Medical staff would receive as much formal instruction as the medical directors of the units deemed appropriate.
     2.4. The test would be conducted for 1–2 months, or until approximately 40–50 patients had been ventilated.
     2.5. Evaluation documents would be kept at the bedside for clinicians to note issues with the instruments.
     2.6. Any staff who had worked at least 5 shifts with the devices would be asked to fill out a formal evaluation.
     2.7. Data from clinical and bench testing would be entered into a decision matrix as described by Chatburn and Primiano in: Decision analysis for large capital purchases: how to buy a ventilator. *Respir Care*. 2001:46(10):1038–1053.
     2.8. This protocol is subject to change.

DOCUMENT G-3: GUIDELINES GOVERNING THE CLINICAL TRIAL

These guidelines were intended to be followed for the clinical trial and were aimed principally at ensuring patient safety and reducing organizational risk.

Guidelines for Use of the Viasys Avea Ventilator During Clinical Trials

1. Patient Selection
     1.1. Patients shall be selected in consultation with IICU or PICU attending physician.
     1.2. Unstable patients will be excluded.

1.3. If a prospective decision is made to exclude a patient, this should be communicated to the clinical supervisor on duty and the Viasys representative.

2. Verbal Consent From Parents
  2.1. Parents should be asked for their verbal consent. They should be informed:
    2.1.1. That this new ventilator is commercially available in the United States.
    2.1.2. That the benefits to their child may include advanced capabilities of the ventilator.
    2.1.3. That we are still gaining experience with the ventilator and that as a result there is a small increased risk to their child of ineffective ventilation, but that their child will be very closely monitored while on the ventilator.
    2.1.4. That the ventilator will be used with their child for only a few hours or at most a few days.

3. Modes Allowed
  3.1. The following modes/features are to be used only with the consent of the NICU/PICU attending physician and Clinical Coordinator or Department Director.
    3.1.1. Flow cycling above 5% in any mode.
    3.1.2. Machine volume in conjunction with volume limitation (e.g., volume targeting with volume limiting).

4. Hours Of Trial
  4.1. Patients shall be put on the Avea or removed from it only between the hours 0700 and 1300. Exceptions require the consent of the attending physician and the Respiratory Therapy Clinical Coordinator or Department Director.

5. Conditions Requiring Intervention
  5.1. The following conditions should be reported to the on-duty Clinical Supervisor, Clinical Coordinator, and the Viasys representative immediately:
  5.2. Any significant deterioration in blood gases that cannot be readily attributed to a nonventilator related cause.
  5.3. Any significant increase in spontaneous respiratory rate or other indication of increased agitation or work of breathing.
  5.4. Any significant increase in levels of ventilatory support or F_1O_2.

6. Indications For Terminating Trial
   6.1. The patient should be removed from the Avea and replaced on the Servo 300 if:
      6.1.1. Any of the conditions in section 5 occur and you are unable to contact the Viasys Representatives or Clinical Coordinator.
      6.1.2. Any time you are concerned that the ventilator might not be operating properly.

DOCUMENT G-4: MEMO TO STAFF ON VENTILATOR IMPLEMENTATION PLANS

After the ventilator selection had been made, this memo was developed to describe how the training and rollout of the new ventilators would occur. A primary guiding principle was, "No just-in-time training at the bedside." All training was done in classroom environments.

Memo

To:	See Distribution List
From:	Director Respiratory Care
Date:	_____
Subject:	New Ventilator Implementation

This memo is to outline our plans for introduction of the new Viasys Avea mechanical ventilators.

1. Guiding Principles
   a. Planned go live date is _____. This is the date we would begin putting patients on the Avea.
   b. We will start patient applications in the PICU first and then move to the IICU.
   c. All RTs and RNs assigned to a patient on the new ventilators will receive training and have demonstrated competency (return demonstration) before being assigned to a patient being ventilated with the Avea.
   d. Initial training will take place in a classroom environment (not at the bedside). RTs and RNs will not be pulled from staffing for initial training to minimize interruptions and give plenty of time for training.
   e. RNs will be required to sign up for at least one training session.

    f. RTs may be required to attend more than one training session depending on demonstrated competency.

    g. The RT department will begin training a group of expert users (Avea Aces) in December. During this ventilator rollout, one of these Avea Aces will always be on duty. This team will also conduct RN training (along with the Viasys team).

    h. No patients will be placed on the new ventilator during this implementation period without the consent of the RT supervisor, nursing supervisor, and attending physician.

    i. The first time any RT staff places a patient on an Avea or cares for a patient already on an Avea, proper ventilator operation must be verified by an Avea Ace or Viasys Clinical Specialist.

    j. All patients placed on the Avea during the initial 1–2 months of ventilator usage will be monitored with either T_CPCO_2 or E_TCO_2 if equipment is available. Exceptions must be cleared with the clinical supervisor or clinical coordinator. RT is arranging for rental of additional E_TCO_2 monitors.

    k. Advanced features will be used only with the consent of the clinical supervisors or clinical coordinator. Advanced features include:

        i. Use of volume limitation feature.

        ii. Use of variable flow cycling during mandatory breaths.

        iii. Use of airway pressure release ventilation.

    l. All ventilator alarms will be set according to the (see below) located in the RT department manual and at the end of this memo.

    m. Standardized patient assessment risk:

        i. As with all ventilated patients, these will be carefully monitored for increased work of breathing, adequacy of ventilation, and adequacy of oxygenation when first placed on the Avea.

        ii. Any changes in the patient status in the immediate period after placing patients on the Avea will be reported to the attending physician and the respirator clinical supervisor.

2. Nursing Training

    a. Training for RNs will provided by:

        i. Viasys clinical trainers.

        ii. Specially trained RTs who have been trained as expert users on the Avea.

        iii. The RT clinical coordinator.

b. Training content:
   i. The focus of this training is intended to highlight the essentials needed to safely operate this ventilator from a nursing perspective.
   ii. Training content is outlined in the appendix of this document.
   iii. Major areas of concentration will be:
      1. Basics of the ventilator
      2. Determination of ventilator settings
      3. Alarm management
      4. Suctioning
      5. F_IO_2 adjustment
      6. Flow sensor management and care
c. Return demonstration for nursing:
   i. Training will include a return demonstration on the essential functions of the ventilator. See the appendix for the return demonstration document. It may be necessary to have some staff attend more than one training session.
d. Record keeping:
   i. The RT Clinical Coordinator will keep track of the class attendance rosters and return demonstration documentation. See the appendix for a class attendance roster. Attendance rosters will be copied to the RT department. All documents will be forwarded to nursing management.

3. RT Training
   a. Avea Ace Training:
      i. We will train all clinical supervisors (full time and relief) and at least two people on night shift and two people on days who mostly work opposite schedules to become Avea Aces or super users.
      ii. This would involve additional advanced training on the Avea. The Aces would provide training and direct support to clinical staff (all disciplines). This would mean spending some extra time at the hospital in December, January, and February helping train nurses and RTs and helping when Aveas are put on patients.
      iii. Avea Ace training will last about 90 minutes, and RTs should attend two sessions.

   b. RT Staff Training
      i. All RTs not identified as an Avea Ace must sign up for at least one training session. After _____ RTs will not be able to work anymore until training is completed.
      ii. Training location to be announced.
      iii. Avea Policy and Manual:
         1. The RT Department Policy Manual has been upgraded to reflect the use of the Avea and includes links to PDF versions of the Avea operating manuals.

4. Medical Staff Training
   a. Respiratory Therapy will coordinate training to include:
      i. Surgeons
      ii. House staff
      iii. NNPs
      iv. PICU and CVIC attending
      v. Neonatologists

Distribution List:

Respiratory Care Staff	Nursing Management	Administration
Clinical Supervisors (RT)	Intensive Care Medical Directors	
Clinical Engineering	Viasys Representatives	

DOCUMENT G-5: OUTLINE FOR NURSING TRAINING ON THE AVEA VENTILATOR

A lot of planning went into what the respiratory therapists, nurses, and physicians would be taught about the operation of the ventilator. Nursing and respiratory therapy training on the new ventilator was mandatory and was not to occur "just-in-time" at the bedside.

Avea Nursing Training Outline

1. Soft Key Review
   • There are 20 soft keys around the outside edge of the ventilator monitor.
   • All of these and their functions will be covered during your nursing in-service.

2. Touch Turn Touch
   - This is the method by which settings are changed on this ventilator, and it will be covered in your nursing in-service.

3. Alarm Silence
   - Will silence audible alarm for 2 minutes.
   - Not functional for a Vent Inop condition.
   - Pressing the alarm silence key again before the 2 minutes are up will cancel the silence.

4. Alarm Reset
   - Cancels visual signals when no longer active.

5. Panel Lock
   - This soft key locks the screen allowing you to prevent accidental setting changes. The RN will still be able to silence and reset alarms, as well as activate the suction/increase O_2 soft keys.
   - The panel lock must be disabled to allow any manipulation of the F_IO_2 setting.

6. Alarm Limits
   - There are 9 alarm limits available and they will be set according to the department's alarm management policy.
   - There are two audible alarm conditions
     - *High Priority:* This category of alarm requires immediate action. For a high priority alarm, the alarm indicator is read and a five toned alarm warning is heard at three low pitched followed by two high pitched sounds. Some examples of High Priority alarms are Circuit Disconnect and High Peak Pressure.
     - *Medium Priority:* A medium priority alarm displays a yellow indicator and sounds three tones, all at the same pitch. Some examples of medium priority alarms are High and Low minute ventilation alarms and High RR alarms.
     - *Low Priority:* Single tone alarm warning, which is not repeated.

7. Manual Breath
   - Delivers single mandatory breath every time it is pushed.

8. Suction
   - This soft key will silence the audible alarm and will pre-oxygenate for 2 minutes. This is intended for use with inline suction catheters.
   - If the suction key is pressed again during the 2 minutes, the maneuver will be cancelled.

9. Increase F_IO_2 Feature
   - When this key is pressed, the ventilator increases the oxygen concentration delivered to the patient for 2 minutes.
   - Alarms will not be silenced.
   - The percent which the F_IO_2 will be increased is set by the RT per policy, but there is a default of 20% increase in neonates and 79% increase in ped/adult size ranges.

10. Adjusting F_IO_2
    - Panel lock must be disabled to make this change.
    - Touch the F_IO_2 setting, turn the thumb wheel to the desired F_IO_2 setting, and confirm by touching the setting again or pushing the ACCEPT soft key.

11. Sensor Care
    - All neonatal patients must have a proximal flow sensor inline at all times.
    - The sensors will allow accurate measurement of volume and graphics at the patient's ET tube.
    - The sensors can be affected by secretions and water accumulation, which may cause auto-cycling and inaccurate flow and volume measurements.
    - The sensor should always be propped above the patient to prevent pooling of fluid in the flow sensor. Special attention should be exercised when using saline to rinse an in-line suction catheter.
    - Whenever sensor function is in question please call the RT responsible for your patient and have them assess the sensor. A backup sensor will always be at the bedside per RT policy.

12. Monitored Parameters
    - These are breath-to-breath measurements that are obtained at the ventilator flow sensor or at the proximal flow sensor with neonatal ventilation.
    - They are displayed as five square boxes on the left hand side of the monitor screen or 15 square boxes in the monitor screen of the ventilator.

13. Set Parameters
    - These are the main ventilator settings for the current mode of operation and can be found at the bottom of the monitor screen. All active settings for the current ventilator mode are displayed in this area.

DOCUMENT G-6: NURSING RETURN COMPETENCY DEMONSTRATION FORM

These were jointly developed by nursing and respiratory therapy, completed by the respiratory therapist doing the training, and then returned to nursing for recordkeeping purposes.

Nursing Return Demonstration Competency for the Viasys Avea Ventilator

Staff Name   _____

Date   _____

Unit   _____

Trainer   _____

Topic	Overview	Return Demonstration	Instructor
Ventilator Layout:			
Soft Key Review:			
Touch Turn Touch:			
Alarm Silence:			
Alarm Reset:			
Panel Lock:			
Alarm Settings:			
Suctioning:			
Increase F_IO_2 Feature:			
Adjusting F_IO_2:			
Sensor Care:			
Monitored Parameters:			
Monitor Screen:			
Set Parameters:			

DOCUMENT G-7: AVEA COMPETENCY CHECKLIST

This form was developed for the new ventilator, in this case the Viasys Avea. It became the competency check-off list for any new employees who become trained on the Avea.

Competency Checklist

Viasys Avea Ventilator

Staff Name: _____

PRIVATE: _____

Item:		Finished?
Select and assemble the ventilator circuit		YES / NO
Complete EST test (leak, circuit compliance & O$_2$ sensor calibration)		YES / NO
Complete the following patient setup for an adult patient		
Patient Size	Adult	YES / NO
Automatic Tube Compensation (ATC)	Off	YES / NO
Leak Compensation	Off	YES / NO
Note Circuit Compliance Compensation (Circ Comp) Test Results	_____ ml/cm H$_2$O	YES / NO
Humidification	Active On	YES / NO
Enter Patient Weight if available (IBW)	_____kg	YES / NO
Primary Controls		
Breath Type/Mode	Volume SIMV	YES / NO
Breath Rate (Rate)	10 bpm	YES / NO
Tidal Volume (Volume)	600 mL	YES / NO
Peak Flow	50 L/min	YES / NO
Inspiratory Pause (Insp Pause)	0.0 sec	YES / NO
Inspiratory Time (I-Time)	Measured	YES / NO

(Continues)

Item:		Finished?
PSV	10 cm H_2O	YES / NO
PEEP	5 cm H_2O	YES / NO
Inspiratory Flow Trigger (Flow Trig)	1.0 L/min	YES / NO
% O_2	30%	YES / NO
Advanced Controls		
Vsync	0 (Off)	YES / NO
Vsync Rise	—	YES / NO
Demand Flow	1 (On)	YES / NO
Waveform	Decelerating	YES / NO
Bias Flow	2.0 L/min	YES / NO
Inspiratory Pressure Trigger (Pres Trig)	3.0 cm H_2O	YES / NO
PSV Rise	5	YES / NO
PSV Cycle	10%	YES / NO
PSV T_{max}	1.5 sec	YES / NO
Machine Volume (Mach Vol)	—	YES / NO
Volume Limit (Vol Limit)	—	YES / NO
Inspiratory Rise (Insp Rise)	—	YES / NO
Flow Cycle	—	YES / NO
Alarm Settings		
High Rate	30 bpm	YES / NO
High Tidal Volume (High Vt)	—	YES / NO
Low Exhaled Minute Volume (Low Ve)	3.0 L/min	YES / NO
High Exhaled Minute Volume (High Ve)	15.0 L/min	YES / NO
Low Inspiratory Pressure (Low Ppeak)	10 cm H_2O	YES / NO
High Inspiratory Pressure (High Ppeak)	55 cm H_2O	YES / NO
Low PEEP	3 cm H_2O	YES / NO

Item:		Finished?
Apnea Interval YES / NO		20 sec

Auxiliary Controls: Locate and verify appropriate function of the following controls:

Manual Breath	—	YES / NO
Suction	—	YES / NO
$\uparrow\%O_2$	—	YES / NO
Nebulizer	—	YES / NO
Inspiratory Hold (Insp Hold)	—	YES / NO
Expiratory Hold (Exp Hold)	—	YES / NO

Employee's Signature: _____   Date:_____

Evaluator's Signature: _____   Date:_____

DOCUMENT G-8: POST-VENTILATOR CLINICAL TRIAL ASSESSMENT SUMMARY

Clinical Ventilator Evaluation-Respiratory

Date _____

Years of PICU or NICU/IICU Experience _____

Number of Shifts Worked with the Ventilator _____

Name (optional) _____

	Viasys Avea	Servo 300
Please rate the ventilators on the following variables	Circle One	Circle One

Size of the Ventilator:

The ventilator fit well at the bedside

Viasys Avea: 1 2 3 4 5 6 7 8 9 10 — Strongly disagree ←→ Strongly agree

Servo 300: 1 2 3 4 5 6 7 8 9 10 — Strongly disagree ←→ Strongly agree

The ventilator was easy to move around

Viasys Avea: 1 2 3 4 5 6 7 8 9 10 — Strongly disagree ←→ Strongly agree

Servo 300: 1 2 3 4 5 6 7 8 9 10 — Strongly disagree ←→ Strongly agree

User Interface:

The ventilator was easy to learn

Viasys Avea: 1 2 3 4 5 6 7 8 9 10 — Strongly disagree ←→ Strongly agree

Servo 300: 1 2 3 4 5 6 7 8 9 10 — Strongly disagree ←→ Strongly agree

The labeling of controls was easy

Viasys Avea: 1 2 3 4 5 6 7 8 9 10 — Strongly disagree ←→ Strongly agree

Servo 300: 1 2 3 4 5 6 7 8 9 10 — Strongly disagree ←→ Strongly agree

The terminology used on the ventilator was easy to understand

Strongly disagree 1 2 3 4 5 6 7 8 9 10 Strongly agree

Strongly disagree 1 2 3 4 5 6 7 8 9 10 Strongly agree

It was easy to adjust the ventilator

Strongly disagree 1 2 3 4 5 6 7 8 9 10 Strongly agree

Strongly disagree 1 2 3 4 5 6 7 8 9 10 Strongly agree

Features:

The ventilator had all the modes I wanted in a ventilator

Strongly disagree 1 2 3 4 5 6 7 8 9 10 Strongly agree

Strongly disagree 1 2 3 4 5 6 7 8 9 10 Strongly agree

I understood all the modes on the ventilator

Strongly disagree 1 2 3 4 5 6 7 8 9 10 Strongly agree

Strongly disagree 1 2 3 4 5 6 7 8 9 10 Strongly agree

The alarms were easy to adjust and reset

Strongly disagree 1 2 3 4 5 6 7 8 9 10 Strongly agree

Strongly disagree 1 2 3 4 5 6 7 8 9 10 Strongly agree

The alarms had a distinctive sound that was easy to identofy

Strongly disagree 1 2 3 4 5 6 7 8 9 10 Strongly agree

Strongly disagree 1 2 3 4 5 6 7 8 9 10 Strongly agree

(Continues)

The alarm volume was loud enough

Strongly disagree 1 2 3 4 5 6 7 8 9 10 Strongly agree

Strongly disagree 1 2 3 4 5 6 7 8 9 10 Strongly agree

The ventilator did not have a lot of nuisance alarms

Strongly disagree 1 2 3 4 5 6 7 8 9 10 Strongly agree

Strongly disagree 1 2 3 4 5 6 7 8 9 10 Strongly agree

The volumes displayed by the ventilator were accurate

Strongly disagree 1 2 3 4 5 6 7 8 9 10 Strongly agree

Strongly disagree 1 2 3 4 5 6 7 8 9 10 Strongly agree

Patients seemed able to trigger the ventilator with relative ease

Strongly disagree 1 2 3 4 5 6 7 8 9 10 Strongly agree

Strongly disagree 1 2 3 4 5 6 7 8 9 10 Strongly agree

The ventilator seemed to perform well in the presence of an airway leak

Strongly disagree 1 2 3 4 5 6 7 8 9 10 Strongly agree

Strongly disagree 1 2 3 4 5 6 7 8 9 10 Strongly agree

The pulmonary graphics features on the ventilator were useful

Strongly disagree 1 2 3 4 5 6 7 8 9 10 Strongly agree

The likelihood of accidental changes of the ventilator settings is low

Strongly disagree 1 2 3 4 5 6 7 8 9 10 Strongly agree

The ventilator settings are easy to read in a low light environment

Strongly disagree 1 2 3 4 5 6 7 8 9 10 Strongly agree

This form was developed for the new ventilator, in this case the Viasys Avea. It became the competency check-off list for any new employees who become trained on the Avea.

Orientation and Training Documents

DOCUMENT H-1: INTENSIVE CARE ORIENTATION CHECKLIST

Intensive Care Unit
In the intensive care unit, orientation will vary according to the workload. Other sources of information are available to assist you through this rotation. At the end of each day, please review the skills list below with your preceptor. Indicate the areas you have covered. Questions or concerns should be addressed at that time. Please use the same checklist throughout your orientation.

Do you have experience with this?		Are you competent in performing?		Learning Module	Learning Options	Evaluation Mechanism	Supervisor, Manager, or Preceptor Signature	Comments
yes	no	yes	no	Airway Maintenance	E = Equipment Manuals	T = Test		
					C = Class	D = Direct Observation		
					P = P and P	C = Competency Module		
					V = Video			
					L = Equipment Lab			
				Manual Ventilation				
				Pressure Manometer				
				self-inflating bags				
				anesthesia bags				

(Continues)

Do you have experience with this?		Are you competent in performing?		Learning Module	Learning Options	Evaluation Mechanism	Supervisor, Manager, or Preceptor Signature	Comments
yes	no	yes	no	**Suctioning**				
				In-line				
				NP/NT				
				Depth measurement				
				Intubation Assist				
				Equipment				
				Location/ preparation				
				Rapid sequence				
				ICU form				
				Documentation review				
				Skin Care				
				Intubated patient				
				Tracheostomy site				
				Noninvasive ventilation				
				TT Stabilization				
				Skin prep				
				Nasal tube				
				Oral tubes with clamp				
				Oral tubes without clamp				

This is only page 1 of 17 pages. Note the different methods of learning and mechanisms of evaluation.

DOCUMENT H-2: MECHANICAL VENTILATION COGNITIVE COMPETENCY

This was from a pediatric hospital and thus is focused on neonatal and pediatric mechanical ventilation. It was accompanied by a very large training document that was studied in preparation of taking the examination. The test was passed out and given to staff and allowed to be taken open book. The minimum passing grade was 80%. The answer key is at the end.

Mechanical Ventilation Cognitive Competency

Instructions: Please print and sign your name on this test, circle or otherwise indicate the correct answers, and turn in to Dave Crotwell or your direct supervisor.

Date:_____

Print Name:_____

Signature:_____

1) Some of the characteristics of ARDS are:
   a) Progressive hypoxemia
   b) Decreased lung compliance
   c) Intrapulmonary shunting
   d) Non-cardiogenic pulmonary edema
   e) All of the above

2) Heterogeneity (nonhomogeneous) in lung injury can best be described as:
   a) Lungs with evenly distributed lung injury but unevenly distributed time constants throughout the lung
   b) Lungs with unevenly distributed lung injury and unevenly distributed time constants throughout the lung
   c) Lungs with unevenly distributed lung injury and evenly distributed time constants throughout the lung

3) ARDS is a nonhomogeneous lung disease.
   a) True
   b) False

4) ARDS is described as diffuse pulmonary infiltrates that occur after acute lung injury from:
   a) Blunt chest trauma
   b) Septic shock
   c) Heart surgery
   d) Both a & b

5) Diagnostic criteria for ARDS include:
   a) PaO_2/F_IO_2 ratio of less than 200
   b) Bilateral infiltrates of noncardiac origin on CXR
   c) Normal pulmonary artery wedge pressure
   d) All of the above

6) It is important to do which of the following when ventilating a patient with ARDS:
   a) Tidal volume set according to predicted body weight
   b) Starting tidal volume of 10ml/kg PBW
   c) Maintain plateau pressure of $\leq$ 30 cmhH$_2$O
   d) Both a & c

7) The arterial pH goal for ARDS is 7.25–7.40.
   a) True
   b) False

8) In patients with ARDS, an I:E ratio goal during conventional ventilation is:
   a) 1:4.0–1:6.0
   b) 1:1.0–1:3.0
   c) 1:0.5–1:1.0
   d) I:E ratio does not matter

9) Flooding of fluid across the alveolar capillary membrane causes:
   a) Increased lung compliance
   b) Decreased airway resistance
   c) Inactivation of natural surfactant
   d) Both a & b

10) The highest respiratory rate recommended for an adult patient in ARDS is:
    a) 20 bpm
    b) 40 bpm
    c) 35 bpm
    d) 60 bpm

11) It is important to set your tidal volume based on predicted body weight and not actual body weight.
    a) True
    b) False

12) After a few hours of mechanical ventilation, the goal in ARDS is to have tidal volume at approximately:
    a) 6 mL/Kg
    b) 8 mL/Kg
    c) 10 mL/Kg
    d) 12 mL/Kg
    e) Whatever volume is needed to achieve minimally acceptable chest rise, not to exceed 10 mL/Kg

13) Beta agonists (albuterol) are an effective treatment for tracheobron-chomalacia crises.
   a) True
   b) False

14) The upper effective range for PEEP or CPAP to treat tracheobron-chomalacia (TBM) is:
   a) 4–8 cm H_2O.
   b) 5–10 cm H_2O.
   c) 6–12 cm H_2O.
   d) 8–15 cm H_2O.

15) TBM is associated with:
   I. BPD, especially in low gestation infants
   II. Cartilage damage in the airway lumen
   III. Congenital heart disease
   IV. Responsiveness to beta agonists
   a) I & II only
   b) II & IV only
   c) III only
   d) I, II, III only

16) The most effective respiratory care treatment of TBM is:
   a) Pressure support ventilation
   b) Tracheal dilation
   c) Antibiotic therapy to prevent tracheitis
   d) Inhaled anti-inflammatants to reduce airway narrowing from edema
   e) Positive pressure during exhalation (PEEP or CPAP)

17) The immature airway is a highly compliant structure that undergoes progressive stiffening with age. Stiffening of up to three-fold occurs in which months of gestation:
   a) Months 4 to 7
   b) Months 5 to 8
   c) Middle 3 months
   d) Last 3 months

18) The indications for initiation of large patients on HFOV are:
   a) Patients requiring an F_1O_2 of $\geq 60\%$
   b) MAP > 24 cm H_2O
   c) Unable to maintain Pplat < 30–35 cm H_2O
   d) All of the above

19) Before transitioning a patient to HFOVs adequate titration of sedation, analgesia, and neuromuscular blockade should be done.
   a) True
   b) False

20) HFOV use in large patients with ARDS is now widely accepted as an important tool in improving survival.
   a) True
   b) False

21) One of the most important things to assess before and during transition to HFOV is:
   a) Minute ventilation
   b) Mean airway pressure and intravascular volume status (BP)
   c) PIP
   d) Tidal volume
   e) None of the above

22) When using the HFOV, blood pressures can drop because of:
   a) Decreased venous return
   b) Increased afterload
   c) Increased preload
   d) Vagal stimulation because of overstimulated stretch receptors

23) The F_1O_2 when transitioning to HFOV is usually started at:
   a) 50%
   b) Same as on conventional
   c) 100%
   d) > 60%

24) The main determinant(s) of oxygenation on HFOV are:
   a) MAP
   b) F_1O_2
   c) Amplitude
   d) a & b

25) The main determinants of ventilation on HFOV are:
   a) Amplitude
   b) Bias flow
   c) Frequency
   d) Both a & c

26) Increasing the frequency on the HFOV will improve CO_2 removal.
   a) True
   b) False

27) Large patients on HFOV should never be taken off for suctioning.
   a) True
   b) False

28) Possible signs that a patient on HFOV has a pneumothorax are:
   a) Decreased breath sounds on the affected side
   b) Decrease chest wiggle
   c) Decreased blood pressure
   d) All of the above
   e) Both b & c

29) A neonate on the oscillator has a chest x-ray that shows rib expansion to 11th rib, and the $PaCO_2$ elevated. This could be because:
   a) Under expansion
   b) Over expansion and decreased pulmonary blood flow
   c) Decreased FRC
   d) Increased pulmonary blood flow

30) Lung hyperinflation can cause:
   I. Increased dead space
   II. Decreased dead space
   III. Increased pulmonary blood flow
   IV. Decreased Q_S/Q_T
   V. Increased $PaCO_2$
   a) I, III, IV
   b) I, IV, V
   c) IV, V
   d) I, III, V
   e) I, V

31) At which patient weight would you consider switching over from a 3100A to a 3100B:
   a) > 35 Kg
   b) 25 Kg
   c) 60 Kg
   d) All patients

32) A neonate with PPHN is placed on the oscillator shortly after admission to the IICU. His mean arterial blood pressure at the time of admission is 53 mmHg, and post ductal S_PO_2 = 82%. After being placed on the oscillator, he is shaking to the hips, the F_IO_2 = 100% and MAP is set at 24 cm H_2O, post ductal S_PO_2 is now 93% and the mean arterial blood pressure has dropped to 30 mmHg. What would you recommend:
a) Increase the MAP on the oscillator
b) Increase the AMP
c) Give a fluid bolus
d) Place on conventional mechanical ventilation in PRVC

33) Two potent pulmonary vasoconstrictors are:
a) Hypoxia and alkalosis
b) Hyperoxyia and acidosis
c) Hypoxia and acidosis
d) Alkalosis and hyperoxia

34) A typical chest x-ray of PPHN will be markedly abnormal.
a) True
b) False

35) A neonate with PPHN has a $PaCO_2$ of 24 mmHg:
a) That is the target $PaCO_2$
b) Is too low because of the risk of decreased cerebral perfusion
c) Is too low because of decreased pulmonary perfusion
d) Is too high because of pulmonary shunting

36) The two main causes of continuing PPHN in the newborn are:
a) Poor lung compliance and low tidal volumes
b) Hyperoxia and hypercarbia
c) Hypoxia and acidosis
d) Hypocarbia and poor lung compliance

37) Which are characteristics of the lungs in BPD patients?
   I. Arrest of lung maturation
   II. Halt in alveolarization
   III. Abnormal capillary bed development
   IV. Lack of surfactant
a) I & II only
b) II & IV only
c) III only
d) All

38) Permissive hypercapnia is a valid ventilator strategy in BPD, keeping the capillary pH:
   a) 7.30 and below
   b) 7.25 and below
   c) 7.20 and above
   d) 7.15 and above

39) There is no consensus whether or not early intervention with HFOV reduces the incidence or severity of BPD.
   a) True
   b) False

40) A neonate with chronic lung disease is having increased work of breathing, increased $PaCO_2$, and breath sounds that reveal increased crackles. The possible problem could be:
   a) Incorrect ventilator settings
   b) Fluid overload
   c) Hypoxia
   d) Cold stress

41) In BPD patients with tracheotomies, the largest possible tube size should always be used to eliminate leaks.
   a) True
   b) False

42) Ventilator strategy in BPD patients should emphasize adequate gas exchange while minimizing VILI.
   a) True
   b) False

43) In the oxyhemoglobin dissociation curve, the horizontal axis is:
   a) SaO_2
   b) PaO_2
   c) Hgb level
   d) SpO_2
   e) None of the above

44) Factors that can cause the pulse oximeter to function poorly include:
   I. Motion artifact
   II. Hypertension
   III. Dyshemoglobinemia
   IV. Poor peripheral perfusion
   a) I, II
   b) I, III
   c) II, III
   d) I, III, IV
   e) II, III, IV

45) O_2 delivery to the cells of the body can be affected by:
   a) Cardiac output
   b) Hemoglobin level
   c) SaO_2
   d) All of the above

46) Venous congestion can cause inaccuracy in oximeters.
   a) True
   b) False

47) A dyshemoglobin is hemoglobin:
   a) That binds with oxygen but then cannot unbind
   b) Can only carry a limited amount of oxygen
   c) Carries an excess amount of oxygen, releasing many oxygen radicals
   d) Cannot chemically interact with oxygen and thus can carry no oxygen

48) Dyshemoglobins include which of the following:
   I. Carboxyhemoglobin
   II. Methemoglobin
   III. Anemic hemoglobin
   IV. Deoxygenated hemoglobin
   V. Inadequate hemoglobin
   a) I,
   b) I, II
   c) I, III, IV
   d) All

49) Which is the most reliable indicator for adequate oxygenation in a post-operative patient?
   a) PaO_2
   b) SVO_2
   c) SaO_2
   d) $TcPO_2$

50) A shift to the right of the oxyhemoglobin dissociation curve has:
   a) Decreased oxygen affinity to hemoglobin
   b) Increased oxygen affinity to hemoglobin
   c) A result of hypothermia
   d) Decrease in $PaCO_2$

51) In a normal patient, E_TCO_2 range values are:
   a) 27–30
   b) 30–55
   c) 30–43
   d) 45–55

52) If minute ventilation is fixed, as the cardiac output goes up, E_TCO_2 goes down.
   a) True
   b) False

53) Which type of capnograph has more dead space?
   a) Mainstream
   b) Sidestream
   c) They are the same

54) Which type of capnograph adds more weight to the airway?
   a) Mainstream
   b) Sidestream
   c) They are the same

55) E_TCO_2 is a valid means of verifying endotracheal intubation during a prolonged cardiac resuscitation.
   a) True
   b) False

56) If the E_TCO_2 waveform becomes more squared off (more flat) over time, that means the patient:
   a) Has more air trapping
   b) Has less air trapping
   c) Has a lower cardiac output
   d) None of the above

57) On which patients is it required that you use an E_TCO_2 monitor:
   I. A stable 14-year-old postoperative patient who has been in the PICU for 10 ten days and is very stable
   II. A 650 gram neonate with a 2.0 ETT who is extremely unstable, agitated, and exhibiting lots of motion
   III. All new ventilated admits, may spot check if ETT unstable
   a) I
   b) I, II
   c) I, II, III
   d) I, III

58) The most likely cause of an increasing gradient between $PaCO_2$ and E_TCO_2 is:
   a) Calibration failure of the E_TCO_2 monitor
   b) Esophageal intubation
   c) Ventilation perfusion derangement
   d) The patient is improving

59) The low E_TCO_2 alarm should be used:
   a) At the discretion of the RT and set 5 mmHg below the E_TCO_2
   b) At all times and set at 5–10 mmHg below the E_TCO_2
   c) Only when accidental extubation is a concern
   d) Rarely because the low E_TCO_2 reading are generally not very accurate.

60) If the patient accidentally extubates the E_TCO_2 will:
   a) Rise suddenly because ventilation has fallen
   b) Rise suddenly because ventilation has risen
   c) Fall to almost zero because alveolar CO_2 has dropped
   d) Rise suddenly because alveolar CO_2 has risen
   e) Fall to almost zero because no exhaled gas is going through the endotracheal tube

61) When placing the sat probe for preductal saturations, the probe must be placed on:
   a) The left hand
   b) The right hand
   c) Either hand
   d) Lower limbs

62) When placing the sat probe for postductal saturations, the best probe placement is:
   a) The left hand or lower limbs
   b) The right hand
   c) Either hand

63) Coarctation of the aorta is a cyanotic heart lesion.
   a) True
   b) False

64) Ventricular septal defect is associated with increased pulmonary blood flow.
   a) True
   b) False

65) A neonate born with a congenital heart defect with decreased pulmonary blood flow, i.e., Tetrology of Fallot, will have clinical presentation of:
   a) Intense cyanosis
   b) Tachypnea without respiratory distress
   c) Strong peripheral pulses
   d) All of the above

66) An infant born with coarctation of aorta can show symptoms of:
   a) Decreased pulses in the lower extremities
   b) Increased pulses in the lower extremities
   c) Cyanotic
   d) Increased perfusion in lower extremities

67) With hypoplastic left heart syndrome, if the ductus closes the infant can exhibit:
   a) Shock
   b) Death
   c) Cyanosis
   d) All of the above

68) Right ventricular hypertrophy is caused by:
   a) Decreased pulmonary vascular resistance
   b) Decreased afterload
   c) Increased pulmonary vascular resistance
   d) Decreased systemic vascular resistance

69) RSV can be transmitted on fomites.
   a) True
   b) False

70) Time constant of the lung is calculated according to which of the following formulas:
   a) $R_{aw} \times C_{lung}$

   b) $\dfrac{R_{aw}}{C_{lung}}$

   c) $T_I \times \left(\dfrac{C_{dyn}}{T_E} \right)$

   d) $R_{aw} \times \sqrt{\dfrac{C_{dyn}}{1 - C_{dyn}}} \times \sum_{\beta}^{i} (C_{lung} + 0.1)$

71) The time constant for Hyaline membrane disease is long.
   a) True
   b) False

72) Preterm neonates weighing 1100 grams would need which size endotracheal tube:
   a) 2.5
   b) 3.0
   c) 3.5
   d) 2.0

73) A neonate weighing 1100 grams would have the ETT taped at:
   a) 9 cm at the lip
   b) 7 cm at lip
   c) 8 cm at the lip
   d) 8.5 cm at the lip

74) During intubation, a neonate's head should be hyperextended to view the vocal chords.
   a) True
   b) False

75) What ventilator measurements would you monitor after administration of surfactant in the PRVC Mode?
   a) PEEP and RR
   b) PS tidal volumes
   c) Tidal volume in cc/kg and PIP
   d) Auto PEEP

76) A neonate on HFOV should be left on the ventilator during administration of surfactant.
   a) True
   b) False

77) Subambient oxygen therapy is used to:
   a) Increase pulmonary blood flow
   b) Decrease pulmonary blood flow
   c) Increase pulmonary compliance
   d) Increase FRC

78) A 27-week premature neonate has just been given a second dose of surfactant. He is on an Avea in SIMV Pressure Control with the following settings:
   $F_IO_2 = 50\%$
   $PIP = 22$ cmH$_2$O
   $PEEP = 4$ PIP
   V_T exhaled 18 mL/Kg
   You would:
      I. Increase the PIP
      II. Decrease the PIP
      III. Decrease the F_IO_2 to keep S_PO_2 88–93%
      IV. Decrease the F_IO_2 to keep S_PO_2 95–100%
      V. Change flow sensor and verify measurements again
   a) I, IV
   b) II, III
   c) II, IV
   d) V

79) A 34-week neonate with RDS has a sharp drop in heart rate to 80, S_pO_2 to 80%. Breath sounds are difficult to assess. Heart rate raises to 115 with positive pressure ventilation via ETT but S_pO_2 are still very low. The therapist should:
   a) Assume the neonate is extubated and pull the tube and begin bag mask ventilation
   b) Visually inspect pharynx with laryngoscope to ensure ETT is passing through the chords
   c) Place a colorimetric E_TCO_2 detector on tube to assess airway status
   d) Increase the ventilator settings

80) A neonate with pulmonary interstitial emphysema that is worse on one side than the other should be placed:
   a) With the most affected side down
   b) With the most affected side up
   c) Supine
   d) Prone

81) For a neonate with PIE, what is a desirable S_pO_2?
   a) > 95% < 99%
   b) > 94% < 98%
   c) > 87% < 95%
   d) > 84% < 90%

82) Which medication cannot be administered via the ETT?
   a) Epinephrine
   b) Atropine
   c) Narcan
   d) Dopamine

83) The medication given to keep the ductus arteriosus patent in neonates with cyanotic congenital heart defects is:
   a) Dopamine
   b) Prostaglandin E
   c) Calcium chloride
   d) Atropine
   e) Prostacylin E

84) A secondary effect of Prostaglandin E is infant apnea.
   a) True
   b) False

Case Study #1

You are working in the NICU and are called to the ER for a high-risk delivery. The mother of this infant did not receive any prenatal care. The delivery was uneventful and a large term (3000 gram) male infant was born. Initially the infant looked okay until he started to cry. During the crying episode he became blue and limp, bradycardic and apneic. Upon assessing the infant you noticed a scaphoid abdomen, and when listening to breath sounds you noticed that the left lung was diminished. On room air the infant's sats are only 75%.

85) What should you do next?
    I. Bag-mask ventilate the baby with 100% F_IO_2
    II. Give O_2 via blow-by
    III. Needle the chest
    IV. Place an NG tube
    a) I, II, IV
    b) II, III
    c) II, IV
    d) All

The infant continues to deteriorate despite blow-by oxygen.

86) What should you do next?
    I. Prepare for intubation
    II. Start CPR
    III. Get an ABG
    IV. Observe
    a) I only
    b) II, III
    c) I, II, III
    d) All

87) What size ETT would you use for this infant?
    a) 2.5
    b) 3.0
    c) 3.5
    d) 4.0

88) The infant is intubated. He is on 100% F_IO_2. Following our protocol, what initial settings are appropriate for this patient?

   a) SIMV   rate 20   PEEP 6   PIP 25 T_I 0.6
   b) SIMV   rate 40   PEEP 5   PIP 20 T_I 0.5
   c) SIMV   rate 45   PEEP 6   TV 10 cc/kg T_I 0.5
   d) SIMV   rate 100   PEEP 5   PIP 25 T_I 0.5

   Your first ABG comes back:

   Ph 7.53 CO_2 29 PaO_2 69

89) Your measured V_T is 5 cc/kg, what ventilator parameter would you adjust?
   a) Reduce rate
   b) Reduce PEEP
   c) Reduce V_T
   d) Increase T_I

90) Which of the following are clinical signs of an infant with a diaphragmatic hernia?
   I. Cyanosis
   II. Severe respiratory distress
   III. Opaque chest x-ray
   IV. Mediastinal shift
   a) I, II
   b) I, III, IV
   c) I, II, III
   d) I, II, IV
   e) All

91) A baby with congenital diaphragmatic hernia will present with the following breath sounds:
   I. Decreased or absent over some or most lung fields
   II. Bowel sounds in chest
   III. Inspiratory rub
   IV. Hyper resonance
   V. Vocal fremitus
   a) I, II
   b) II only
   c) I, II, III
   d) All

92) Where would you want to keep the $PaCO_2$s for congenital diaphragmatic hernia with PPHN?
   a) 80–100 mm Hg
   b) 60–80 mm hg
   c) 40–65 mm Hg
   d) 30–40 mm Hg

93) Which ventilator parameter would you *avoid if possible* when treating a patient with CDH?
   a) Low PEEP
   b) High PIP
   c) Hyperventilation
   d) Nitric oxide

94) Where would you want to keep your PaO_2 for CDH with PPHN?
   a) 40–50 mm Hg
   b) 50–60 mm Hg
   c) 60–70 mm Hg
   d) 80–100 mm Hg

95) What is the most important thing to avoid when initially treating a diaphragmatic hernia patient:
   a) Placement of a nasogastric tube
   b) Manual ventilation with a face mask
   c) Auscultation
   d) Chest x-ray

96) CDH x-ray will show the following:
   I. Ground glass appearance
   II. Air-filled bowel seen in thorax
   III. Displaced mediastinum to unaffected side
   IV. Lung hypoplasia
   a) III
   b) I, III
   c) II, III, IV
   d) IV

97) Which side of the lung is most often affected in CDH?
   a) Right
   b) Left

98) Infants with CDH are often hypoxemic. Calculate the oxygen index of this infant: MAP = 12, F_IO_2 = 80, PaO_2 = 60, HR = 120, PIP = 28
   a) 30
   b) 16
   c) 40
   d) 18

99) If a patient's oxygen index is *over 30* what might that indicate?
   a) Patient needs surfactant
   b) Patient needs CPR
   c) Patient is poorly oxygenating and may need ECMO
   d) Patient needs more tidal volume

100) The prognosis of a patient with CDH depends on which of the following?
   I. The size of the defect
   II. The degree of hypoplasia
   III. The condition of the unaffected lung
   IV. Success of surgical procedure
   a) I & II
   b) I & IV
   c) I, II, & III
   d) All

101) A Ph of < 7.20 in an infant with CDH may increase pulmonary vascular resistance.
   a) True
   b) False

Case Study #2

A 40-week gestational age infant weighing 4.5 kg is admitted via airlift for meconium aspiration. There was thick meconium present at birth and suctioned from the patient's trachea. Baby is intubated for tachypnea, profound hypercarbia and hypoxia.

102) Choose the most appropriate vent settings:

a) SIMV/PC/PS	RR 40	V_T 10 cc/kg	PEEP 5	F_IO_2 60%
b) SIMV/PC/PS	RR 50	V_T 8 cc/kg	PEEP 6	F_IO_2 50%
c) SIMV/PC/PS	RR 40	V_T 5 cc/kg	PEEP 5	F_IO_2 100%
d) SIMV/PC/PS	RR 45	V_T 5 cc/kg	PEEP 10	F_IO_2 100%

103) Your first gas after placing the patient on the ventilator at the settings above are: pH = 7.26, PaCO$_2$ = 71 mmHg, PaO$_2$ = 60 mmHg.
What change would you make?
a) Increase your rate by 6
b) Increase your PEEP by 2
c) Make no ventilator changes, suction patient if required, and repeat ABG in 1 hour
d) Push ETT in 1 cm

104) An hour later you get another ABG and it is:
pH 7.09   CO$_2$ 98   PO$_2$ 55
Your chest x-ray shows significant air trapping and atelectasis. What would you suggest?
a) Increase V$_T$
b) Increase PEEP
c) Recommend changing to HFOV
d) Suction patient and give more surfactant

105) When transitioning this patient from conventional ventilation to HFOV you want to start the MAP at:
a) 5 cm H$_2$O above conventional MAP
b) 2 cm H$_2$O below conventional MAP
c) 2 cm H$_2$O above conventional MAP

106) Your patient is stable on the oscillator, but the chest shake has decreased from your last check and the S$_P$O$_2$ has decreased from 96% to 89%. You should consider:
a) Increasing the AMP
b) Increasing the F$_I$O$_2$
c) Increasing the MAP
d) Suctioning using in-line catheter
e) Suctioning using open suctioning technique

107) Aspiration of meconium in utero or during the first breaths at birth can cause which of the following?
  I. Airway obstruction
  II. Chemical pneumonitis
  III. PPHN
  IV. Increased pulmonary vascular resistance
a) I & II
b) I & III
c) I, II, & III
d) All

108) A typical x-ray of a baby who has meconium aspiration would show all the following except:
    a) Areas of consolidation
    b) Tracheal deviation to the left
    c) Atelectasis
    d) Hyperinflation

109) What effect does meconium have on surfactant?
    a) It increases the production of surfactant
    b) It inactivates the surfactant
    c) It has no effect on surfactant production
    d) It increases surfactant

110) In neonates with meconium aspiration and air trapping you want to set your frequency at:
    a) 12–15 Hz
    b) 8 Hz or as low as 5 Hz
    c) 10 Hz

111) The 3100A HFOV is only approved by the FDA for rescue ventilation of neonates.
    a) True
    b) False

112) When ventilating patients with air leak you want to set your MAP at:
    a) 2–4 cmH$_2$O above your conventional MAP
    b) 1–2 cmH$_2$O below conventional MAP
    c) 0–1 cmH$_2$O above conventional MAP
    d) 4 cmH$_2$O below your conventional MAP

113) Two goals for all ventilation strategies is:
    I. Get the patient back to conventional ventilation as soon as possible
    II. Establish and maintain an adequate FRC
    III. Improve gas exchange
    a) I, II, III
    b) I, III
    c) II, III

114) What are the units of measure for compliance of the respiratory system?
    a) L/cm/s
    b) mL/cm/s
    c) cm/mL
    d) mL/cmH$_2$O
    e) cm/L/s

115) What are the units of measure for resistance of the respiratory system?
   a) L/cm/s
   b) mL/cm/s
   c) cm/mL
   d) L/s
   e) $cmH_2O/L/s$

116) List the normal values for each of the following:
   a) CaO_2 _____ _____
   b) Hemoglobin _____
   c) Base excess _____
   d) HCO_3 _____

117) Calculate the CaO_2 for the following patient:
   Hgb 14, SaO_2 92%, PaO_2 78 mmHg
   a) 14.8
   b) 17.5
   c) 19.0
   d) 16.9

118) Which best describes oxygen delivery?
   a) C.O. $\times$ CaO_2
   b) CaO_2 − CvO_2
   c) A − aDO_2
   d) SaO_2 $\times$ Hgb $\times$ 1.34

119) An increase in the difference between arterial and venous oxygen content can be indicative of what?
   a) Right to left pulmonary shunting
   b) Increase cardiac output
   c) Decreased cardiac output
   d) Decreased oxygen extraction
   e) Lower cellular PO_2 levels

Mechanical Ventilation Cognitive Competency Answer Key

1. e	6. d	11. a	16. e
2. b	7. a	12. a	17. d
3. a	8. b	13. b	18. d
4. d	9. c	14. d	19. a
5. d	10. c	15. a	20. b

21. b	49. a	77. b	105. c
22. a	50. a	78. b	106. d
23. c	51. c	79. c	107. d
24. d	52. b	80. a	108. b
25. d	53. a	81. c	109. b
26. b	54. a	82. d	110. b
27. b	55. b	83. b	111. b
28. d	56. b	84. a	112. c
29. b	57. d	85. c	113. c
30. e	58. c	86. a	114. d
31. a	59. b	87. c	115. e
32. c	60. e	88. b	116. a) 20 mL/dL
33. c	61. b	89. a	b) 12–15 g/dL
34. b	62. a	90. d	c) 0–2
35. b	63. b	91. a	d) 2–26
36. c	64. a	92. c	117. b
37. d	65. b	93. b	118. a
38. c	66. a	94. d	119. c
39. a	67. d	95. b	
40. b	68. c	96. c	
41. b	69. a	97. b	
42. a	70. a	98. b	
43. b	71. a	99. c	
44. d	72. b	100. d	
45. d	73. b	101. a	
46. a	74. b	102. c	
47. d	75. c	103. c	
48. b	76. b	104. c	

DOCUMENT H-3: VIASYS AVEA COGNITIVE COMPETENCY

The answer key is at the end.

Viasys Avea Competency Exam

Name:_____
Date:_____

1) In neonatal mode the maximum deliverable volume is:
   a) 39 ml
   b) 150 ml
   c) 250 ml
   d) 300 ml

2) A rise time of 9 provides a slower, less turbulent, lower total peak flow to your patient than a rise time of 1.
   a) True
   b) False

3) The machine (Mach) volume is?
   a) The minimum volume delivered to your patient
   b) The maximum volume delivered to your patient
   c) The minimum volume delivered from the ventilator
   d) The maximum volume delivered from the ventilator

4) With which patient is it appropriate to use the heated wire anemometer?
   a) Any patient
   b) Neonatal patients
   c) Adult patients
   d) Patients receiving 80/20 Heliox therapy

5) Tubing compliance is active in the neonatal mode.
   a) True
   b) False

6) What is the lowest level the bias flow can be effectively set at?
   a) 0.5 lpm above the flow trigger
   b) 2 lpm above the flow trigger
   c) It is set to an appropriate level regardless of the flow trigger
   d) It should be set the same as the flow trigger

7) In neonatal, pediatric, and adult mode the ventilator will always increase the F_iO_2 by 20% when the suction button is depressed.
   a) True
   b) False

8) When connecting a Heliox source gas to the back of the Avea it requires a special hose.
   a) True
   b) False

9) Where in the hospital is the Heliox mixture located?

10) When setting machine volume in the neonatal mode what is the name of the value that you use in the monitoring window to ensure that an appropriate minimum tidal volume is set?

11) In which mode or modes of ventilation can you enable the machine volume advanced feature?

12) Explain how a flow cycled breath type would terminate.

13) The vent is set in Pressure AC with an I-Time set at .4 seconds and the flow cycle is turned on to 40%. The measured I-Time could be .17 seconds.
   a) True
   b) False

14) In a Pressure Support breath, flow cycle can be turned off.
   a) True
   b) False

15) How do you determine an appropriate setting for the TiMax for a pressure support breath?

16) Both machine volume and flow cycle features are active on a patient. The machine volume will be guaranteed before the flow cycle is allowed to function.
   a) True
   b) False

17) In the neonatal mode you are looking at a monitored display of exhaled Vte and you notice there is an asterisk in the display window. What would you suspect is the problem?

18) How would you fix the problem from Question 17?

19) You are performing an EST on the Avea prior to putting it on a patient and it consistently fails the leak test. You then bypassed the humidifier and the circuit is rechecked but you still have a leak. What would you suspect was the source of the problem?

20) When performing an EST with the circuit connected to the humidifier, should you perform the EST with a dry or a wet humidifier?

21) Why is it important to set the patient weight when in the setup mode?

22) While volume ventilating a patient with the demand flow turned on (advanced setting), the patient can receive a larger tidal volume than what is set.
   a) True
   b) False

23) If the ventilator is auto cycling and you turn the flow trigger control all the way to 20 and it is still auto cycling, what value would you next check to determine if you have set the trigger sensitivity inappropriately?

24) In an 800-gram patient receiving Survanta, which of these ventilator settings decrease the likelihood of over distention from rapidly improving lung compliance?
   a) Set a tight High PIP alarm
   b) Set a tight High Minute Ventilation alarm
   c) Set a tight High Tidal Volume alarm
   d) All of the above

25) In the three ventilator settings below, which has the most noticable alarm?
   a) Volume Limit
   b) High Minute Ventilation alarm
   c) High Tidal Volume alarm

26) There are three different priority alarms that can be heard on the Avea.
   a) True
   b) False

27) When changing the V_T in Volume Control what other parameter is affected?
   a) The Rise time
   b) The flow
   c) The I time
   d) None of the above

28) PRVC is available in NEO, PEDS, and ADULT.
   a) True
   b) False

29) Machine Volume/VDEL can be used in Volume Control.
   a) True
   b) False

30) Choose the most appropriate answer concerning leak compensation:
   I. Compensates for loss of PEEP in the presence of a leak
   II. Compensates for loss of PIP in the presence of a leak
   III. Should always be turned on
   IV. Should only be turned on in the event of a leak
   a) II, IV
   b) II, III
   c) I, IV
   d) III

31) Does machine Volume base the V_T on the inspiratory or expiratory volumes?

32) The default values for the O_2 percent increase function is:
   a) Pediatric 20%, neonatal 79%
   b) Pediatric 79%, neonatal 20%
   c) Pediatric 79%, neonatal 79%

33) What are the weight criteria for selecting circuit size?
   a) It's not weight specific
   b) Neo < 20 kg, Ped > 20 kg, < 60 kg, Adult > 60 kg
   c) Neo ≤ 7 kg, Ped > 7 kg, < 25 kg, Adult > 25 kg

34) What parameters are most likely to change if flow cycle is on?
   a) Decreased MAP
   b) Decreased Inspiratory Time
   c) a & b

35) A flow sensor must be used in the NEO modes. The best way to monitor CO_2 when concerned about dead space will be:
   a) E_TCO_2 via mainstream sampling
   b) TCM and/or E_TCO_2 Spot check
   c) Arterial Sticks

36) Please number the step sequence correctly to activate machine volume:
___Take note of volume in Vdel during a controlled breath
___ Dial Inspiratory pressure to get Target V_T in cc/kg
___ Dial inspiratory pressure down equal to Pressure support
___ Locate the Vdel parameter
___ Place pt in Pressure A/C or Pressure SIMV mode
___ Under the Advanced Settings of Insp. Pressure set the Mach Volume to match Vdel
___ Set PIP 10–15 cmH$_2$O above peak pressure

37) In the pediatric or adult mode, you wish to activate the Machine volume. You would do which of the following:
a) Dial in the desired V_T to be delivered as Machine volume
b) Take note of the VDel currently being delivered and dial that number in as Mach.Vol.
c) Calculate your V_T exh by using V_T – PIP/PEEP

38) The volume limit function is an advanced feature that allows you to limit the amount of volume delivered to the patient. This function will be most useful in what type(s) of patient:
a) RDS post surfactant administration
b) Patients with history of PIE
c) Patients with pneumothorax
d) All of the above

39) Machine Volume breaths are compliance compensated in Pediatric and Adult modes.
a) True
b) False

40) In Neonatal modes, where would you set the Mach Vol in relation to the Vdel measurement?
a) Set both the same
b) Set Mach Volume above Vdel
c) Set Mach Volume to or slightly below Vdel

41) In Volume Control and PRVC, why is there a difference in set and monitored I-Time?

42) The Vdel is a parameter that can be adjusted.
a) True
b) False

43) You notice the V_T cc's/kg drop on a patient in Pressure Control, Machine Volume. What would you do to correct this?
   a) Increase the machine volume to targeted V_T
   b) Suction patient and increase Vdel
   c) Increase Vdel to targeted V_T
   d) Change flow sensor and suction patient; if V_T does not increase, adjust Machine Vol to obtain targeted mL/kg

44) In PS/CPAP mode, what screen do you access to set the back-up rate?

45) You are in PS/CPAP, the apnea setting is 20 seconds and the back-up rate is 10 bpm. Which parameter will respond first if the patient becomes apneic?

46) What are the criteria to terminate Apnea ventilation?
   a) The patient initiates a spontaneous breath
   b) A manual breath is delivered
   c) The mandatory respiratory rate is increased above the apnea interval setting
   d) All of the above

Avea Competency Exam Answer Key

1. d
2. a
3. c
4. b
5. b
6. a
7. b
8. a
9. PICU hallway closet, RT equipment room, loading dock
10. Vdel
11. Pressure SIMV, Pressure A/C
12. The breath is terminated when the set % deceleration in flow has been reached

13. a
14. b
15. Set PSTimax equal to or up to 2× higher than set Ti
16. a
17. Measurement is out of range
18. Check flow sensor, check dialed in patient weight
19. Leak in the filter or in the circuit
20. Wet
21. Vent uses weight to calculate measurements such as cc/kg and compliance
22. a
23. Pressure Trigger

24. d
25. b
26. a
27. c
28. b
29. b
30. c
31. Inspiratory at machine
32. b
33. c
34. c
35. b
36. 4/2/6/3/1/5/7

37. a
38. d
39. a
40. c
41. There is a lag time related to the tubing compliance compensation
42. b
43. d
44. Under mode section, select Apnea Settings
45. 20 seconds
46. a

DOCUMENT H-4: ACUTE CARE COGNITIVE COMPETENCY

The answer key is at the end.

Acute Care Cognitive Competency

Name: _____
Date: _____

Asthma Protocol

1) Albuterol given via nebulization has been shown to:
    I. Be very effective in preventing and treating post-operative atelectasis
    II. Be slightly more effective than albuterol administered by MDI
    III. Have no clinical effectiveness on most bronchiolitis patients
    IV. Helps to reduce airway edema in asthma patients
    V. Help relieve bronchospasm in asthmatics
    a) All of the above
    b) None of the above
    c) I, III, IV
    d) III, IV, V
    e) II only
    f) III, V

2) The Aero chamber Max is a valved holding chamber made of a special polymer that:
    a) Reduces the likelihood of lower respiratory tract infections
    b) Makes the chamber easier to clean
    c) Reduces the static charge on the inside of the chamber
    d) Increases the static charge on the inside of the chamber

3) How many puffs should you give to be equivalent to 5 mg of nebulized albuterol?
    a) 2
    b) 4
    c) 6
    d) 8
    e) 10

4) When using an albuterol MDI with a valved holding chamber, what is the optimal time for holding the mask to a patient's face?
   a) About 1–2 minutes
   b) Between 20 and 30 seconds
   c) Until the patient has taken between 5–10 spontaneous breaths
   d) Until no more aerosol is visible in the chamber

5) Infants and toddlers get better deposition of an inhaled aerosol if they are crying than they do if they are breathing quietly because when crying they are taking bigger breaths.
   a) True
   b) False

6) Which of the following affect the deposition of an aerosol in the human airway?
   I. Patient position
   II. Respiratory rate
   III. Depth of breathing
   IV. Sustained inspiration
   V. Aerosol characteristics
   a) I
   b) I, II
   c) I, III, IV
   d) II, V
   e) All

7) What is the percent of drug that typically gets to the lung of a spontaneously breathing child when administering albuterol via blow-by technique?
   a) < 5%
   b) 10%
   c) 20%
   d) 30%

8) To prevent medication errors, you should throw out all MDI caps before placing the MDI in the valved holding chamber.
   a) True
   b) False

9) Using the Respiratory Scoring Tool, what is the Respiratory Score for the following:
5-year-old female, BS coarse with an end expiratory wheeze bilaterally. RR 30 HR 120, Substernal retractions and Nasal flaring noted, complains of chest pain unable to count to 10 but uses 4–5 words between breaths.   Score_____

10) You have an RCU patient that receives eight puffs albuterol Q2. It has been 2 hours since their last Q2 treatment and it is time for you to assess them. Your pretreatment score of the patient is 5, what is the next step?
a) Give eight puffs albuterol
b) Give four puffs albuterol
c) Space patient to Q4, at that time give eight puffs albuterol
d) Space patient to Q4, at that time give four puffs albuterol

11) Asthmatic patients not on the RCU do not require a pre- and post-Respiratory Score.
a) True
b) False

12) Asthma education with patients and families will cover which of the following topics?
 I. Asthma medications and administration of medications
 II. Causes of asthma
 III. How to minimize risk
 IV. CPR
 V. When to contact their primary care providers
a) I
b) I, II
c) I, II, III, V
d) All

13) If you are asked to provide asthma education to a family that does not speak English, you need to contact interpreter services to assist or find personnel who can interpret for you.
a) True
b) False

14) It is expected that RTs deliver what percentage of MDIs on the asthma pathway?
    a) 10–20%
    b) 30–40%
    c) 50–60%
    d) 100%

15) It is the beginning of your shift and your Q2 RCU patient is due at 9:00. How do you establish with the RN the plan of care for this patient?
    a) Just do all the treatments
    b) Touch base with the RN, and arrange a schedule to share the responsibilities for this patient
    c) Ask the RN to do all the treatments
    d) Just wing it and see how it goes

16) The MAR is a legal document. It is imperative that you check it for accuracy and sign off your meds at the time of treatment.
    a) True
    b) False

17) It's a really busy day and the RN has the patient chart open to the MAR, she kindly offers to sign off the eight puffs of albuterol that you just gave to the patient. Per hospital policy, you must sign off the medication yourself.
    a) True
    b) False

18) If you are having a really busy day it's okay to sign off your meds and do your charting at the end of the day.
    a) True
    b) False

19) Before starting any procedure it is important to identify the patient by looking at the name placard outside the room.
    a) True
    b) False

Bronchiolitis

20) Albuterol has been shown in studies to be a benefit to most bronchiolitis patients who receive it.
    a) True
    b) False

21) Naso-pharyngeal suctioning has been shown to benefit the majority of bronchiolitis patients.
    a) True
    b) False

22) Albuterol generally should be used for these patients even though they have no documented response to the drug because many of the benefits of the drug cannot be seen immediately but come later.
    a) True
    b) False

23) You are admitting a new bronchiolitis patient. Per the protocol, you should assess and score your patient, suction them (if needed), and then repeat a score after suction. An albuterol trial should only be attempted if the suctioning did not improve the patient score.
    a) True
    b) False

24) Nasal washes to get a Fluorescent Assay (FAs) and NP suctioning are a/n:
    a) Shared responsibility between RNs and RTs
    b) RT only duty
    c) RN only duty
    d) MD only duty

25) When you obtain a nasal wash, it is important to obtain cells of the mucosa and not just mucus because mucus alone will not show a virus or virus infected cells.
    a) True
    b) False

26) How many cc's of specimen do you need for the lab to perform the test on a nasal wash?
    a) 1 cc
    b) 2 cc
    c) 3 cc
    d) 4 cc

27) You need to obtain a nasal wash for an active 4-year-old. Choose the correct procedure:
   a) Have patient blow nose to clear mucus, tilt head back and instill saline into one nare while holding their breath. Then bend forward and blow nasal contents into a cup.
   b) Place a catheter into the nare, rapidly instill saline into the opposite nare, and immediately aspirate.
   c) Place patient on their side and swaddle or restrain. Place catheter in bottom nare and instill saline into the superior nare, immediately aspirate from the downside nare.

CPT

28) Which of the following are considered a contra-indication to CPT:
   a) Pleural effusion
   b) Large untreated pneumothorax
   c) Cardiac arrythmias
   d) Brittle bones
   e) All of the above

29) All new CPT orders must have a recent CXR (within 24 hours) that you and the doctor have viewed.
   a) True
   b) False

30) Chest physiotherapy has been shown in studies to be effective in improving pulmonary function and/or symptoms in which of the following diseases:
   I. Pneumonia
   II. Asthma
   III. Diffuse atelectasis
   IV. Lobar atelectasis or lobar consolidation
   V. Cystic Fibrosis
   VI. Bronchiectasis
   a) All of the above
   b) I, II, III
   c) V only
   d) IV, V, VI

31) To reduce the risk of aspiration, it is best policy to perform CPT prior to feeding or 1–2 hours postfeeding.
   a) True
   b) False

Ventilator Dependent Patients

32) RNs are allowed to turn ventilators on and off as necessary.
    a) True
    b) False

33) RNs will do all of the trach care for these patients.
    a) True
    b) False

34) After the parents of a patient have seen trach care being done they can do this on their own if they feel comfortable.
    a) True
    b) False

35) Cardio-respiratory monitors are not necessary on this unit.
    a) True
    b) False

36) Your patient is desaturating and your ventilator is alarming patient disconnect. You cannot find the leak. Your best option is to:
    a) Call a code 188
    b) Silence the alarm
    c) Hand bag your patient and call for back-up
    d) Give albuterol

37) You enter your patient's room due to a ventilator alarm and discover the patient was accidentally decannulated. Your patient is not breathing, SpO_2 is reading 30%, and the heart rate is 75 bpm. Which of the following are acceptable courses of action:
    a) Call a code 188
    b) Attempt to reinsert the trach tube
    c) Bag mask ventilated with a gauze covering the stoma if you cannot get the trach back in
    d) All of the above

38) The RN for a ventilated patient on T11 calls you frantically stating the machine is alarming and the patient is not ventilating. Your response to her should be:
    a) I'm coming right down
    b) Take the patient off the vent and manually bag the patient until I get there
    c) Silence the alarms
    d) a & b

Monitoring

39) Pulse oximetry that is exposed to a lot of daylight or bright lights will:
   a) Stop reading
   b) Read falsely low
   c) Read falsely high
   d) Need recalibration

40) Your patient is pink, warm, well perfused, and kicking his or her feet. The saturation monitor is reading 80% with a poor tracing. The appropriate action is to:
   a) Silence the alarm
   b) Check probe placement, change probe site if required
   c) Strongly hold feet down
   d) All of the above

41) You have a patient who is being monitored Q4 with an E_TCO_2 monitor. The patient has a moderate leak around their stoma. You can expect the E_TCO_2 to read:
   a) Erroneously low
   b) Erroneously high
   c) Be very accurate
   d) None of the above

Airways

42) Artificial airways include which of the following:
   I. Tracheostomy
   II. Nasal prongs
   III. Nasal stints
   IV. Nasopharyngeal tube
   a) I only
   b) I, II, III
   c) All
   d) I, III, IV

43) Artificial airways are to be assessed Q4.
   a) True
   b) False

44) Nostril retainers used in patients for cleft lip repair are not considered an artificial airway.
   a) True
   b) False

45) Choose the best answer. Tracheostomy care is:
   a) Done by the parents at their discretion
   b) A shared responsibility between RN and RT, performed Q shift and prn
   c) An RN only responsibility

46) It is imperative to verify that there is a spare trach, along with a trach one size smaller, and resuscitative equipment at the bedside. When do we check for this?
   a) At the beginning of every shift
   b) Monday, Wednesday, and Friday
   c) Once a week

47) Your patient has a 4.5 Bivona TTS for an artificial airway and needs to be transported to MRI for a test. Identify what will be an issue for this patient.
   a) Patient cannot receive oxygen while in the MRI
   b) Bivona trach tubes are reinforced with metal and they need to be changed out to a Shiley trach of similar size before leaving the room
   c) Patient needs frequent suctioning
   d) There are no problems with this scenario

48) You are performing tracheostomy care with a fellow RT. You are holding the tracheostomy in place and the patient starts coughing and turning red in the face. The appropriate action is to:
   a) Let go of the trach so as not to harm the patient
   b) Continue holding the trach, ask your fellow RT to pause until the coughing spell stops
   c) Place your finger over the trach outlet to stop the patient from coughing
   d) Change the trach out altogether because it's in the esophagus

49) Choose the equipment and supplies required for a patient with an artificial airway traveling in-house.
   I. Bag and mask
   II. Spare artificial airway
   III. Oxygen
   IV. Cardio-respiratory monitor
   V. Feeding supplies
   a) I
   b) I, II
   c) I, II, III, IV
   d) All

50) It is appropriate to fill a pediatric 4.0 Shiley tracheostomy cuff with water.
   a) True
   b) False

51) Your patient has a 4.5 cuffed Shiley trach with the cuff inflated. The speech therapist has requested we help with the trial of a Passy-Muir Valve. What action is most appropriate:
   a) Auscultate your patient
   b) Ensure the cuff is inflated
   c) Ensure the cuff is deflated
   d) Bag and suction your patient

52) Circuit changes on ventilators and HATC are due Q30 days; this includes changing out the Resuscitator bag.
   a) True
   b) False

53) An R1 calls you about a patient on G3 that he would like to start on Bipap. He is in moderate respiratory distress and has no history of Bipap use. You agree that the patient requires Bipap but are unsure of how to proceed. You try to access the computer to look up our policy but the computers are down hospital wide. What is the most appropriate action?
   a) Start the Bipap as ordered
   b) Call your shift supervisor to request assistance
   c) Request a CXR
   d) Obtain a CBG

Cardiac

54) Some cardiac patients do not require oxygen even with saturations of 80%.
   a) True
   b) False

55) Fluid balance is commonly an important factor to consider when assessing a cardiac patient in respiratory distress.
   a) True
   b) False

CBGs

56) How many times should you attempt to draw a CBG before asking another therapist for assistance?
   a) 1 time
   b) 2 times
   c) 5 times
   d) 10 times

57) The heel is an appropriate puncture site for a 3-year-old patient.
   a) True
   b) False

58) When performing a CBG on the heel it is preferred to use the crown area of the heel.
   a) True
   b) False

59) How many capillary tubes does the lab require for a CBG?
   a) 1 tube
   b) 2 tubes
   c) 3 tubes
   d) 4 tubes

60) How many capillary tubes does the lab require for a CBG and electrolytes?
   a) 1 tube
   b) 2 tubes
   c) 3 tubes
   d) 4 tubes

Case Study

61) The RN for a patient on G2 calls and tells you her patient is in respiratory distress, has an SpO$_2$ of 85%, and has been suctioned without relief. She would like to know if you could come and assess the patient. The appropriate response is:
   a) Call the MD
   b) Tell the RN to do a CBG and call you back with the results
   c) Say that you'll be right there
   d) Tell the RN to give an albuterol and that you'll be there as soon as you can

62) Your assessment of the patient is an RR 42 with substernal, intercostal, and suprasternal retractions. The patient is lying supine with his chin to his chest. Patient looks mottled, is on a non-rebreather with saturations still in the 80s. Choose the most appropriate next step.
a) Reposition patient to ensure a patent airway
b) Get a STAT CXR
c) Give an albuterol treatment
d) NP suction patient

63) Auscultation reveals coarse rhonchi throughout with diminished breath sounds in the right upper and middle lobes. The RN states patient was fed about two hours ago and vomited prior to the onset of this episode. Choose the most appropriate action:
a) Start nasal CPAP
b) Get a CXR
c) Transfer patient to ICU
d) NP suction

64) The physician arrives and requests you obtain a CBG. The results are: pH 7.24/ CO_2 79/ PCO_2 54/ BE 4/ HCO_3 28. How would you classify this CBG?
a) Respiratory alkalosis with hyperoxia
b) Metabolic alkalosis with hypoxemia
c) Respiratory acidosis with hypoxemia
d) Respiratory acidosis with hyperoxia

65) The physician decides to transfer the patient to the ICU. What supplies would you bring with you?
   I. Bag and mask
   II. Oxygen
   III. Defibrillator
   IV. Cardio-respiratory monitor
   V. Chest tube supplies
a) I, II
b) I, II, IV
c) I, II, III, IV
d) IV only
e) All of the above

Acute Care Competency Exam Key:

1. f	18. b	35. b	52. a
2. c	19. b	36. c	53. b
3. d	20. b	37. d	54. a
4. c	21. a	38. d	55. a
5. b	22. b	39. b	56. b
6. e	23. a	40. b	57. b
7. a	24. a	41. a	58. b
8. a	25. a	42. d	59. a
9. 6	26. b	43. a	60. b
10. c	27. c	44. a	61. c
11. b	28. e	45. b	62. a
12. c	29. a	46. a	63. d
13. a	30. d	47. b	64. c
14. c	31. a	48. b	65. b
15. b	32. b	49. c	
16. a	33. b	50. b	
17. a	34. b	51. c	

Index

A

absenteeism
case study, 141–142
cross–industry comparisons,
144–145
episodic, 140
illness–related, 140–141
measurements of, 141–145
mixed messages concerning,
141
unplanned absences measurements, 143–144
academic preparation, for respiratory therapy management,
2–4
accountability–respect–teamwork
(ART) management
theory, xi
accounts payable detail reports,
operating budgets and, 212
accuracy measurements
in billing practices, 120–121,
123
technology evaluation and,
233–240
tidal volume accuracy, bench
testing of, 262–266
active listening skills
for respiratory therapy management, 8–12
staff development and, 277–285
Adams, Scott, 68–70
administrative assistants, hospital
structure and role of, 31
advertising, as recruiting tool, 294
agency staffing
reduced dependency on, 220
staffing systems' use of,
160–163

aging workforce, staffing systems
management and, 140–141
airway management systems,
medical errors management
and, 132–134
alarm systems, medical errors
management and, 132–134
American Association for
Respiratory Care (AARC)
benchmarking services, 95
conferences sponsored by, 255
expert opinion panels of, 247
Human Resource Study of
2005, 140, 160–161
in-service training and education programs, 308–309
membership in, 13–14
performance evaluation metrics, 113
respiratory therapy staffing levels and, 149–150
utilization studies resources at,
113
American Association of
Critical–Care Nurses
(AACN), communication
guidelines of, 280–285
ancillary service departments,
hospital organization, 21
angioplasty, expert opinion evaluation of, 246–247
animal studies, technology evaluation with, 247–249
Annals of Improbable Research, 232
annualization techniques, operating budgets and, 210–211
antibiotics, overuse of, 113
appearances, hiring process and
importance of, 291–292

application process, hiring practices and, 290–293
arterial blood gas (ABG)
monitoring
pricing charges for, 179–183
respiratory therapists and, xvii
utilization measurements of,
115–118
asthma education, clinical quality
metrics and role of, 120, 122
authority gradients, communication failures and, 281–285
automated billing systems, characteristics of, 186

B

banners for staff recognition, 299
benchmarking
performance evaluation, respiratory therapy depart-
ment, 92–96
pricing policies and, 176–183
process control charts, 134–136
severity of illness adjustments,
101–103
bench testing
resuscitation bags, 258–262
technology evaluation using,
232, 247–249, 257–270
tidal volume accuracy, 262–266
bias, randomized controlled trials
and, 241–244
Bierce, Ambrose, ix
billing practices
accuracy metrics for, 120–121,
123
charting compliance metrics,
121, 124